The Molecular Basis for the Link between Maternal Health and the Origin of Fetal Congenital Abnormalities:
An Overview of Association with Oxidative Stress

Editor:

Bashir M. Matata

Liverpool Heart & Chest Hospital NHS Foundation Trust
United Kingdom

Co- Editor:

Maqsood M. Elahi

Prince of Wales and Sydney Children Hospital
Australia

CONTENTS

FOREWORD

When I was a medical student taking biochemistry, a professor and an expert in protein folding explained from the lecture. "I don't expect you to remember how proteins fold. I am here to show you a window by which you judge the world." I am a busy clinical cardiovascular surgeon and not a molecular biochemist but I often look through his window and postulate how protein conformation could relate to antigen presentation in transplantation immunology, how proteins stick to surfaces of our extracorporeal membrane oxygenation circuits, and how genetic alterations result in abnormal protein conformations affecting tissue integrity.

Effective translational research requires that clinicians frequently refresh their view through many basic science windows. I have witnessed many successful translational research efforts in various institutions that I have been fortunate to be a part, e.g. Johns Hopkins Hospital, Mayo Clinic, University of Pittsburgh Medical Center, and Heart Science Center at Harefield, UK.

This book attempts to provide a similar integrative window view to a problem with international research interests larger than any institution. It is a collection of precise research into the mechanism of fetal oxidative stress, temporal susceptibility to the insult, and long-term sequelae. It is only through forums, like this, that the work of various laboratories is inextricably linked towards the common goal of disease prevention.

There are much epidemiological evidences that various environmental factors are associated with an increased incidence of fetal congenital abnormalities. These include maternal alcohol and cocaine abuse, exposure to radiation, exposure to pesticides, temporal exposure to certain medications (teratogens), advanced maternal age, maternal morbid obesity, and markedly elevated maternal hemoglobin $A_{1c.}$ The understanding of these and other associations have contributed greatly towards improved maternal and fetal health in the 20th century on individual basis. In summary, a real prevalence of fetal congenital abnormalities in the 21st century remains there. The key link remains undefined. Is it fetal oxidative stress?

In allopathic medicine, we treat end stage disease at an organ level medically or surgically often decades after the causative insult. This represents an enormous disconnect. It is quite inefficient and certainly not cost effective. Drs. Matata and Elahi present a laudable effort in reducing this disconnection. The search for prevention continues in many disease processes. Ultimately, the understanding requires a molecular approach for a complete picture. I applaud the contributing authors for their most valuable insights.

Kenton J. Zehr, M.D.

Chief, Division of Cardiothoracic Surgery
Director, Center for Aortic Disease
Scott & White Clinic
Professor of Surgery
Texas A & M University, Health Science Center, School of Medicine
Temple, Texas

PREFACE

Reactive oxygen species (ROS) are produced as by-products of mitochondria electron transport chain. At moderate concentrations (yet unknown acceptable ranges at various developmental phases), ROS functioned in normal physiology by regulating enzymes and redox-sensitive gene expression. The cell utilizes a body of machinery to balance oxidative molecules, including ROS scavengers (e.g., thiols, vitamin C and E) and detoxifying enzymes (e.g., superoxide dismutase, glutathione reductase). Excessive ROS can cause oxidation of proteins, lipids, and DNA. It is known that such unbalanced oxidative capacity may lead to oxidative stress that is implicated in the aetiology of many diseases such as aging, cancer, diabetes, and cardiovascular disease.

Oxidative stress is a common feature of many commonly known or suspected risk factors of or conditions associated with adverse (poor or excessive) fetal growth and/or preterm birth, such as preeclampsia, diabetes, smoking, malnutrition or excessive nutrition, infection or inflammation. Plausibly, oxidative stress might be the key link, underlying the superficial "programming" associations between adverse fetal growth or preterm birth and later elevated risks of the metabolic syndrome, type 2 diabetes and other disorders. Adverse programming may occur without affecting fetal growth, but more frequently among low birth weight infants, merely because they more frequently experience known or unknown conditions with oxidative insults.

Oxidative stress programming may operate either directly through the modulation of gene expression or indirectly through the adverse effects of oxidized lipids or other molecules at critical developmental windows and therefore resetting/programming the susceptibility to the metabolic syndrome and other disorders. Because the placenta serves as a barrier against or quencher of oxidative insults to maintain the homeostasis of foetus' intrauterine environments, it is not a surprising observation that preterm infants are more susceptible to programming in early postnatal life, because preterm infants have to experience equivalent intrauterine development stage during postnatal development in an oxygen-rich environment. This fact justifies the main goal of this book: to investigate the susceptibility of biological systems to oxidative insults that likely depends on its resilience and maturity stage at the time of insult. And develop that there could be different critical time windows (prenatal or even postnatal) in "programming" different diseases. Plausibly, prenatal and early postnatal periods are the most critical "windows" to oxidative stress programming insults.

The first chapter offers to the reader a self-contained theory of the role of maternal nutrition and associated oxidant stress in the development of the fetal cardiovascular system. Chapters 2-4 contain new and in our opinion, important concepts on the effects of maternal nutrition on a number of areas: offspring fertility; the importance of the peri-conceptional period on long-term development; fetal programming and hypothalamic-pituitary-adrenal axis outcome and epigenetics and epigenetic dysregulation and cell growth retardation. In chapter 5, the authors discuss more precisely the endothelial dysfunction during cardiac development and the significance of cardiovascular disease risk factors associated with increased ROS and the subsequent decrease in vascular bioavailability of nitric oxide. A detailed body of evidence is presented for the impact of oxidative-nitrosative stress during maternal pregnancy on fetal development in animal models and also the association with the onset of cardiovascular conditions in adult humans. Specifically the presence of ROS in circulating blood as the key intermediary related to vascular injury and organ dysfunction has been highlighted. In addition, the evidence that describes the unique nature of relationship between cell-signalling, transcriptional mechanisms and oxidative-nitrosative stress in the progression of coronary heart disease have also been discussed.

In chapters 6-9, the focus is on the fetal and neonatal programming based on evidence from clinical practice. In particular, the discussion revolves around the probability of oxidative stress and its contribution to the pre-pubertal environment. As mentioned earlier the aim if this monograph is two folds: first to discuss the issues around maternal and fetal metabolic dysfunction in pregnancy disease and its association with vascular oxidative and nitrosative stress. Second to introduce this textbook as an avenue for future discussion on possibilities of further developments in this area, with a view that a diversity of opinions have been covered particularly in the direction in which the current research is moving.

The first editor (BM) would like to dedicate this book to his wife Aliya, children Luqman, Leila and Claire for their support. In addition, this editor would like to acknowledge the help of Ms Shirley Ratcliffe for assistance in editing the manuscripts.

The second editor (ME) would like to dedicate this book to his mother Mrs Fehmida Sultana who always helped him, not only in overcoming many difficulties in his personal life, but she also encouraged him to broaden his fields of interest and to enrich his personal experiences. The present book is the outcome of this wonderful cooperation and friendship between the two authors which, hopefully, will continue for still many years to come.

We would like to thank Prof. Kenton Zehr for writing the foreword and Bentham Science Publishers, for their support and efforts.

Bashir M. Matata
Department of Cardiothoracic Surgery
Prince of Wales and Sydney Children Hospital
Randwick, NSW
Australia

Maqsood M. Elahi
The Liverpool Heart & Chest Hospital NHS Foundation Trust
Thomas Drive, Liverpool
United Kingdom

List of Contributors

Maqsood M. Elahi Cardiothoracic Surgeon, Department of Cardiothoracic Surgery, Prince of Wales and Sydney Children Hospital, Randwick, NSW, Australia.

Bashir M. Matata Director of Clinical Trials Unit/Lecturer (Hon), Liverpool Heart & Chest Hospital NHS Foundation Trust, Liverpool, L14 3PE, United Kingdom.

Pascalle Chavatte-Palmer Assistant Professor, UMR INRA/ENVA/INA P-G 1198 biologie du développement et reproduction, 78350 Jouy-en-Josas, France.

Gunther Meinlschmidt Full Professor, Department of Clinical Psychology and Psychotherapy, Faculty of Psychology University of Basel, Birmannsgasse 8, CH-4055 Basel, Switzerland.

Hany Aly Department of Newborn Services, The George Washington University and the Children's National Medical Center, Washington, DC, USA.

Kaoru Nagai Assistant Professor, Department of Epigenetic Medicine, Interdisciplinary Graduate School of Medicine and Engineering, University of Yamanashi, Yamanashi, 409-3898, Japan.

Angelica Mohn Associate Professor, Departments of Pediatrics, University of Chieti, 66100 Chieti, Italy.

Luis Sobrevia Associate Professor, Cellular and Molecular Physiology Laboratory (CMPL), Division of Obstretics and Gynaecology, Medical Research Centre (CIM), School of Medicine, Faculty of Medicine, Pontificia Universidad Catolica de Chile, Marcoleta 391, Santiago, Chile.

Umberto Simeoni Full Professor, Chair on Infancy, Environment and Health, The University Foundation, Université de la Méditerranée, Marseille, France.

Cha Dupont Service d'Histologie-Embryologie-Cytogenetique-Biologie de la Reproduction-CECOS, Hôpital Jean Verdier (AP-HP), F-93143 Bondy, France.

Rachel Levy Service d'Histologie-Embryologie-Cytogenetique-Biologie de la Reproduction-CECOS, Hôpital Jean Verdier (AP-HP), F-93143 Bondy, France.

Anne-Gael Cordier INRA, UMR 1198 Biologie du développement et reproduction, F-78350 Jouy en Josas, France.

Claudine Junien INRA, UMR 1198 Biologie du développement et reproduction, F-78350 Jouy en Josas, France.

Marion Tegethoff   Division of Clinical Psychology and Psychiatry, Department of Psychology, University of Basel, Switzerland.

Tetyana H. Nesterenko   Department of Newborn Services,

The George Washington University and the Children's National Medical Center, Washington, DC, USA.

Valentina Chiavaroli   Department of Pediatrics, University of Chieti, 66013 Chieti, Italy.

Francesco Chiarelli   Department of Pediatrics, University of Chieti, 66013 Chieti, Italy.

Marcelo González   Cellular and Molecular Physiology Laboratory (CMPL)

Division of Obstetrics and Gynecology

School of Medicine

Pontificia Universidad Católica de Chile

P.O. Box 114-D, Santiago, Chile.

Ernesto Muñoz   Cellular and Molecular Physiology Laboratory (CMPL)

Division of Obstetrics and Gynecology

School of Medicine

Pontificia Universidad Católica de Chile

P.O. Box 114-D, Santiago, Chile.

Carlos Puebla   Cellular and Molecular Physiology Laboratory (CMPL)

Division of Obstetrics and Gynecology

School of Medicine

Pontificia Universidad Católica de Chile

P.O. Box 114-D, Santiago, Chile.

Enrique Guzmán-Gutiérrez   Cellular and Molecular Physiology Laboratory (CMPL)

Division of Obstetrics and Gynecology

School of Medicine

Pontificia Universidad Católica de Chile

P.O. Box 114-D, Santiago, Chile.

Fredi Cifuentes   Cellular and Molecular Physiology Laboratory (CMPL)

Division of Obstetrics and Gynecology

School of Medicine

Pontificia Universidad Católica de Chile

P.O. Box 114-D, Santiago, Chile.

Fernando Abarzúa   Cellular and Molecular Physiology Laboratory (CMPL)

Division of Obstetrics and Gynecology

School of Medicine
Pontificia Universidad Católica de Chile
P.O. Box 114-D, Santiago, Chile.

Andrea Leiva   Cellular and Molecular Physiology Laboratory (CMPL)
Division of Obstetrics and Gynecology
School of Medicine
Pontificia Universidad Católica de Chile
P.O. Box 114-D, Santiago, Chile.

Paola Casanello   Cellular and Molecular Physiology Laboratory (CMPL)
Division of Obstetrics and Gynecology
School of Medicine
Pontificia Universidad Católica de Chile
P.O. Box 114-D, Santiago, Chile.

2

CHAPTER 1

Fetal Programming of Disease Process in Later Life- Mechanisms beyond Maternal Influence

Maqsood M. Elahi[1] and Bashir M. Matata[2*]

[1]*Department of Cardiothoracic Surgery, Prince of Wales and Sydney Children Hospital, Randwick, NSW, Australia and* [2]*The Liverpool Heart & Chest Hospital NHS Foundation Trust, Thomas Drive, Liverpool, United Kingdom*

Abstract: Cardiovascular disease (CVD) is the leading cause of death worldwide and is the principal cause of early death in developing countries. The acceleration of the epidemic of early CVD is thought to include genetic factors as well as demographic factors such as lifestyle changes and nutritional transitions. CVD prevalence is a consequence of the interaction between the distribution of relative genotype frequencies and environmental exposures of a particular population. Although, the biological determinants of CVD and metabolic disorders in low and middle income countries are likely to be similar to those in affluent countries, the drivers of these determinants are likely to differ. In accordance with the developmental origin of health and disease (DOHaD) hypothesis adverse intrauterine influences such as poor maternal nutrition lead to impaired fetal growth, resulting in low birth weight, short birth length, and small head circumference. These adverse influences are postulated to also induce the fetus to develop adaptive metabolic and physiological responses. These responses, however, may lead to disordered reactions to environmental challenges as the child grows, with an increased risk of glucose intolerance, hypertension, and dyslipidaemia in later life and adult CVD as a consequence. This chapter discusses some of the possible links between programmed development and oxidative stress as one of the underlying mechanisms involved in the DOHaD phenomenon.

Keywords: Antioxidants, Fetal origin, congenital anomalies, premature birth, diabetes, cardiovascular disease, metabolic syndrome.

INTRODUCTION

As the first decade of 21st century draws to a close, it is clear that cardiovascular disease (CVD) is still a ubiquitous cause of morbidity and a leading contributor to mortality in the world [1,2]. It is now widely realized that at present, the developing countries contribute a greater share to the global burden of CVD than the developed countries [3,4]. It is estimated that 5.3 million deaths attributable to CVD occurred in the developed countries in 1990, whereas the corresponding figure for the developing countries ranged between 8 to 9 million (*i.e.*, a relative excess of 70%) [3,4]. Regional estimates of CVD mortality indicate that the difference would be even higher if the term "developed countries" is restricted to established market economies only and excludes the former socialist economies (Table 1).

Table 1: Regional Differences in Burden of CVD (1990). DALY Indicates Disability-Adjusted Life Year

Region	Population, millions	CVD Mortality, thousands	Coronary Mortality, thousands	Cerebrovascular Mortality, thousands	DALYs Lost, thousands
Developed regions	1144.0	5328.0	2678.0	1447.9	39 118
Developing regions	4123.4	9016.7	2469.0	3181.2	108 802
Established market economies	797.8	3174.7	1561.6	782.0	22 058
Former socialist economies	346.2	2153.3	1116.3	665.9	17 060
India	849.5	2385.9	783.2	619.2	28 592
China	1133.7	2566.2	441.8	1271.1	28 369

*Address correspondence to Bashir M. Matata: Liverpool Heart & Chest Hospital NHS Foundation Trust, Thomas Drive, Liverpool, L14 3PE, UK; Tel +44 151 600 1380; E-mail: matata_bashir@hotmail.com

Table 1: cont....

Other Asian countries and islands	682.5	1351.6	589.2	350.4	17 267
Sub-Saharan Africa	510.3	933.9	109.1	389.1	12 252
Middle Eastern crescent	503.1	992.3	276.6	327.4	12 782
Latin America	443.3	786.7	269.1	224.1	9538

Adopted from Murray and Lopez [3].

This high, yet inadequately recognized, contribution of developing countries to the absolute burden of CVD is illustrated by the fact that 78% of the 49.9 million global deaths from all causes occurred in regions other than the established market economies or former socialist economies (Table **2**).

Table 2: Shows Regional Contributions to Mortality (1990). Values are Given as Percentage of World Total

Region	All causes %	CVD %
Established market economies	14	22
Former socialist economies	8	15
India	19	17
China	18	18
Other Asian countries and islands	11	9
Sub-Saharan Africa	10	7
Middle Eastern Crescent	9	7
Latin America	6	5
World	100	100

Adopted from Murray and Lopez [3].

During last decade of 20th century, the projected relative contribution of CVD deaths to total mortality was higher in the developed countries (nearly 49%) than that in the developing countries (nearly 23%). Yet the developing countries actually contributed 68% to the total global deaths due to non-communicable diseases and 63% of world mortality due to CVD. This is because the excess total mortality in the developing countries was translated into excess absolute CVD mortality due to the large populations involved [3,4]. Moreover, a greater cause for concern is the early age of CVD deaths in the developing countries compared with the developed countries *e.g.* the proportion of CVD deaths occurring below the age of 70 years is 26.5% in the developed countries compared with 46.7% in the developing countries3-4 and even larger for India (52.2%) [3,4].

Therefore, the contribution of the developing countries to the global burden of CVD, in terms of disability adjusted years of life lost, is 2.8 times higher than that of the developed countries (Table **1**).

Although there are inadequacies and imperfections of cause-specific mortality ascertainment methods currently used in many developing countries, the conservative assumptions made by the analysts suggest that this pattern will become even more pervasive as the CVD epidemic accelerates in many developing regions of the world, even as it retains its primacy as the leading public health problem in the developed regions [5-8]. A considerable cause for alarm is the projected rise in both proportional and absolute CVD mortality rates in the developing countries over the next 25 years [6-9]. Reasons for this anticipated acceleration of the epidemic includes genetic factors as well as demographic factors including lifestyle changes and nutritional transitions.

GENETIC FACTORS

It is increasingly recognized that CVD prevalence is a consequence of the interaction between the distribution of relative genotype frequencies and environmental exposures of a particular population [10,11]. It is suggested that distribution of such relative frequencies of genotypes involved in determining the distribution of individual susceptibilities to CVD is dependent on the number of segregating susceptibility genes, the number of alleles of each gene, their relative frequencies, and the correlation between alleles of each gene and alleles of different genes [12-14]. There are hundreds of genes known to have functional allelic variations that might contribute to determining an individual's susceptibility to CVD and all functional variations in a particular gene are not expected to be present in all populations [10-14]. Because new DNA variations arise in isolation and their chance, selection, and migration work as "filters" in each population to modify the relative frequencies of genetic variations in evolutionary time, different populations will have different combinations of DNA variations [15,16]. Therefore different combinations of susceptibility genes will be involved in determining CVD risk in different individuals in different families and is always difficult to relate such different combinations of susceptibility genes to the CVD risk. However, only few genetic studies of common multifactorial diseases recognize the importance of this question [17,18].

In 2004, the INTERHEART study examined the influence of nine risk factors for CVD [19] and reported that smoking, diabetes, hypertension, obesity, diet, inactivity, no alcohol intake, ApoB: ApoA1 ratio and psychosocial factors accounted for 90-94% of population-attributable risk. Based on this model, the authors [19] suggested that populations with all these risk factors are 337 times more likely to suffer cardiac disease than populations with none. In addition to these risk factors (which may themselves be genetically determined), a positive family history increases coronary artery disease (CAD) and myocardial infarction (MI) risk to 2-3.9 fold [20].

Until recently, such attempts to identify the genetic associations used either candidate gene or linkage studies. The former examines variations in a low number of known, plausibly associated genes in affected cases and controls, and while linkage studies assess affected families/sibling pairs using microsatellite markers to define a genomic region linked to the phenotype. So far, these approaches have been applied with great success to identifying causative mutations in monogenic cardiovascular diseases, such as hypertrophic cardiomyopathy and long QT syndrome [21-24]. However, the complex interplay between environment and genetics demonstrated in INTERHEART made it clear that similar approaches are unlikely to identify the poorly penetrant and multiple causative genes that account for non-Mendelian diseases, such as CVD. Although in rare occasions CVD can also be inherited in a Mendelian fashion (predominantly in conditions leading to elevated LDL), this only accounts for a small proportion of incident cases [25], most of which are likely to be polygenic. Linkage studies of non-Mendelian CVD have provided some biased associations [26-34], conspicuously lacked reproducibility between cohorts, suffered from poor statistical power and lacked detailed genomic mapping provided by conventional microsatellite markers.

Recent technological advancement, coupled with greater understanding of the structure of the human genome derived from genome sequencing projects [35-37], now make unbiased whole-genome association studies (GWAS) possible [38]. The International Haplotype Mapping project [39] identified hundreds of thousands of single nucleotide polymorphisms (SNPs), assessed their degree of linkage disequilibrium (the degree to which a SNP predicts the DNA flanking it). It is reported that genotyping 0.008% of an individual's nucleotides (250 000-350 000 in total) is able to identify an individual genome [40]. This technological advance led the Wellcome Trust Case Control Consortium and others to perform SNP-based GWAS on patients with CAD compared with matched controls [41]. For example the most reproducible locus conferring increased risk of CAD is situated on chromosome 9 (locus 9p21.3) [42-44] and increases risk by approximately 1.2 for a single copy (1.5 in the 25% of the population who carry two copies) [45]. Interestingly, unlike other regions associated with surrogate risk factors for CAD, such as C-reactive protein (CRP) [46], adiposity [47] and left ventricle (LV) mass [48], the 9p21.3 locus does not affect such risk factors, suggesting that it promotes CAD in a non-canonical manner. However, studies are suggesting that SNP-based GWAS knowledge provides no additional benefit [49], despite the availability of genotyping via the internet. First because loci such as 9p21.3 confers effect by altering the regulatory region of DNA [42]; second the involved region that overlaps a non-coding RNA named ANRIL, only conserve in primates and not other mammals or lower organisms and third the associations of some loci (*e.g.* 9p21.3 locus) are also present in conditions such as dementia [50] and stroke [51], rather than specifically CAD. Therefore, incorporation of risk-conferring alleles such as 9p21.3 and others into a CAD prediction algorithm is still not clear and thus remains to be substantiated in terms of its true importance under the current models and on clinical parameters [52].

DEMOGRAPHIC FACTORS

In the second half of the twentieth century, most developing countries experienced a major surge in life expectancy [53]. For example, the life expectancy in India rose from 41.2 years in 1951-1961 to 61.4 years in 1991-1996. This was principally due to a decline in deaths occurring in infancy, childhood, and adolescence.

This was also related to more effective public health responses to perinatal, infectious, and nutritional deficiency disorders and to improved economic indicators such as per-capita income and social indicators such as female literacy in some areas. Although much remains to be done in these areas, the demographic shifts have augmented the ranks of middle-aged and older adults.

The increasing longevity provides longer periods of exposure to the risk factors of CVD resulting in a greater probability of clinically manifest CVD events [54]. The concomitant decline of infectious and nutritional disorders (competing causes of death) further enhances the proportional burden due to CVD and other chronic lifestyle-related diseases.

This shift, representing a decline in deaths from infectious diseases and an increase in those due to chronic diseases, is often referred to as the modern epidemiological transition [8,9]. The ratio of deaths due to pre-transitional diseases (related to infections and malnutrition) to those caused by post-transitional diseases (*e.g.*, CVD and metabolic disorder) varies among regions and between countries, depending on factors such as the level of economic development and literacy as well as availability and access to health care.

The direction of change towards a rising relative contribution of post-transitional diseases is, however, common to and consistent among the developing countries [9]. The experience of urban China, in which the proportion of CVD deaths rose from 12.1% in 1957 to 35.8% in 1990, is illustrative of this phenomenon [55].

The United Kingdom itself is a diverse society with 7.9% of the population from minority ethnic groups (Africa, Middle-East, Indian Subcontinent, South America and Chinese region) [56]. The causes of the excess CVD and metabolic disorder morbidity and mortality in minority ethnic groups are incompletely understood by socio-economic factors.

However, the role of classical CVD risk factors is clearly important despite the patterns of these risk factors varying significantly by ethnic group. Moreover, the CVD epidemiology of African Americans does not represent well the morbidity and mortality experience seen in black Africans and black Caribbean's, both in Britain and in their native African countries.

In particular, atherosclerotic disease and coronary heart disease are still relatively rare in the latter groups. This is unlike the South Asian Diaspora which has prevalence rates of CVD in epidemic proportions both in the Diaspora and on the subcontinent [56].

Data for population surveillance of CVD and metabolic disorders are limited in many countries. The World Health Organization (WHO) has set up a range of projects aimed at improving the amount and quality of relevant data [57]. The Surveillance of Risk Factors (SuRFs) project, launched in 2003, presents chronic disease risk factor profiles from 170 WHO member states. These data include patterns of physical inactivity, low fruit/vegetable intake, obesity, blood pressure, cholesterol, and diabetes [58].

The most recent report SuRF2 enables country comparisons for these data [59]. Fig. (**1**) shows data on the percentage of adults in the different countries of Southeast Asian Nations with body mass index (BMI) >30 kg/m^2.

The variation is marked and it is interesting to note that two of the poorest countries in the region, Laos and Myanmar, have severe obesity rates comparable with some of the wealthiest. On the other hand, Singapore, the most developed country in the region does not suffer from obesity epidemic.

Although, the biological determinants of CVD and metabolic disorders in low and middle income countries are likely to be similar to those in affluent countries, [60] the drivers of these determinants are likely to differ. For example, rural-urban migration may be an important factor in promoting the adoption of Western dietary habits and activity patterns, leading to an increased CVD risks.

Socioeconomic patterns of disease risk, so well established in affluent countries, are more complex in some low and middle income countries [60-62]. New opportunities to use large demographic surveillance projects as tools to study CVD and metabolic disorders are emerging rapidly as part on the work of INDEPTH (International Network of field sites with continuous Demographic Evaluation of Populations and their Health in developing countries) [63].

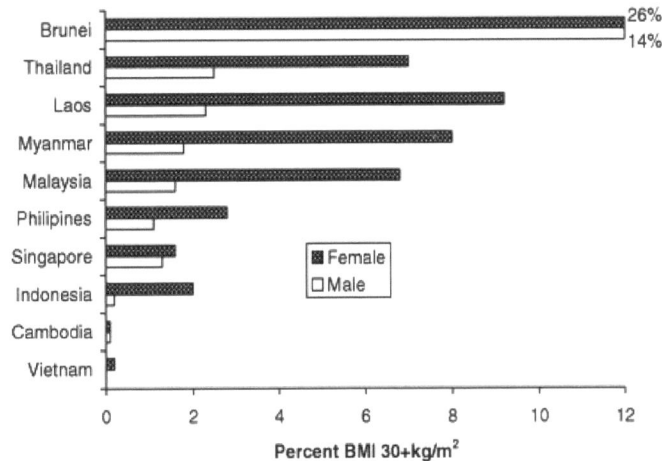

Figure 1: Use of WHO web Global InfoBase [58,59]: Obesity (BMI $\geq$ 30 kg/m^2) in the Association of Southeast Asian Nations in 2002.

Even with such studies of understanding of determinants for rising CVD/ metabolic disorder epidemic and explaining such differences as to how rural-urban migration increases risks of obesity, diabetes, and CVD- will not be possible. One important caveat to looking at such data is to study the role of impaired early growth, resulting from fetal and infant nutrition operating at different stages of the life course [64,65] an issue that particularly applies to when defining the causality of this problem.

NUTRITIONAL TRANSITION AND LIFE STYLE CHANGES

Another concern is that if population levels of CVD risk factors rise as a consequence of adverse lifestyle changes accompanying industrialization and urbanization, the rates of CVD mortality and morbidity could rise even higher than the rates predicted solely by demographic changes.

It is suggested that both the degree and the duration of exposure to CVD risk factors would increase due to higher risk factor levels coupled with a longer life expectancy. An increase in body weight (adjusted for height), blood pressure, and cholesterol levels in Chinese population samples aged 35 to 64 years, between the two phases of the Sino-MONICA study (1984 to 1986 and 1988 to 1989) and the substantially higher levels of CVD risk factors in urban population groups compared with rural population groups in India provide evidence of such trends [54,55,66,67].

A cross-sectional survey of urban Delhi and its rural environs revealed that a higher prevalence of CHD in the urban sample was associated with higher levels of body mass index, blood pressure, fasting blood lipids (total cholesterol, ratio of cholesterol to HDL cholesterol, triglycerides), and diabetes.54 The increasing use of tobacco in a number of developing countries will also translate into higher mortality rates of CVD, CHD and other tobacco-related diseases [68,69].

As reviewed by Drewnowski and Popkin [70] the global availability of cheap vegetable oils and fats has resulted in greatly increased fat consumption among many countries.

The transition now occurs at lower levels of the gross national product than previously and is further accelerated by rapid urbanization. For example, the proportion of upper-income persons who were consuming a relatively high-fat diet (>30% of daily energy intake) rose from 22.8% to 66.6% between 1989 and 1993 in China. The lower- and middle-income classes also showed a rise (from 19% to 36.4% in the former and from 19.1% to 51.0% in the latter) [68].

These countries, with a diet that is traditionally high in carbohydrates and low in fat, have shown an overall decline in the proportion of energy from complex carbohydrates along with the increase in the proportion of fat [71]. The globalization of food production and marketing is also contributing to the increasing consumption of energy-dense foods poor in dietary fibre and several micronutrients [71].

THE COMPLEXITY OF THE PROBLEM

The prior discussion in sections 1.1 -1.4 hence shows that CVD has a complex multifactorial aetiology leading to a reappraisal of the ways in which three key factors- genome, development and environment- influence the adult phenotype, including the individual's susceptibility to disease. Neither genetic makeup nor exposures to adverse environments predict with certainty the onset, progression, or severity of CVD. Disease develops as a consequence of interactions between the "initial" conditions, coded in the genotype, and exposures to environmental agents indexed by time and space [72-74] that are integrated by dynamic, regulatory networks at levels above the genome [75].

The interaction of an individual's environmental experiences with her/his genotype determines the history of her/his multidimensional phenotype, beginning at conception and continuing through adulthood (Fig. **2**).

At a particular point in time, each genotype has a range of possible phenotypes determined by the range of possible environmental histories. The phenotype of an individual to react to contemporary environments in a particular environmental niche, at a particular point in time, is influenced by the phenotype produced by previous genotype-phenotype combination. The figure illustrates this relationship, by collapsing an individual's phenotype into single dimension, showing two of the many possible phenotype histories for a given genotype. The consequence of these interactions with exposures to environmental agents indexed by time and space is that many individuals who have a genotype that predicts an increased risk of CVD will remain healthy because of exposures to compensatory environments. The converse will also be true: individuals who have a genotype that has a low risk of CVD might develop disease because of an adverse environmental history.

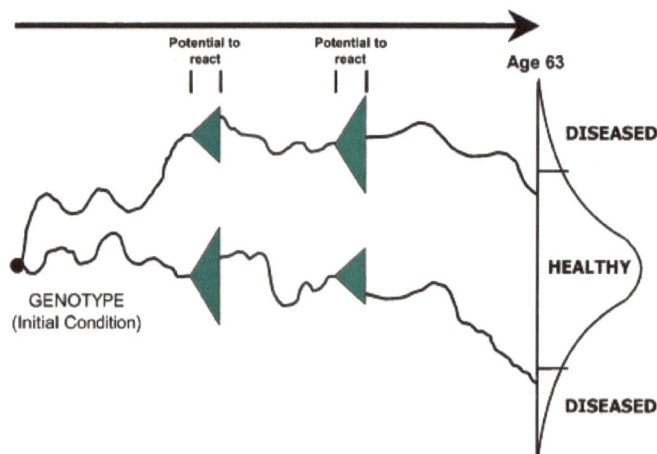

Figure 2: Adopted with Permission from Sing *et al.,* [76].

CVD research has revealed tens of high-risk environmental factors and hundreds of genes, each with many variations that influence disease risk. The phenotypic measures of health are constantly being shaped, changed, and transposed as a consequence of epigenetic networks of cellular and organismal dimensions that change over the lifetime of the individual. At the level of the cell, these networks influence DNA methylation and repair; they also serve to organize coordinated responses to heat-shock, oxygen deprivation, and other environmental changes [77]. The relationships between these subsystems influence the trajectory of an individual's phenotype to influence the expression of the participating genes [78-80] (Fig. **3**).

This figure shows how a particular multigene genotype is connected to the domain of potential CVD phenotypes through the primary biochemical and physiological subsystems. The important role that biochemistry and physiology play in the connections between the genome and disease phenotypes brings into question the utility of the overused, simplistic view that the genome produces an independent, isolated, and fixed one-way flow of information from genome to phenotype.

Studies have suggested that different ethnic groups that live in the same geographic areas and share similar environmental risks have different profiles of disease markers and prevalence, which may propose a genetic cause for differences in disease susceptibility [81,82]. Yet, with some notable exceptions [83] few ancestry-specific alleles have been discovered that can explain particular pathologies. Other explanations of both inter-individual and ethnic differences in disease risk, therefore, need to be considered. Of note, high incidences of metabolic disease are found in those ethnic groups in which the average birthweight is low84 or the rates of gestational diabetes and maternal obesity are high [85].

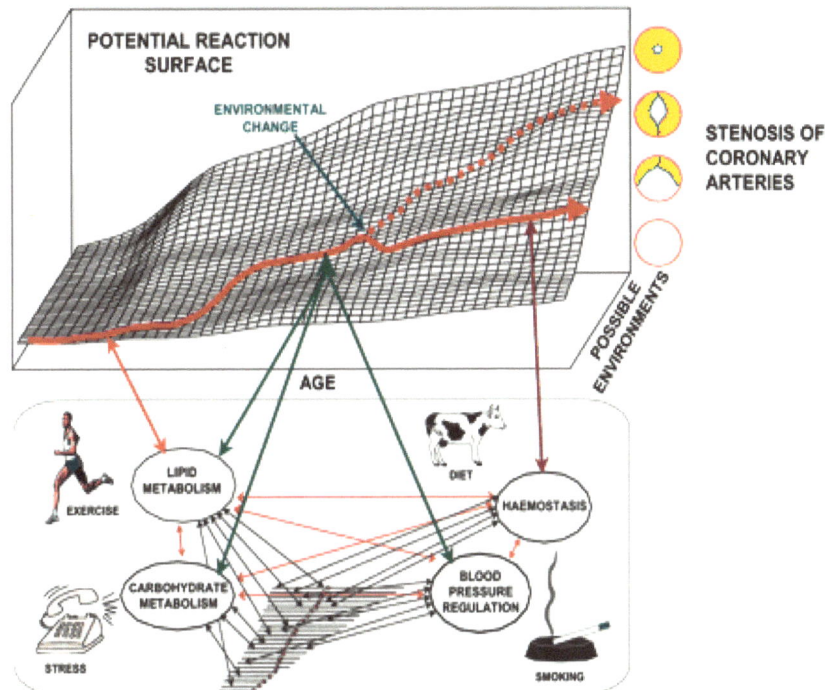

Figure 3: Adopted with Permission from Sing *et al.,* [76]. A Model for an Individual's Propensity to Develop CVD such as Coronary Artery Disease

Untangling the effects of genes from those of environmentally determined developmental processes is not straightforward. Importantly, fetal nutrition does not equate to maternal food intake, but rather is dependent on maternal metabolism, cardiovascular function and, particularly, placental function [86]. The long-lasting changes in developmental trajectory that underpin altered susceptibility to disease may arise, at least in part, from epigenetically mediated alterations in gene expression. Whereas compelling evidence supports both the developmental origins of health and disease and the underlying epigenetic mechanisms, [87] many features of the latter remain insufficiently understood.

These elements include the differences among epigenetic mechanisms across species and between patterns of epigenetic modifications on paternal and maternal genomes, the mechanisms that regulate the establishment, stability and flexibility of epigenetic changes, and the precise connection between an epigenetic change, altered gene expression and the resultant phenotype for CVD epidemic in countries [72-80]. The hypothesis is currently recognised as "Developmental origins of Health and Disease" (DOHaD) and requires particular understanding before proceeding further with this subject.

DEVELOPMENTAL ORIGINS OF HEALTH AND DISEASE

DOHaD hypothesis states that adverse intrauterine influences such as poor maternal nutrition lead to impaired fetal growth, resulting in low birth weight, short birth length, and small head circumference. These adverse influences are postulated to also induce the fetus to develop adaptive metabolic and physiological responses. These responses, however, may lead to disordered reactions to environmental challenges as the child grows, with an increased risk of glucose intolerance, hypertension, and dyslipidaemia in later life and adult CVD as a consequence [88-94]. Although some supportive evidence for the hypothesis has been provided by observational studies, [95-99] it awaits further evaluation for a causal role. If it does emerge as an important risk factor for CVD, the populations of developing countries will be at an especially enhanced risk because the vast numbers of poorly nourished infants who have been born in the past several decades now suffer a threat through an over-nourished rich environment. The steady improvement in child survival will lead to a higher proportion of such infants surviving to adult life, when their hypothesized susceptibility to vascular disease may manifest itself [100-109].

ORIGINS OF THE HYPOTHESIS- HISTORICAL PERSPECTIVE

The "*early or fetal origin of adult disease hypothesis*" originally proposed by Barker and colleagues in Southampton, United Kingdom, suggested that environmental factors, particularly nutrition, act in early life to program the risks for the early onset of cardiovascular and metabolic disease in adult life and premature death [88,89, 93,94, 110,111].

Before the fetal origins hypothesis was articulated, an association between early life events and later cardiovascular disease had been proposed on more than one occasion. In 1934, Kermack *et al.* [112] demonstrated that death rates from all causes in the United Kingdom and Sweden fell between 1751 and 1930. The authors concluded that this was the result of better childhood living conditions during this period. Subsequently, Forsdahl [113] reported that there was a correlation within different geographical regions of Norway between coronary heart disease in 1964-1967 and infant mortality rates some 70 years earlier.

Forsdahl [113] postulated that poverty may act through a nutritional deficit to result in a life-long vulnerability to disease with a more affluent adult life-style. In 1985, Wadsworth *et al.* [114] in the United Kingdom reported that adult blood pressure was inversely related to birth weight in men and women born in 1946. In 1986, Barker and colleagues suggested that poor health and physique of mothers were important determinants of the risk of stroke in their offspring [93]. Soon afterwards, they proposed that environmental influences, which impair growth and development in early life, result in an increased risk for ischemic heart disease [94]. This then led to a worldwide series of epidemiological studies that extended the initial observations on the association between pre- and postnatal growth and cardiovascular disease to include associations between early growth patterns and an increased risk for hypertension, impaired glucose tolerance, non-insulin-dependent or type-2 diabetes, insulin resistance, and obesity in adult life [115-124].

THE THRIFTY PHENOTYPE HYPOTHESIS, DEVELOPMENTAL PLASTICITY AND PREDICTIVE ADAPTIVE RESPONSES

To explain the biological basis of the associations observed between early growth patterns and health outcomes in the epidemiological studies, number of mechanistic frameworks such as "*thrifty genotype*" [125,126] and then "*thrifty phenotype*" [127] derived from thrifty genotype, were proposed. "Thrifty genes" were proposed to be selected during evolution at a time when food resources were scarce and they resulted in a "fast insulin trigger" and thus an enhanced capacity to store fat, which placed the individual at risk of insulin resistance and type-2 diabetes [126].

In contrast the thrifty phenotype hypothesis suggested that when the fetal environment is poor, there is an adaptive response, which optimizes the growth of key body organs to the detriment of others and leads to an altered postnatal metabolism, which is designed to enhance postnatal survival under conditions of intermittent or poor nutrition [128-129]. It was proposed that these adaptations only became detrimental when nutrition was more abundant in the postnatal environment, than it had been in the prenatal environment [127].

Lucas suggests that that there are embryonic and fetal adaptive responses to a suboptimal intrauterine environment which result in permanent adverse consequences either via the induction, deletion, or impaired development of a permanent somatic structure or the physiological system [129]. In fact closing the critical window early in development allows the preservation of maternal strategy in offspring phenotype, which in humans benefits the mother by constraining offspring demand after weaning. The offspring gains by being buffered against environmental fluctuations during the most sensitive period of development, allowing coherent adaptation of organ growth to the state of the environment. The critical window is predicted to close when offspring physiology becomes independent of maternal physiology, the timing of which depends on offspring trait [130-133]. All this highlight the relationship between intrauterine nutritional experiences and subsequent health outcomes [134,135].

Researchers working with humans and animal models of human diseases often view the effects of early life events as the developmental plasticity. This embodies the idea that developmental plasticity is the ability of a single genotype to produce more than one alternative form of structure, physiological state, or behaviour in response to environmental conditions [135-

137]. Consistent with this, it is thought that CVD may be a consequence of fetal adaptations to under nutrition that are beneficial for short-term survival, even though they are detrimental to health in post reproductive life [112].

Although some effects of nutrition may be direct consequences of alterations in substrate availability, McCance and Widdowson demonstrated that early under nutrition had a permanent effect on the subsequent growth of rats, whereas later under nutrition only had a transient effect [138].

It is clear from a range of diverse fields including evolutionary ecology and molecular biology that a given genotype can give rise to different phenotypes, depending on environmental conditions [139-141].

There are many different species where the impact of an environment experienced by one generation determines the development and behaviour of the next generation. Female birds are able to alter many aspects of the composition of the egg in response to a range of environmental factors including food availability, levels of sibling competition, and the quality of their mates [139]. Such maternal effects can result in the effects of a specific environmental factor persisting across several generations [135-137, 141].

If the effects of the past conditions produce mismatches with current, changed conditions, however, then developmental plasticity may have a detrimental effect on survival and reproductive success [142]. Thus Bateson *et al.* [141] propose that for individuals whose early environment has predicted a high level of nutrition in adult life and who develop a large phenotype, the better the postnatal conditions the better will be their adult health. For individuals whose conditions in fetal life predicted poor adult nutrition and who develop a small phenotype, the expected outcomes may vary, although they are predicted to be worse off when there is a relative excess of nutrition in postnatal life.

There has also been a proposal to separate those homeostatic responses that represent fetal adaptations to changes in the intrauterine environment and that may have long-term consequences, from those which need not confer immediate advantage but are induced in the expectation of future adaptive changes [143]; this latter group of responses has been defined as "predictive adaptive" [90,92,137,141]. In this model of predictive adaptive response, selection across generations operates to favour protection of those predictive adaptive responses that aid survival to reproductive age.

The programmed or plastic responses made during development that have immediate adaptive advantage might also act to limit the range of postnatal adaptive responses to a new environment and would be considered to be "inappropriate" predictive adaptive responses. This general model is therefore consistent with the original thrifty phenotype hypothesis which stated that fetal adaptations to a poor intrauterine environment may have adverse consequences if there is a relative excess of nutrition available in adult life.

The use of the term "predictive adaptive response" must be clarified because it is used in two very different ways in the literature. In a physiological context it refers to adjustments made by an individual in response to current conditions. For example, in conditions of severe intrauterine deprivation, there is the capacity to lose structural units such as nephrons, cardiomyocytes, or pancreatic β-cells within developing organ systems. Such decreases in structural and hence the life-long functional capacity of an organ system may be an inadvertent consequence of a decrease in energy supply across the placenta or a selective trade off to maintain the development of more important tissues, such as the brain [144-146].

In an evolutionary context it refers to changes in the characteristics of populations or species resulting from natural selection, mainly promoting Darwinian fitness and adaptive according to the evolutionary criteria of enhancing survival or reproductive success [147].

In case of fetal origins of disease, this would require that environmental conditions present early in life are predictive of the conditions the individual will encounter in the future over a range of timescales (Fig. **4**).

It is suggested that at one extreme, rapid and reversible homoeostatic mechanisms counter an immediate challenge. Then, stressors or exposures during critical developmental periods can affect growth, tissue differentiation, and physiological set-points, affecting responses to environmental challenges for life. New evidence suggests that epigenetic mechanisms could contribute to such challenges [148,149].

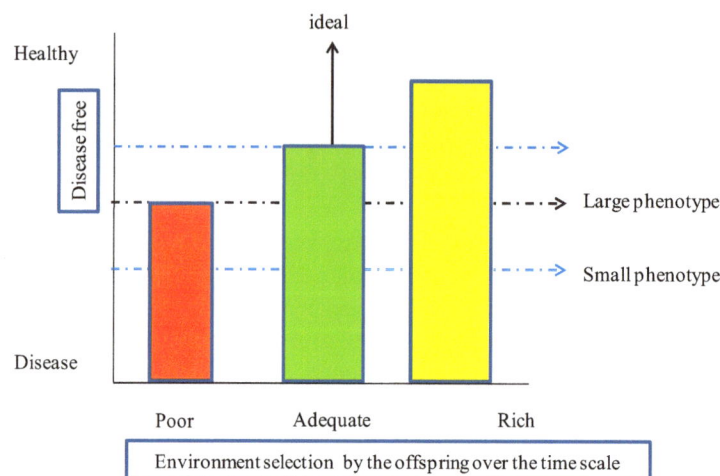

Figure 4: Modes of Human Adaptability.

On a long timescale, the genomes of populations can change over many generations as a result of selection or drift, and there are many examples of responses to environmental change becoming integrated into the human genome [141,150-152]. Clinical medicine and public health research have focused largely on causation and intervention at the short-term end of this spectrum. In this context consideration of the outcomes of developmental plasticity acting over the intermediate timescale is now important [141]. In humans, development plasticity can induce responses that have short-term benefits for the mother or the fetus but on longer term costs reduced fitness leading to disease process [152,153]. It is suggested that when environmental conditions change strikingly between conception and adulthood, as has happened in most current human populations, the potential for a substantial mismatch is especially great, and this difference contributes to increased disease risk [135].

ENVIRONMENTAL CUES AFFECTING HUMAN DEVELOPMENT

These broad considerations are relevant to understanding of some critical variations such as developmental adaptations that permanently change structure, physiology, and metabolism, thereby predisposing individuals to cardiovascular, metabolic, and endocrine disease in adult life [154,155]. The human baby responds to under nutrition, placental dysfunction and other adverse influences by changing the trajectory of his or her development and slowing growth. Although the fetus was thought to be well-buffered against fluctuations in its mother's condition, a growing body of evidence suggests that the morphology and physiology of the human baby is affected by the state of the mother [156,157].

It is possible therefore, that human development may involve induction of particular patterns of development by cues that prepare the developing individual for the type of environment in which he or she is likely to live. Individuals may be affected adversely if the environmental prediction provided by the mother and the conditions of early infancy prove to be incorrect [113].

Thus, people whose birth weights were towards the lower end of the normal range and who subsequently grows up in affluent environments are at increased risk of developing coronary heart disease, type-2 diabetes and hypertension [39,40, 156,158]. Those born as heavier babies and brought up in affluent environments enjoy a much reduced risk. The long-term influences may arise from cues acting from before conception to infancy [159].

The ill effects of being small, which in the short term include high death rates and childhood illness, are usually treated as yet another inevitable consequence of adversity. However, a functional and evolutionary approach suggests that the pregnant women in poor nutritional condition may signal to her unborn baby that help it to cope with a shortage of food. When sufficiently high levels of nutrition are available after the development of a small phenotype has been initiated, marginal benefits of rapid growth may offset the costs [160], but they may also trigger the health problems arising in later life. This concept is illustrated in Fig. (**5**).

Although adaptive responses may explain some variation in human development, it would be implausible to argue that all responses to the environment should be explained in these terms. Under nutrition, stress or hypoxia may impair normal development. Babies with low birth weight have a reduced functional capacity and fewer cells [161]. The latter may be part of a general reduction in cell numbers or a selective trade-off in the development of tissues that are less important to the baby, such as the kidney [162]. Reduced numbers of nephrons at birth is a life-long deficit, as all nephrons are formed during a sensitive period of development in late gestation. The resulting increased functional demand on each individual nephron, for example by increased blood flow through each nephron, may lead to acceleration of the nephron's death that accompanies normal ageing, with a consequent rise in blood pressure [163,164].

The diversity in past and present ecological conditions of humans is also likely to introduce complexity into the relationship between developmental prediction and later health outcome. For example, some populations may have adapted genetically to conditions of nutritional stress, especially seasonal food shortages, over a long time span, while others will have been buffered from such local evolutionary effects. The sharp increase in glucose intolerance leading to type-2 diabetes might arise from genetic differences between populations [165-167]. The possibility of a thrifty genotype well adapted to harsh conditions is not incompatible with the plastic induction of thrifty phenotypes from a pool of uniform genotypes. However, the hypothesis that differences in susceptibility to diabetes are explained by genetic differences would not readily account for the evidence from the Dutch famine of 1944-45 that glucose intolerance is induced by maternal malnutrition during the final three months of pregnancy [167]. However, persisting into adult life, insulin resistance leads to increasing blood glucose and type-2 diabetes develops, especially in people who have become overweight. 'Thrifty' handling of sugar becomes maladaptive if under nutrition in the womb is followed by excess in later life 168.

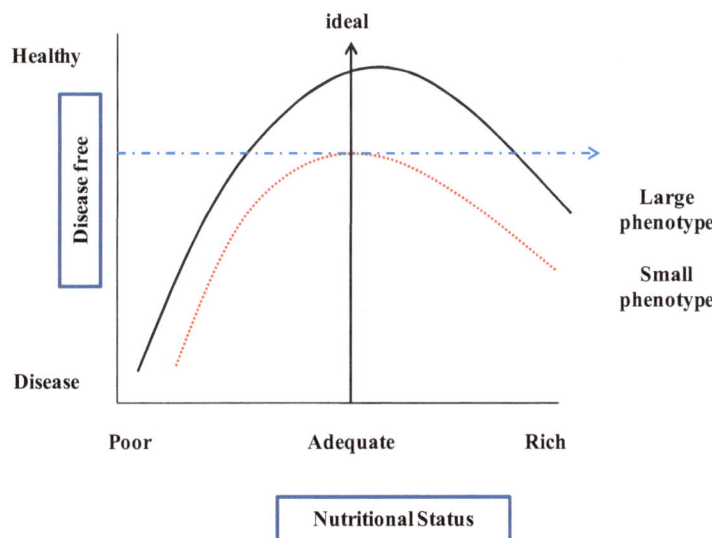

Figure 5: The Hypothetical Relationship Between Adult Health and Nutritional Level During Later Development for Two Extreme Human Phenotypes that were Initiated by Cues Received by the Fetus. Reprinted by Permission from Macmillan Publishers Ltd: Bateson *et al.,* Nature, 430: 419-421, 2004 [141].

Conversely, individuals with large bodies may be particularly at risk in harsh environments such as prison camps or during famines [153,168-169]. Especially striking is the evidence from a famine-exposed Ethiopian population, where the incidence of rickets was nine times greater in children who had been reported as having high birth weights than in age-matched control children [170]. No such differences were found in children with normal birth weights.

CONCLUSION

Numerous epidemiological and animal studies discussed so far have shown an association between altered maternal nutrition and cardiovascular or metabolic disease in the offspring. Namely, alterations in fetal nutrition (either under- or over-nutrition) may result during critical periods when offspring are most vulnerable to developmental adaptations that permanently change the structure, physiology and metabolism of the offspring, thereby predisposing individuals to metabolic and cardiovascular diseases in adult life.

Today the most common maternal dietary imbalance in populations is an excessive intake of dietary fat. There is growing body of evidence that significant health problems for women of reproductive age result from being overweight or obese due to overeating. Extensive studies have shown that maternal over nutrition retards placental and fetal growth, and increases fetal and neonatal mortality in animal models. Results of epidemiological studies indicate that almost 65% of the adult population in the U.S. is overweight (defined as a body mass index (BMI) > 25 kg/m², while 31% of the adult population is obese (defined as BMI > 30 kg/m²). Many overweight and obese women unknowingly enter pregnancy and continue overeating during gestation. These women usually gain more weight during the first pregnancy and accumulate more fat during subsequent pregnancies. Maternal obesity or over-nutrition before or during pregnancy may result in fetal growth restriction and increased risk of neonatal metabolic syndrome and cardiovascular risk factors.

Previously, studies have demonstrated abnormalities in plasma lipids, vascular fatty acids, and evidence for reduced endothelium-dependent relaxation in adult offspring of rodent models fed on a lard-rich diet during pregnancy, suckling or lactation. However neither the designs of these studies carried out nor the fat intake mimic the typical high-fat Western diet and human situation. Moreover, to date no one has determined the role of early pharmacological intervention in mothers and its effects on offspring in terms of cardiovascular control using the animal model.

REFERENCES

[1]   Nissen SE. Cardiovascular outcomes in randomized trials: should time to first event for "hard" end points remain the standard approach? J Am Coll Cardiol 2009; 54(25): 2363-65.

[2]   Tai ES, Poulton R, Thumboo J, *et al.* An update on cardiovascular disease epidemiology in South East Asia. Rationale and design of the LIFE course study in CARdiovascular disease Epidemiology (LIFECARE). CVD Prevent Control 2009; 4(2): 93-102.

[3]   Murray CJL, Lopez AD. Global comparative assessments in the health sector. Geneva, Switzerland: World Health Organization 1994.

[4]   Lopez AD. Assessing the burden of mortality from cardiovascular disease. World Health Stat Q 1993; 46: 91-6.

[5]   Reddy KS, Yusuf S. Emerging epidemic of cardiovascular disease in developing countries. Circulation 1998; 97 (6): 596-601.

[6]   Thom TJ, Epstein FH, Feldman JJ, *et al.* Total Mortality and Mortality From Heart Disease, Cancer, and Stroke From 1950 to 1987 in 27 Countries: Highlights of Trends and Their Interrelationships Among Causes of Death. Washington, DC: US DHHS PHS, National Institutes of Health; NIH publication No. 1992; 92-3088.

[7]   Whelton PK, Brancati FL, Appel LJ, *et al.* The challenge of hypertension and atherosclerotic cardiovascular disease in economically developing countries. High Blood Pressure Cardiovasc Prevent 1995; 4: 36-45.

[8]   Pearson TA, Jamison DT, Tergo-Gauderies J. Cardiovascular disease. In: Jamison DT, Mosley WH, Eds. Disease Control Priorities in Developing Countries. New York, NY: Oxford University Press 1993.

[9]   Omran AR. The epidemiologic transition: a key of the epidemiology of population change. Milibank Memorial Fund Q. 1971; 49: 509-38.

[10]   Scriver CR, Byck S, Prevost L, Hoang L. PAH mutation analysis consortium. In: Chadwick DJ, Cardew G, Eds. Variation in the Human Genome (Ciba Foundation Symposium 197). Chichester, UK: John Wiley and Sons 1996: pp. 73-96.

[11]   Weatherall D. The genetics of common diseases: the implications of population variability In: Chadwick DJ, Cardew G, Eds. Variation in the Human Genome (Ciba Foundation Symposium 197). Chichester, UK: John Wiley and Sons 1996: pp. 300-11.

[12]   Clark AG, Weiss KM, Nickerson DA, *et al.* Haplotype structure and population genetic inferences from nucleotide sequence variation in human lipoprotein lipase. Am J Hum Genet 1998; 63 (2): 595-612.

[13]   Fullerton SM, Clark AG, Weiss KM, *et al.* Apolipoprotein E variation at the sequence haplotype level: implications for the origin and maintenance of a major human polymorphism. Am J Hum Genet 2000; 67 (4): 881-900.

[14]   Stengård JH, Clark AG, Weiss KM, Kardia S, *et al.* Contributions of 18 additional DNA sequence variations in the gene for apolipoprotein E to explaining variation in quantitative measures of lipid metabolism. Am J Hum Genet 2002; 71(3): 501-17.

[15]   Gluckman PD, Hanson MA. Living with the past: evolution, development, and patterns of disease. Science 2004; 305 (5691): 1733-36.

[16]   Charles F. Sing, Jari H. Stengård, and Sharon L.R. Kardia. Genes, environment, and cardiovascular disease. Arterioscler Thromb Vasc Biol 2003; 23 (7): 1190- 96.

[17]   Elahi MM, Asotra K, Matata BM, *et al.* Tumor necrosis factor alpha -308 gene locus promoter polymorphism: an analysis of association with health and disease. Biochim Biophys Acta 2009 (3);1792: 163-72

[18]   Elahi MM, Gilmour A, Matata BM, *et al.* A variant of position -308 of the Tumour necrosis factor alpha gene promoter and the risk of coronary heart disease. Heart Lung Circ 2008; 17 (1): 14-8.

[19]   Yusuf S, Hawken S, Ounpuu S, *et al.* Effect of potentially modifiable risk factors associated with myocardial infarction in 52 countries (the INTERHEART study): case-control study. Lancet 2004; 364 (9438): 937-52.

[20]   Shea S, Ottman R, Gabrieli C, *et al.* Family history as an independent risk factor for coronary artery disease. J Am Coll Cardiol 1984; 4 (4): 793-801.

[21]   Watkins H, Ashrafian H, McKenna WJ. The genetics of hypertrophic cardiomyopathy: Teare redux. Heart 2008; 94 (10): 1264-8.

[22]   Shimizu W. The long QT syndrome: therapeutic implications of a genetic diagnosis. Cardiovasc Res 2005; 67 (3): 347-56.

[23]   Fatkin D, Graham RM. Molecular mechanisms of inherited cardiomyopathies. Physiol Rev 2002; 82 (4): 945-80.

[24]   Spooner PM. Sudden cardiac death: the larger problem...the larger genome. J Cardiovasc Electrophysiol 2009; 20 (5): 585-96

[25]   Dandona S, Roberts R. Creating a genetic risk score for coronary artery disease. Curr Atheroscler Rep 2009; 11 (3): 175-81.

[26]   Pajukanta P, Cargill M, Viitanen L, *et al.* Two loci on chromosomes 2 and X for premature coronary heart disease identified in early- and late-settlement populations of Finland. Am J Hum Genet 2000; 67 (6): 1481-93.

[27]   Francke S, Manraj M, Lacquemant C, *et al.* A genome-wide scan for coronary heart disease suggests in Indo-Mauritians a susceptibility locus on chromosome 16p13 and replicates linkage with the metabolic syndrome on 3q27. Hum Mol Genet 2001; 10 (24): 2751-65.

[28]   Broeckel U, Hengstenberg C, Mayer B, *et al.* A comprehensive linkage analysis for myocardial infarction and its related risk factors. Nat Genet 2002; 30 (2): 210-14.

[29]   Harrap SB, Zammit KS, Wong ZY, *et al.* Genome-wide linkage analysis of the acute coronary syndrome suggests a locus on chromosome 2. Arterioscler Thromb Vasc Biol 2002; 22 (5): 874-78.

[30]   Wang Q, Rao S, Shen GQ, Li L, *et al.* Premature myocardial infarction novel susceptibility locus on chromosome 1P34-36 identified by genomewide linkage analysis. Am J Hum Genet 2004; 74 (2): 262-271.

[31]   Hauser ER, Crossman DC, Granger CB, *et al.* A genomewide scan for early-onset coronary artery disease in 438 families: the GENECARD Study. Am J Hum Genet 2004; 75 (3): 436-47.

[32]   Helgadottir A, Manolescu A, Thorleifsson G, *et al.* The gene encoding 5-lipoxygenase activating protein confers risk of myocardial infarction and stroke. Nat Genet 2004; 36 (3): 233-39.

[33]   Helgadottir A, Manolescu A, Helgason A, *et al.* A variant of the gene encoding leukotriene A4 hydrolase confers ethnicity-specific risk of myocardial infarction. Nat Genet 2006; 38 (1): 68-74.

[34]   Samani NJ, Burton P, Mangino M, *et al.* A genomewide linkage study of 1,933 families affected by premature coronary artery disease: The British Heart Foundation (BHF) Family Heart Study. Am J Hum Genet 2005; 77 (6): 1011-20.

[35]   McPherson JD, Marra M, Hillier L, *et al.* A physical map of the human genome. Nature 2001; 409 (6822): 934-41.

[36]   Lander ES, Linton LM, Birren B, *et al.* Initial sequencing and analysis of the human genome. Nature 2001; 409 (6822): 860-921.

[37]   Venter JC, Adams MD, Myers EW, *et al.* The sequence of the human genome. Science 2001; 291 (5507): 1304-51.

[38]   Hirschhorn JN, Daly MJ. Genome-wide association studies for common diseases and complex traits. Nat Rev Genet 2005; 6 (2): 95-108.

[39]   International HapMap Consortium. The International HapMap Project. Nature 2003; 426 (6968): 789-96.

[40]   Topol EJ. The genetics of heart attack. Heart 2006; 92 (6): 855-61.

[41]   WTCCC. Genome-wide association study of 14,000 cases of seven common diseases and 3000 shared controls. Nature 2007; 447 (7145): 661-78.

[42]   McPherson R, Pertsemlidis A, Kavaslar N, *et al.* A common allele on chromosome 9 associated with coronary heart disease. Science 2007; 316 (5830): 1488-91.

[43]   Helgadottir A, Thorleifsson G, Manolescu A, *et al.* A common variant on chromosome 9p21 affects the risk of myocardial infarction. Science 2007; 316 (5830): 1491-3.

[44]   Samani NJ, Erdmann J, Hall AS, *et al.* Genomewide association analysis of coronary artery disease. N Engl J Med 2007 357(5): 443-53.

[45]   Samani NJ, Deloukas P, Erdmann J, *et al.* Large scale association analysis of novel genetic loci for coronary artery disease. Arterioscler Thromb Vasc Biol 2009; 29 (5): 774-80.

[46]   Elliott P, Chambers JC, Zhang W, *et al.* Genetic loci associated with C-reactive protein levels and risk of coronary heart disease. J Am Med Assoc 2009; 302 (1): 37-48.

[47]   Lindgren CM, Heid IM, Randall JC, *et al.* Genome-wide association scan meta-analysis identifies three loci influencing adiposity and fat distribution. PLoS Genet 2009; 5 (6): e1000508.

[48]   Vasan RS, Glazer NL, Felix JF, *et al.* Genetic variants associated with cardiac structure and function: a meta-analysis and replication of genome-wide association data. J Am Med Assoc 2009; 302 (2): 168-78.

[49]   Paynter NP, Chasman DI, Buring JE, Shiffman D, Cook NR, Ridker PM. Cardiovascular disease risk prediction with and without knowledge of genetic variation at chromosome 9p21.3. Ann Intern Med 2009; 150 (3): 65-72.

[50] Emanuele E, Lista S, Ghidoni R, *et al.* Chromosome 9p21.3 genotype is associated with vascular dementia and Alzheimer's disease. Neurobiol Aging 2011;32(7):1231-5.

[51] Gschwendtner A, Bevan S, Cole JW, *et al.* Sequence variants on chromosome 9p21.3 confer risk for atherosclerotic stroke. Ann Neurol 2009; 65 (5): 531-9.

[52] van der Net JB, Janssens AC, Sijbrands EJ, *et al.* Value of genetic profiling for the prediction of coronary heart disease. Am Heart J 2009; 158 (1): 105-10.

[53] World Bank. World Development Report: Investing in Health. New York, NY: Oxford University Press 1993.

[54] Reddy KS. Cardiovascular disease in India. World Health Stat Q. 1993;46: 101-7

[55] Yao C, Wu Z, Wu J. The changing pattern of cardiovascular diseases in China. World Health Stat Q 1993; 46: 113-8.

[56] Lip GY, Barnett AH, Bradbury A, *et al.* Ethnicity and cardiovascular disease prevention in the United Kingdom: a practical approach to management. J Hum Hyperten 2007; 21(3): 183-211.

[57] World Health Organisation. World Health Report 2003. Shaping the Future. Geneva: WHO 2003.

[58] World Health Organisation. World Health Report 2002. Reducing Risks, Promoting Healthy Life. Geneva: WHO, 2002.

[59] World Health Organisation. Surveillance for Chronic Disease Risk Factors. Country Level Risk Factors and Comparable Estimates. SuRF2 Report. Geneva: WHO, 2005. Available at: http://www.who.int/ncd_surveillance/infobase/web//surf2/start.html

[60] Yusuf S, Hawken S, Ôunpuu S, *et al.* Effect of potentially modifiable risk factors associated with myocardial infarction in 52 countries (the INTERHEART study): case-control study. Lancet 2004; 364 (9438): 937-52.

[61] Bovet P, Ross AG, Gervasoni JP, *et al.* Distribution of blood pressure, body mass index and smoking habits in the urban population of Dar es Salaam, Tanzania, and associations with socioeconomic status. Int J Epidemiol 2002 ; 31(1): 240-7.

[62] Ezzati M, Hoorn SV, Rodgers A, *et al.* Estimates of global and regional potential health gains from reducing multiple major risk factors. Lancet 2003; 26 (9380): 271-80.

[63] INDEPTH. Population and Health in Developing Countries. Volume 1, Population, Health, and Survival at INDEPTH Sites. INDEPTH Network. Ottawa: International Development Research Centre, 2002. Available at: http://www.indepth-network.org/default.asp

[64] Bhargava SK, Sachdev HS, Fall CH, *et al.* Relation of serial changes in childhood body-mass index to impaired glucose tolerance in young adulthood. N Engl J Med 2004; 350 (9): 865-75.

[65] Barker DJP. Mothers, Babies and Health in Later Life, 2nd ed. Ediburgh: Churchill Livingstone 1998.

[66] Wu Z, Yao C, Zhao D, *et al.* Sino-MONICA project: a collaborative study on trends and determinants in cardiovascular diseases in China, Part i: morbidity and mortality monitoring. Circulation 2001; 103 (3): 462-8.

[67] Wu Z, Yao C, Zhao D. Cardiovascular disease risk factor levels and their relations to CVD rates in China--results of Sino-MONICA project. Eur J Cardiovasc Prev Rehabil 2004; 11 (4): 275-83.

[68] Peto R. Tobacco: the growing epidemic in China. JAMA 1996; 275 (21): 1683-84.

[69] Peto R, Lopez AD, Boreham J, Thun M, Heath C Jr, Doll R. Mortality from smoking worldwide. Br Med Bull 1996; 52(1): 12-21.

[70] Drewnowski A, Popkin BM. The nutrition transition: new trends in the global diet. Nutr Rev 1997; 55 (2): 31-43.

[71] Lang T. The public health impact of globalisation of food trade. In: Shetty PS, McPherson K, Eds. Diet, Nutrition and Chronic Disease: Lessons from Contrasting Worlds. Chichester, UK: Wiley 1997: pp. 173-87.

[72] Zerba KE, Sing CF. The role of genome type-environment interaction and time in understanding the impact of genetic polymorphisms on lipid metabolism. Curr Opin Lipidol 1993; 4: 152-62.

[73] Zerba KE, Ferrell RE, Sing CF. Genotype-environment interaction: apolipoprotein E (*Apo E*) gene effects and age as an index of time and spatial context in the human. Genetics 1996; 143 (1): 463-78.

[74] Zerba KE, Ferrell RE, Sing CF. Complex adaptive systems and human health: the influence of common genotypes of the *apolipoprotein E (ApoE)* gene polymorphism and age on the relational order within a field of lipid metabolism traits. Hum Genet 2000; 107: 466-75.

[75] Lusis AJ. Atherosclerosis. Nature 2000; 407 (6801): 233-41.

[76] Delles C, McBride MW, Padmanabhan S, *et al.* The genetics of cardiovascular disease. Trends Endocrinol Metab 2008; 19(9): 309-16.

[77] Davidson EH, McClay DR, Hood L. Regulatory gene networks and the properties of the developmental process. Proc Natl Acad Sci USA 2003; 100 (4): 1475-80.

[78] Strohman RC. Maneuvering in the complex path from genotype to phenotype. Science 2002; 296 (5568): 701-3.

[79] Dennis C. Altered states. Nature 2003; 42 (6924): 686-88.

[80] Gottesman II, Gould TD. The endophenotype concept in psychiatry: etymology and strategic intentions. Am J Psychiatry 2003; 160 (4): 636-45.

[81] Whincup PH, Gilg JA, Papacosta O, *et al.* Early evidence of ethnic differences in cardiovascular risk: cross sectional comparison of British south Asian and white children. BMJ 2002; 324(7338): 635.

[82]   McKeigue PM. Metabolic consequences of obesity and body fat pattern: lessons from migrant studies. Ciba Found Symp 1996; 201: 54-64.

[83]   Dhandapany PS, Sadayappan S, Xue Y, *et al.* A common MYBPC3 (cardiac myosin binding protein C) variant associated with cardiomyopathies in south Asia. Nat. Genet 2009; 41 (2): 187-91.

[84]   Yajnik CS, Fall CH, Coyaji KJ, *et al.* Neonatal anthropometry: the thin-fat indian baby. The Pune maternal nutrition study. Int J Obes Relat Metab Disord 2003; 27 (2): 173-180.

[85]   Dabelea D, Knowler WC, Pettitt DJ. Effect of diabetes in pregnancy on offspring: follow-up research in the Pima indians. J Matern Fetal Med 2000; 9 (1): 83-88.

[86]   Gluckman PD, Hanson MA. Maternal constraint of fetal growth and its consequences. Semin. Fetal Neonatal Med 2004; 9: 419-42.

[87]   Gluckman PD, Hanson MA. Developmental Origins of Health and Disease. Cambridge University Press: Cambridge 2006.

[88]   Barker DJP. Fetal origins of coronary heart disease. BMJ 1995; 311 (6998): 171-4.

[89]   Barker DJP, Martyn CN, Osmond C, Haleb CN, Fall CHD. Growth *in utero* and serum cholesterol concentrations in adult life. BMJ 1993; 307 (6918): 1524-27.

[90]   Wells JC. Historical cohort studies and the early origins of disease hypothesis: making sense of the evidence. Proc Nutr Soc 2009; 68(2): 179-88.

[91]   Gluckman PD, Hanson MA, Pinal C.The developmental origins of adult disease. Matern Child Nutr 2005; 1: 130-41.

[92]   Gluckman PD, Hanson MA, Buklijas T, Low FM, Beedle AS Epigenetic mechanisms that underpin metabolic and cardiovascular diseases. Nat Rev Endocrinol 2009; 5 (7): 401-8.

[93]   Barker DJ, Osmond C. Infant mortality, childhood nutrition, and ischaemic heart disease in England and Wales. Lancet 1986; 1 (8489): 1077-81.

[94]   Gluckman PD, Hanson MA. The developmental origins of the metabolic syndrome. Trends Endocrinol Metab 2004; 15 (4): 183-7.

[95]   Veena SR, Krishnaveni GV, Wills AK, *et al.* Association of birthweight and head circumference at birth to cognitive performance in 9-10 year old children in South India: prospective birth cohort study. Pediatr Res 2009; 67(4): 424-9.

[96]   Martorell R, Horta BL, Adair LS, *et al.* Weight Gain in the First Two Years of Life Is an Important Predictor of Schooling Outcomes in Pooled Analyses from Five Birth Cohorts from Low- and Middle-Income Countries. J Nutr 2010; 140 (2): 348-54.

[97]   Whincup PH, Kaye SJ, Owen CG, *et al.* Birth weight and risk of type 2 diabetes: a systematic review. JAMA 2008; 300 (24): 2886-97.

[98]   Owens S, Fall CH. Consequences of poor maternal micronutrition before and during early pregnancy. Trans R Soc Trop Med Hyg 2008; 102 (2): 103-4.

[99]   Victora CG, Adair L, Fall C, *et al.* Maternal and Child Undernutrition Study Group. Maternal and child undernutrition: consequences for adult health and human capital. Lancet 2008; 371 (9609): 340-57.

[100] Martyn CN, Barker DJP, Jespersen S, Greenwald S, Osmond C, Berry C. Growth *in-utero*, adult blood pressure and arterial compliance. Br Heart J 1995; 73 (2): 116-21.

[101] Law CM, Shiell AW. Is blood pressure inversely related to birth weight? The strength of evidence from a systematic review of the literature. J Hypertens 1996; 14 (8): 935-41.

[102] Joseph KS, Kramer MS. Review of evidence on fetal and early childhood antecedents of adult chronic disease. Epidemiol Rev 1996; 18 (2): 158-74.

[103] Verschuren WMM, Jacobs DR, Bloemberg BPM, *et al.* Serum total cholesterol and long-term coronary heart disease mortality in different cultures: twenty-five year follow-up of the Seven Country Study. JAMA 1995; 274 (2): 131-6.

[104] McKeigue PM, Ferrie JE, Pierpont T, *et al.* Association of early-onset coronary heart disease in South Asian men with glucose intolerance and hyperinsulinemia. Circulation 1993; 878 (1): 152-61.

[105] Enas EA, Mehta JL. Malignant coronary artery disease in Young Asian Indians: thoughts on pathogenesis, prevention and treatment. Clin Cardiol 1995; 18 (3): 131-5.

[106] Elahi M, Chetty G, Matata B. Ethnic differences in the management of coronary heart disease patients: lessons to be learned in Indo-Asians. Med Princ Pract 2006; 15 (1): 69-73.

[107] Reddy KS. Cardiovascular disease and diabetes in migrants: interaction between nutritional changes and genetic background. In: Shetty PS, McPherson K, Eds. Diet, Nutrition and Chronic Disease: Lessons from Contrasting Worlds. Chichester, UK: Wiley 1997: pp. 71-5.

[108] Pais P, Pogue J, Gerstein H, *et al.* Risk factors for acute myocardial infarction in Indians: a case-control study. Lancet 1996; 348 (9024): 358-363.

[109] Bhatnagar D, Anand IS, Durrington PN, *et al.* Coronary risk factors in people from the Indian Subcontinent living in West London and their siblings in India. Lancet 1995; 345 (8947): 404-9.

[110] Barker DJP. Mothers, babaies and health in later life, 2nd ed. London: Churchill Livingstone 1998.

[111]   Barker DJP, Gluckman PD, Godfrey KM, *et al.* Fetal nutrition and cardiovascular disease in adult life. Lancet 1993; 341 (8850): 938-41.

[112]   Kermack WO, McKendrick AG, *et al.* Death-rates in Great Britain and Sweden. Some general regularities and their significance. Lancet 1934: 698-703.

[113]   Forsdahl A. Are poor living conditions in childhood and adolescence an important risk factor for arteriosclerotic heart disease? Br J Prev Soc Med 1977; 31 (2): 91-5.

[114]   Wadsworth ME, Cripps HA, Midwinter RE, *et al.* Blood pressure in a national birth cohort at the age of 36 related to social and familial factors, smoking, and body mass. Br Med J 1985; 291 (6508): 1534-8.

[115]   Elwood PC, Pickering J, Gallacher JE, *et al.* Long term effect of breast feeding: cognitive function in the Caerphilly cohort. J Epidemiol Commun Health 2005; 59 (2): 130-3.

[116]   Eriksson JG. Gene polymorphisms, size at birth, and the development of hypertension and type-2 diabetes. J Nutr 2007; 137 ($): 1063-5.

[117]   Martin RM, Gunnell D, Pemberton J, *et al.* Cohort profile: The Boyd Orr cohort--an historical cohort study based on the 65 year follow-up of the Carnegie Survey of Diet and Health (1937-39). Int J Epidemiol 2005; 34 (4): 742-9.

[118]   Lumey LH, Stein AD, Kahn HS, *et al.* Cohort profile: the Dutch Hunger Winter families study. Int J Epidemiol 2007; 36 (6): 1196-204.

[119]   Leon DA, Lawlor DA, Clark H, *et al.* Cohort profile: the Aberdeen children of the 1950s study. Int J Epidemiol 2006; 35 (3): 549-52.

[120]   Wadsworth M, Kuh D, Richards M, Hardy R. Cohort Profile: The 1946 National Birth Cohort (MRC National Survey of Health and Development). Int J Epidemiol 2006; 35 (1): 49-54.

[121]   Antonisamy B, Raghupathy P, Christopher S, *et al.* Cohort Profile: the 1969-73 Vellore birth cohort study in South India. Int J Epidemiol 2009; 38 (3): 663-9.

[122]   Richter L, Norris S, Pettifor J, *et al.* Cohort Profile: Mandela's children: the 1990 Birth to Twenty study in South Africa. Int J Epidemiol 2007; 36 (3): 504-11.

[123]   Eriksson JG, Osmond C, Kajantie E, Forsén TJ, Barker DJ. Patterns of growth among children who later develop type-2 diabetes or its risk factors. Diabetologia 2006; 49 (12): 2853-58.

[124]   Neel JV. Diabetes mellitus: a "thrifty" genotype rendered detrimental by "progress"? Am J Hum Genet 1962; 14: 353-62.

[125]   Neel JV. The "thrifty genotype" in 1998. Nutr Rev 1999; 57 (5): 2-9.

[126]   Hales CN and Barker DJ. Type 2 (non-insulin-dependent) diabetes mellitus: the thrifty phenotype hypothesis. Diabetologia 1992; 35 (7): 595-601

[127]   Dulloo AG Thrifty energy metabolism in catch-up growth trajectories to insulin and leptin resistance. Best Pract Res Clin Endocrinol Metab 2008; 22 (1): 155-71.

[128]   Gardiner HM. Early environmental influences on vascular development. Early Hum Dev 2007; 83 (12): 819-23.

[129]   Lucas A. Programming by early nutrition in man. Ciba Found Symp 1991; 156: 38-50.

[130]   Wiesel TN, Hubel DH. Comparison of the effects of unilateral and bilateral eye closure on cortical unit responses in kittens. J Neurophysiol 1965; 28 (6): 1029-40.

[131]   Thoman EB, Levine S. Hormonal and behavioral changes in the rat mother as a function of early experience treatments of the offspring. Physiol Behav 1970; 5 (12): 1417-21.

[132]   Ferguson MW and Joanen T. Temperature of egg incubation determines sex in Alligator mississippiensis. Nature 1982; 296 (5860): 850-53.

[133]   Waterland RA and Garza C. Potential mechanisms of metabolic imprinting that lead to chronic disease. Am J Clin Nutr 1999; 69 (2): 179-97.

[134]   Barker DJP. Developmental origins of adult health and disease. J Epidemiol Commun Health 2004; 58 (2): 114-5.

[135]   Gluckman PD, Hanson MA, Bateson P, *et al.* Towards a new developmental synthesis: adaptive developmental plasticity and human disease. Lancet 2009; 373 (9675): 1654-57.

[136]   Gluckman PD, Lillycrop KA, Vickers MH, *et al.* Metabolic plasticity during mammalian development is directionally dependent on early nutritional status. Proc Natl Acad Sci USA 2007; 104 (31): 12796-800.

[137]   Gluckman PD, Hanson MA. Developmental plasticity and human disease: research directions. J Intern Med 2007; 261 (5): 461-71.

[138]   McCance RA, Widdowson EM. The determinants of growth and form. Proc R Soc Lond B Biol Sci 1974; 185 (78): 1-17.

[139]   Lindstrom J. Early development and fitness in birds and mammals. Trends Ecol Evol 1999; 14 (9): 343-48.

[140]   Waterland RA, Jirtle RL. Early nutrition, epigenetic changes at transposons and imprinted genes, and enhanced susceptibility to adult chronic diseases. Nutrition 2004; 20 (1): 63-8.

[141]   Bateson P, Barker D, Clutton-Brock T, *et al.* Developmental plasticity and human health. Nature 2004; 430 (6998): 419-21.

[142]   Gillman MW. Developmental origins of Health and Disease. N Engl J Med 2005, 353 (17): 1848-50.

[143] Horton TH, fetal origins of developmental plasticity: animal models of induced life history variation. American J. Hum Biol 2005; 17 (1): 34-43.

[144] Harding JE. The nutritional basis of the fetal origins of adult disease. Int J Epidemiol 2001; 30 (1): 15-23.

[145] Hattersley AT, Beards F, Ballantyre E, Appleton M, Harvey R, Ellard S. Mutations in the glucokinase gene of the fetus result in reduced birthweight. Nat Genet 1998; 19 (3): 268-70.

[146] Hattersley AT, Tooke JE. The fetal insulin hypothesis: an alternative explanantion of the association of low birthweight with diabetes and vascular disease. Lancet 1999; 353 (9166): 1789-92.

[147] West-Eberhard MJ, Developmental plasticity and evolution. Oxford University Press, New York 2003.

[148] Jablonka E, Lamb MJ. Evolution in four dimensions: genetic, epigenetic, behavioral and symbolic variation in the history of life. MIT Press: Cambridge 2005.

[149] Gluckman PD, Hanson MA, Beedle AS. Non-genomic transgenerational inheritance of disease risk. Bioessays 2007; 29 (2); 149-54.

[150] Enattah NS, Jensen TG, Nielsen M, *et al.* Independent introduction of two lactase-persistence alleles into human populations reflects different history of adaptation to milk culture, Am J Hum Genet 2008; 82(1); 57-72.

[151] Hancock AM, Witonsky DB, Gordon AS, *et al.* Adaptations to climate in candidate genes for common metabolic disorders, PLoS Genet 2008; 4 (2); 32.

[152] Hales CN, Barker DJ. Type- 2 (non-insulin-dependent) diabetes mellitus: the thrifty phenotype hypothesis. Diabetologia 1992; 35 (7); 595-601.

[153] Gluckman PD, Hanson MA, Spencer HG, Bateson P. Environmental influences during development and their later consequences for health and disease: implications for the interpretation of empirical studies, Proc Biol Sci 2005; 272; 671-77.

[154] Bateson, P. Fetal experience and good adult design. Int J Epidemiol 2001: 26 (5); 561-70.

[155] Vitzthum VJ. A number no greater than the sum of its parts: the use and abuse of heritability. Hum Biol 2003; 75 (4), 539-58.

[156] Barker DJP. Mothers, Babies and Health in Later Life. Churchill Livingstone: Edinburgh 1998.

[157] Barker DJP, Eriksson JG, Forsen T, *et al.* Fetal origins of adult disease: strength of effects and biological basis. Int J Epidemiol 2002; 31 (6): 1235-39.

[158] Godfrey KM, Barker DJ, Robinson S, *et al.* Maternal birthweight and diet in pregnancy in relation to the infant's thinness at birth. Br J Obstet Gynaecol 1997; 104 (6): 663-7.

[159] Eriksson JG, Forsén T, Tuomilehto J, Winter PD, Osmond C, Barker DJ. Catch-up growth in childhood and death from coronary heart disease: longitudinal study. Br Med J 1999; 318 (7181): 427-31.

[160] Metcalfe NB, Monaghan P. Compensation for a bad start: grow now, pay later? Trends Ecol Evol 2001; 16 (5): 254-60.

[161] Widdowson EM, Crabb DE, Milner RD. Cellular development of some human organs before birth. Arch Dis Child 1972; 47 (254): 652-55.

[162] Hinchliffe SA, Lynch MR, Sargent PH, Howard CV, Van Velzen D, *et al.* The effect of intrauterine growth-retardation on the development of renal nephrons. Br J Obstet Gynaecol 1992; 99 (4): 296-301.

[163] Mackenzie HS, Brenner BM. Fewer nephrons at birth: a missing link in the etiology of operational hypertension. Am J Kidney Dis 1995; 20(1): 91-8.

[164] in the etiology of essential hypertension? Am J Kidney Dis 1995; 26 (1): 91-8.

[165] Keller G, Simmer G, Mall G, Ritz E, Amann K. Nephron number in patients with primary hypertension. N Engl J Med 2003; 348 (2): 101-8.

[166] Neel JV, Diabetes mellitus; a thrifty genotype rendered detrimental by progress. Am J Hum Genet 1962; 14: 353-62.

[167] Diamond J. The double puzzle of diabetes. Nature 2003; 423 (6940), 599-602.

[168] Ravelli ACJ, *et al.* Glucose tolerance in adults after prenatal exposure to famine. Lancet 1998; 351 (9097): 173-77.

[169] Hales CN, Desai M, Ozanne SE. The thrifty phenotype hypothesis: how does it look after 5 years? Diabet Med 1997; 14 (3): 189-95.

[170] Chali D, Enquselassie F, Gesese M. A case control study on determinants of rickets. Ethiop Med J 1998; 36 (4): 227-34.

CHAPTER 2

Maternal Nutrition and its Effects on Offspring Fertility and Importance of the Periconceptional Period on Long-Term Development

Cha Dupont[1,2,3*], Anne-Gael Cordier[1,4], Claudine Junien[1], Rachel Levy[2,3] and Pascale Chavatte-Palmer[3,5]

[1]*INRA, UMR 1198 Biologie du développement et reproduction, F-78350 Jouy en Josas, France;* [2]*Service d'Histologie-Embryologie-Cytogenetique-Biologie de la Reproduction-CECOS, Hôpital Jean Verdier (AP-HP), F-93143 Bondy, France;* [3]*Unité de Recherche en Epidémiologie Nutritionnelle, UMR U557 INSERM; U1125 INRA, CNAM, Université Paris 13, CRNH IdF, F-93017 Bobigny, France;* [4]*Service de Gynécologie-Obstétrique et Médecine de la Reproduction, Hôpital Antoine Béclère (AP-HP), F-92141 Clamart, France and* [5]*Premup Foundation (Fondation pour la prévention de la prématurité et la protection du nouveau-né prématuré), 4 av. de l'Observatoire, F-75006 Paris, France*

Abstract: The effects of adult lifestyle and environmental chemicals are important factors affecting the fertility of men and women. Many studies have shown that nutritional and hormonal status during fetal development is decisive for long-term control of energy metabolism. Obesity, type 2 diabetes (T2D) and hypertension may take root during early development, throughout gestation and lactation, as stated in the "Developmental Origins of Health and Disease" (DOHaD) hypothesis. Recent data demonstrated that adult lifestyle factors can also impact the fertility of offspring. Among these factors, nutrition plays a major role. In humans, links between birthweight and fertility have been established, but little data on the relationship between maternal nutrition and fertility of offspring are yet available. In animals, studies have shown that both maternal undernutrition and maternal overnutrition can affect the reproductive function of offspring. Maternal nutrition can influence the development of the fetal reproductive system at all stages of development. Indeed, maternal body composition before conception may influence oocyte maturation. Preimplantation embryos are sensitive to environmental conditions that can affect future growth and developmental potential. Furthermore, embryogenesis, cellular differentiation, placentation and organ maturation can be affected by a wide range of mechanisms involved in metabolic programming. Maternal nutrition may affect circular and local concentrations of endogenous hormones that are essential during fetal development and may also affect oxidative balance with consequences on oocyte maturation, follicular steroidogenesis, implantation, embryo cell function and further development. Various exposures to altered maternal nutrition are associated with epigenetic modifications in the offspring, inducing long-term changes in gene expression, potentially leading to disease in later life and infertility. Finally, micronutrient unbalance, alcohol and tobacco exposure during gestation are known to have detrimental effects on offspring development and further studies are required to establish links with fertility. Whereas the role of the maternal environment has been so far mostly studied, it now becomes clearly evident from very recent work that metabolic effects can also be mediated through the paternal gametes.

Keywords: Maternal nutrition, fetal development, energy metabolism, reproductive function, offspring, maternal environment.

I-INTRODUCTION

Context

The effects of adult lifestyle - generally diet and sedentary habits - and environmental chemicals are important factors affecting the fertility of men and women. Recent data demonstrated that adult lifestyle factors can also impact the fertility of their children. Among these factors, nutrition plays a major role.

Malnutrition is the state produced by an inadequate intake of a good quality diet. This can mean undernutrition (intake of not enough nutrients), overnutrition (intake of too many nutrients, too many lipids, and glucids or too many calories). Malnutrition can also be defined by vitamin, mineral or proteins unbalance and excessive amounts of inappropriate substances (alcohol).

*Address correspondence to Cha Dupont: Service d'Histologie-Embryologie-Cytogenetique-Biologie de la Reproduction-CECOS, Hôpital Jean Verdier (AP-HP), F-93143 Bondy, France; E-mail: pascale.chavatte@jouy.inra.fr

In the nineties, Barker's epidemiological studies underlined an increased risk of non-transmittable metabolic diseases in people born small for gestational age (SGA) [1]. Obesity, type 2 diabetes (T2D) and hypertension may take root during early development, throughout gestation and lactation, as stated in the "Developmental Origins of Health and Disease" (DOHaD) hypothesis. Many studies have now shown that nutritional and hormonal status during fetal development and early life determine long-term control of energy metabolism [2]. There is also convincing experimental evidence to suggest that epigenetic marks serve as a memory of exposure, in early life, to inadequate or inappropriate chemical/nutritional/metabolic or non-chemical/social environments.

Many organs are involved in this process and effects of habits during pregnancy can also impact the fertility of the offspring. Since gametogenesis takes place during pregnancy, the maternal dietary intake may also have an impact on children's fertility, thus creating an inter-generational effect [3].

Influence of Gestation on Adult Fertility (Offspring)

Substrate availability is essential for embryo and fetal growth and development. Recently, increasing literature reviews have focused on the effects of maternal diet during each phase of gestation on the health of the offspring, including effects on fertility [4-6]. Maternal body composition before conception may influence oocyte maturation, oviductal environment and endocrine maternal response to early embryo signals. Blastocyst differentiation leads to the inner cell mass formation (resulting in fetus development), and to the trophoblast formation (from which the placenta originates): this differentiation will impact on implantation, placentation and pregnancy evolution. Fetal growth and survival depend on the placenta which forms the interface between the maternal and fetal bloodstreams, facilitating gaseous, nutrients, antibodies, hormones exchanges and the disposal of fetal waste products and contributes to adaption to an altered uterine milieu and to programming [7-10].

In terms of female development, the major events of the ovarian development, which are critical for ovarian function, occur during fetal life such as prophase I meiosis of germ cells and formation of the follicular reserve. In humans and other mammalian species, the pool of resting primordial follicles serves as the source of developing follicles and fertilizable oocyte during the female reproductive lifespan. In terms of male development, Sertoli cells play a central role in the development of a functional testis and their numbers are highly correlated with both adult testicular size and sperm production [11]. These cells proliferate during fetal and neonatal life and the peripubertal period, coordinating testicular development. Alterations of Sertoli cells development impact on other testicular cells such as Leydig cells and fetal gonies, leading to disorders in adulthood [11]. Sertoli cell proliferation may be disturbed during pregnancy through alterations of the development of the hypothalamic–pituitary–gonadal axis during fetal life linked to the concentration of key hormones, such as FSH, T3, T4, GH and estrogens [12]. After birth, programming effects can be emphasized by the neonatal nutritional status, particularly when prenatal and postnatal status differs significantly, as illustrated by the "Predictive Adaptive response" hypothesis. Indeed, it has been suggested that the fetus uses nutritional signals to anticipate its future energetic environment, and through developmental plasticity, adjusts its phenotype accordingly, leading to a thrifty phenotype [13, 14].

II- EFFECTS OF MATERNAL NUTRITION ON OFFSPRING FERTILITY

A- Epidemiological Studies: Human Birth Weight and Subsequent Fertility in Adulthood

Epidemiological studies about maternal nutrition and effects on offspring's fertility are scarce. In human adults, most studies are based on birth weight as an index of nutrition during fetal life [15] because it is difficult to assess *in utero* nutrition retrospectively. Nevertheless, intra-uterine growth retardation (IUGR) may result from different causes including undernutrition, overnutrition and many environmental factors [16]. Moreover, the effects of fetal nutrition on subsequent health are not necessarily associated with birth weight, probably because the critical window of development during which the fetus is sensitive to nutrition occurs before measurable effects on fetal mass are expressed [17].

De Bruin *et al.* (1998) observed in human that IUGR due to placental insufficiency leads to impaired ovarian development, characterized by a decrease volume of primordial follicles in ovarian cortical tissue [18]. At puberty, the prevalence of anovulation seems higher among SGA girls compared to those born with an appropriate weight for gestational age. In the relatively small fraction of ovulating SGA girls, the ovulation rate is lower than in controls, and adolescent SGA girls are at risk for FSH and insulin resistance [19]. It has also been observed that in girls born SGA, prenatal growth restraint is associated with high FSH levels and with small internal genitalia in adolescence [20]. Furthermore, the onset of puberty and the age at menarche are advanced by about 5–10 months. Current evidence suggests that insulin resistance is a key mechanism linking a post-SGA state to early menarche; hence, insulin sensitization may become a valid approach to prevent early menarche and early growth arrest in SGA girls [21]. A link between prenatal environment and polycystic ovary syndrome (PCOS) in adolescence has often been tested but to date, results remain contradictory [22]. Nevertheless, it was suggested that prenatal growth restriction coupled with spontaneous catch-up growth during infancy results in increased insulin resistance and visceral adiposity, associated with elevated plasma Dehydroepiandrosterone Sulfate (DHEAS) and low plasma concentrations of Sex Hormone Binding Globulin (SHBG) at 8 years of age, thus predisposing girls to PCOS [22-24]. Furthermore, high or low maternal birth weight is associated with prolonged time to conceive [25].

Similarly, SGA boys have an increased risk for high FSH and low inhibin B plasma concentrations and reduced testicular volume in adolescence [24, 26]. Cryptorchidism is common in boys born with IUGR and is associated with low sperm count [27]. Ramlau-Hansen *et al.*, however, failed to observe any effects of birth weight on semen quality [28].

Nevertheless, fertility effects may also be the direct consequences of adult metabolic syndrome and overweight, which are often associated with low birth weight. In studies on the developmental origins of health and disease, low birth weight is often used as a proxy for a compromised prenatal development [29], although birth weight is a poor surrogate for nutritional status during gestation and is clearly not a sufficient criterion for testing the involvement of epigenetic modifications [30]. Moreover, factors leading to IUGR are rarely well documented; the use of animal models remains a necessary tool to focus on maternal nutrition and its effects on offspring fertility, as well as to perform invasive tests and study parameters that can not be investigated in humans.

B -Maternal Undernutrition

Undernutrition is known to affect female fertility. Thus, insufficient energy stores may negatively affect ovulation, menses and challenge to initiate and maintain pregnancy [31]. The health and fertility of the offspring can also be affected.

1- Female Effects

Maternal food deprivation in mice induces a small but significant effect on the reproductive success of the daughters. Thus, the mean litter size of the second pregnancy is reduced in the daughters of restricted dams [32]. Puberty delay and reduced ovulation rates have been observed in several species when females were submitted to undernutrition during the fetal period [33]. The reduced ovulation rates were not associated with a change in gonadotropin profiles or pituitary responsiveness [34].

The effect of undernutrition during each critical stage of ovarian development was assessed in sheep fetuses by measuring the granulosa cell layer development, showing a delay in ovarian follicular development when undernutrition was applied from mating to day 50 of gestation [15]. Furthermore, it has recently been shown on rats that maternal undernutrition significantly reduced primordial, secondary and antral follicle numbers in adult offspring. This decrease was associated with decreased mRNA levels of genes, known as critical for follicle maturation and ovulation, and with an increased oxidative stress in the ovary [35].

In humans, maternal exposure to nutritional deprivation specifically during early gestation, as experienced during the late period of the five month Dutch Hunger Winter of 1944–45, increased the risk of early-onset cardio-vascular disease (CVD) and hypertension, increased BMI and glucose intolerance in the offspring [17]. *In utero* exposure to famine, however, did not reduce the fertility of females nor males, but, in contrast, appeared to improve female fertility [36, 37].

2- Male Effects

With regards to males, lambs are frequently used as models to assess the effects of fetal undernutrition on the male reproductive system.

There was no effect of maternal nutrient restriction (31 to 100 days of gestation) on the time of onset of puberty in male lambs. However, altered pituitary responsiveness was observed, together with a significantly lower Sertoli cell number and reduced seminiferous tubules diameter compared to controls [38]. Testis tended to be lighter in newborn lambs whose dams were underfed during gestation compared to lamb that were overnourished [39]. Lately, it was reported in rats that undernutrition during the fetal and post natal periods, until puberty, is associated with lower testicular weight and lower Sertoli cell numbers in adult life. This study did not define which was the critical period for gonadal development [40].

In conclusion, there is clear evidence in both males and females, that maternal under nutrition during pregnancy affects gonadal development and function. Direct effects on fertility have not been fully explored, although available data suggests that these effects may not result in a dramatic decrease in fertility in otherwise healthy animals. More exploratory work is definitely needed both in humans and in animal models.

C- Maternal Overnutrition

The impact of maternal nutrition has been assessed mainly in cases of food restriction in humans, rodents or domestic animals, but significantly fewer studies have focused on the consequences of over-nutrition on offspring fertility.

The increased consumption of energy-dense foods (excessive caloric intake, high fat diets) with low physical activity has led to an epidemic of obesity (http://ec.europa.eu/health/). Overweight affects 30-80% of adults in the WHO European Region and up to one third of children.

1- Female Effects

A high proportion of obese women are infertile or sub-fertile, suffering from anovulatory cycles, increased abortion rates and/or gestational diabetes. Excessive fat stores may inhibit conception by affecting ovulation because of insulin insensitivity, excess of male sex hormones and excess leptin secretion (The ESHRE Capri Workshop Group). These affect the regulation of hypothalamo-pituitary and ovarian hormonal levels. Pregravid obesity increases both maternal and fetal morbidity and mortality.

Of current concern in developed countries is the rising incidence of obesity and type 2 diabetes, which results in offsprings at increased risk of developing obesity, thus inducing a vicious cycle leading to transgenerational transmission and increasing prevalence of these disorders [41]. Part of this transmission is conveyed through the gametes, as evidenced by studies showing an effect of paternal obesity [22].

In humans, high maternal BMI was shown to be associated with younger menarcheal age among daughters [42].

In agriculture, it is common practice to increase the dietary energy intake of ruminants (by increasing fatty acid diet ratio) just prior to breeding as a means to improve ovulation rates and optimize the reproduction performance. This practice, often referred to as "flushing", is particularly efficient on thin animals [43]. The administration of high lipid diets to cows during the peri-conceptional period has also been shown to reduce the number of small and middle size ovarian follicles without affecting oocyte quality or in vitro cleavage [44, 45]. Nevertheless, major excess leads to adverse effects. In the obese ovine model developed by Wallace J, (1996), peri-conceptional maternal over nutrition in adolescent ewes induces fetal IUGR [46]. Using this same model, Da Silva *et al.* observed a delay in ovarian development (2001) [47] and a reduction in the number of primordial follicles on the fetal ovary (2002) [48]. The pituitary expression of LHβ mRNA was also higher in growth-restricted fetuses from dams offered a high nutrient intake in the last days of gestation [48]. Finally, maternal exposure to a high fat diet led to early pubertal onset in rats [49].

2- Male Effects

In men, epidemiological studies have shown a link between overweight or obesity and male infertility [50-52]. High BMI is often associated with altered sperm parameters such as sperm concentration, mobility and morphology, with commonly observed DNA damages [53, 54].

One epidemiological study conducted on 328 men from the Danish pregnancy cohort has shown an influence of high maternal BMI on the sons' semen quality and inhibin B plasma concentrations [51].

In sheep, Da Silva *et al.,* highlighted that prenatal growth restriction delayed the onset of puberty in male lambs [47]. Indeed, growth restricted fetuses from dams offered a high nutrient intake had lower plasma testosterone concentrations and testicular volume compared to normally developed lambs, from birth until 28-35 weeks of age. No significant effects of maternal nutrition were observed, however, on testicular weight, seminiferous cord, or Sertoli cell numbers of male fetuses [55].

It remains unclear whether the observed changes in gonadal development are a direct result of maternal under or overfeeding during the preconceptional period or during pregnancy or if they are a consequence of maternal nutrition on placental development and fetal growth.

D- Micronutrients

Micronutrients deficiencies have been associated with significantly high reproductive risks. Thus, micronutrients unbalance may play a critical role in fertility, conception, implantation, fetal organogenesis and placentation [56]. An inadequate dietary folate intake results in a reduction in DNA biosynthesis and thereby in cell division [56]. Furthermore, folic acid and B12 vitamin, acting as methyl donors, are important contributors to DNA and protein modifications, contributing to long-term effects (reduced incidence of neural tube defects later in development) [57]. Peri-conceptional folic acid intake by mothers is also associated with epigenetic changes in IGF2 in their children [58] and may contribute to intrauterine programming of growth and later disease risks as demonstrated in animal models [59, 60]. However, maternal folic acid inappropriate supplementation significantly increased the risk of mammary adenocarcinomas in the offspring, accelerated the rate of mammary adenocarcinoma appearance and increased the multiplicity of mammary adenocarcinomas in the offspring [61].

Furthermore, vitamin B12 deficiency during gestation inhibits development of seminiferous tubules with decrease of spermatogenic cells and induces apoptosis of spermatocytes in F1 male rats [62].

Changes in the amino acid environment of embryos may lead to abnormal epigenetic effects [63]. Maternal low-protein diet fed to rodents during the peri-conceptional period led to elevation in maternal serum homocysteine levels [64], which may cause folate deficiency and interfere with methyl group donation required for DNA methylation [65].

Excessive perinatal supplementation with micronutrients may be detrimental for fetal development and programming. High level of antioxidant vitamins C and E may affect both maternal endothelial and placental functions and could explain the observed fetal growth restriction [66]. In rats, excess omega-3 fatty acid consumption during pregnancy and lactation leads to lower body weights in adulthood offspring and a shorter lifespan associated with sensory/neurological abnormalities (presbycousis) [67]. Despite effect of micronutrient unbalance on gonadal function has not been explored yet, there is a strong risk that excess or lack of micronutrients also impact offspring fertility.

III. MECHANISMS AND CRITICAL SPATIOTEMPORAL ONTOGENIC PERIODS

A- Mechanism

Maternal nutrition can influence development of the fetal reproductive system at all stages of development. A wide range of mechanisms are involved.

1-Endocrinology

Endogenous hormones are essential during fetal development [3]. The reproductive system and many components of the hypothalamic-pituitary-gonadal system may not develop correctly if exposed to the wrong inappropriate (both in quantity and quality) hormones, resulting in fertility problems in adulthood. Furthermore, hormone receptors, which are physiologically linked to gene expression, represent a mechanism through which endocrine signals can potentially modify gene expression and early life development [6]. Thus, maternal undernutrition during gestation alters maternal steroid hormone levels, including elevation of glucocorticoids (corticosterone, cortisol), the stress hormones, which can profoundly influence the physiological conditions of the conceptus [68].

2-Oxidative stress

Essential fatty acids and their oxygen-derived elements control many metabolic pathways by adapting intracellular signalling, including apoptosis. Antioxidants are necessary for homeostasis: an imbalance in the equilibrium of antioxidants and pro-oxidants (ROS) can result in OS damage, a key element in the pathogenesis of several diseases [69]. While excessive ROS production clearly damages DNA, low levels of ROS affect cell signalling, particularly at the level of redox modulation [70].

Free radicals are essential for the acquisition of fertilizing ability and contribute to chromatin condensation, membrane remodelling. They play a key role in the origin of life and biological evolution, such as signal transduction and gene transcription [56]. Nutritional changes affecting oxidative balance will have consequences on oocyte maturation, follicular steroidogenesis, implantation, and embryo cell function and further development [71]. Consequently, DNA damages by ROS are transmitted to offspring and may affect its fertility.

3-Epigenetic

In recent months, numerous studies focusing on the developmental origin of health and disease (DOHaD) and metabolic programming have identified links between early nutrition, epigenetic processes, and long-term illness. Epigenetic marks are candidates for bearing the memory of early life exposure to inadequate chemical/nutritional or non-chemical/social environments by long-term alterations of gene expression programming. The epigenome serves as an interface between the environment and the genome [72, 73]. The ability of environmental factors to promote a phenotype or disease state not only in the individual exposed but also in subsequent progeny for successive generations is termed transgenerational inheritance. Various exposures such as maternal food restriction, periconceptional folic acid intake or maternal obesity are associated with epigenetic modifications in offspring [29, 59]. The induction of adverse developmental programming in embryos by malnutrition appears to be mediated by altered metabolic signalling within the maternal reproductive tract, leading to changes in embryo metabolism and epigenetic. These latter changes are propagated through development. Epigenetic marks induce long-term changes in gene expression, potentially leading to disease in later life. The genes involved in the regulation of glucose metabolism, adipogenesis, corticoid's answers and adrenal function are particularly suspected.

In animals the developmental environment induces altered phenotypes through epigenetic mechanisms including DNA methylation by DNA methyltransferases (DNMTs), covalent modifications of histones (methylation, acetylation, phosphorylation, ubiquitinylation), and non-coding RNAs. Genome-wide epigenetic reprogramming occurs during ovogenesis stage and early embryo development [74-76]. Therefore, susceptibility to programmation exists before pregnancy and during the periconceptional period [63, 77-80]. Hence, the gamete and the embryo are vulnerable to altered nutritional environment both *in vivo* and *in vitro*, leading to altered epigenetic regulation of imprinted and non-imprinted genes which persist through fetal and postnatal life [81-88].

Epigenetic changes during gametogenesis and early embryo development are better known. Briefly, during gametogenesis, the epigenetic program is strongly modified, for example DNA methylation is erased in primordial germ cells and reapposed during gametic differentiation with specific timing in spermatogenesis and ovogenesis. After fertilization, the acquisition of pluripotency involves the epigenetic resetting of the gamete genome, to allow the activation of essential genes, such as pluripotency-associated genes. The erasure of DNA methylation is achieved in the preimplantation blastocyst [89, 90]. During proliferation and cell differentiation of the different tissues of the embryo, new epigenetic programs are established in a cell-type specific manner, called maternal-to-zygotic transition by Tadros [91]. Whatever the time frame effects on fertility are mediated by the alteration of the expression of key genes involved in ovarian development and function (oocyte maturation, endocrinology), and in hypothalamic and pituitary regulation.

One of the rare opportunities for studying the relevance of such findings to humans is presented by individuals who were prenatally exposed to famine during the Dutch Hunger Winter. Heijmans [30] report that periconceptional exposure to famine is associated with lower methylation of the IGF2 DMR 6 decades later. Data from animal models are consistent with the interpretation that famine underlies the IGF2 hypomethylation and may be related to a deficiency in methyl donors, such as the amino acid methionine [92].

Finally, studies have demonstrated the existence of an on-going self-propagating epigenetic cycle [93, 94], of metabolic memories [95-97] and ageing epigenetic processes [98, 99]. Epimutations in the germline that become permanently programmed can allow then transmission of epigenetic transgenerational phenotypes [100].

Despite recent progress, we are still a long way from understanding how, when and where environmental stressors disturb key epigenetic mechanisms. Since these machineries clearly function in a sequential manner, identifying the original key marks and their changes throughout development, during an individual's lifetime or over several generations, remains a challenging issue [101].

B- Spatiotemporal ontogenic periods

The peri-conceptional period consists of preconception, conception, implantation, placentation and embryo- or organogenesis stages (Fig. **1**), and specific cellular events that occur during the distinct stages of embryogenesis. Each of these steps may be affected by maternal nutrition [56], leading to lasting morbidity including infertility in offspring.

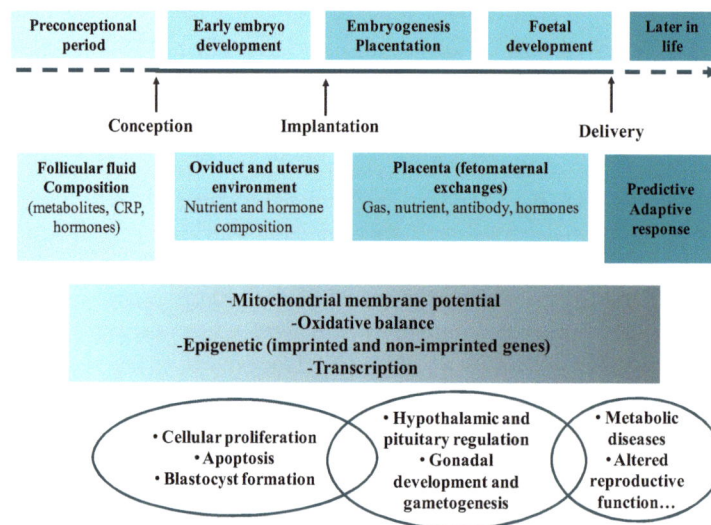

Figure 1: Maternal Nutrition Target During Peri-Conceptional Period.

1 - Preconceptional Period

Maternal obesity could have adverse effects as early as the oocyte and these effects may contribute to effects later in life [102]. Obesity is associated with intrafollicular changes in multiple cellular systems such as increased metabolite, C-reactive protein, and androgen activity levels that influence oocyte developmental competence [103].

Pre-mating nutrition is associated with alteration in the mRNA content in oocytes. Lower amount of glucose transporter 3 (SLC2A3), sodium/glucose cotransporter 1 (SLC5A1), and NaC/KC ATPase mRNAs was detected in oocyte of ewes underfed two weeks before slaughter [104].

Furthermore, it has recently been observed that maternal obesity is associated with altered mitochondrial activity in oocytes that are transmitted to zygotes [105] and to offspring later in life. Indeed, in obese adolescent, a mitochondrial dysfunction was observed and was more pronounced in adolescents borne from obese mother [106]. Then, generation of reactive oxygen species (ROS) was raised while glutathione was depleted and the redox state became more oxidised, suggesting that oxidative stress may alter oocytes DNA in obese females [105].

2 - Preimplantation Period

Preimplantation embryos are sensitive to environmental conditions that can affect future growth and developmental potential [63].

The oviduct and uterus provide the environments for the earliest stages of mammalian embryo development. Nutrient and hormone composition of the oviduct and uterus may be influenced by maternal nutrition and play a key role in embryo uptake of nutrients and its development. So, female reproductive tract fluids should have an important role in the "developmental origins of health and disease" during preimplantation period [107].

Environmental factors commonly influence embryo proliferation or apoptosis and blastocyst ICM and trophectoderm cell numbers [63]. In mice, maternal high and low-protein diets reduce the number of inner cell mass (ICM) cells, lower the mitochondrial membrane potential and elevate reactive oxygen species levels in blastocysts [108]. Kwong and co-workers [109] demonstrated that submitting pregnant rats to a low protein diet during the pre-implantation period (0-4.25 days after mating) was sufficient to disturb subsequent embryo development. Blastocysts showed significantly reduced cell numbers, first within the ICM, and later within both blastocyst cell lineages (ICM/embryoblast and trophectoderm/trophoblast). These changes induced by a slower rate of cellular proliferation and not by increased apoptosis, were subsequently followed by sex-dependent long-term effects such as excess growth and hypertension in adulthood [109-112]. Moreover, blastocyst development in mice is negatively correlated with leptin rates that are increased in obesity [113]. Finally, in rabbits submitted to hyperlipidic diet embryonic gene expression was affected as early as the 8–16 cells stage (especially Adipophilin expression which was confirmed by qRT-PCR) and subsequently fetuses developed IUGR [114].

3. Embryogenesis and Placentation

Metabolic programming can occur during embryogenesis and placentation. Thus, the extra-embryonic lineages derived from the blastocyst show changes in proliferation and functional activity in response to maternal diet treatment or obesity, causing altered nutrient transport to the fetus throughout the gestation period [108,109,112,115,116].

Total placentome mass was significantly lower in overfed ewes compared to control [55] and fetal LHβ mRNA expression was negatively correlated with total placentome weight [55]. Gonadal ridge already appears at the time of gastrulation. Gametogenesis and early development are critical period for erasure, acquisition, and maintenance of genomic imprints [117]. So, maternal micronutrient intake peri-conceptionally, particularly folic acid and B12 vitamin, which act as methyl donors, are important in DNA methylation process and preservation of imprinted gene methylation.

4- Fetal Period

Hormonal secretion is affected by peri-conceptional undernutrition. In ovine fetus undernourished in late gestation, IGF-1 and IGFBP-3 profiles during gestation are modified with possible consequences on reproductive organs development [118]. Maternal undernutrition affects cellular proliferation and gene expression, in particular genes regulating apoptosis in the fetal ovary. This mechanism varies according to the time of exposure to undernutrition during gestation (usually referred to as "critical periods") [119, 120]. Furthermore, the DNA damage in the fetal ovary is increased though the overexpression of anti-tumoral protein p53 and anti apoptotic factor Bcl-2 [121]. Measurements of specific mRNA contents indicated that the physiology of the developing testes in sheep fetuses was significantly altered by nutrient restriction. Undernutrition during the first 50 days of fetal development was clearly associated with increased expression of the key steroidogenically rate-limiting cholesterol transporter StAR [122].

5- Birth

Testis descent, which is a hormone-dependant process, normally occurs by birth. Incomplete descent of one or both testes (cryptorchidism) is associated with lower sperm counts in adulthood [27].

Thus, maternal peri-conceptional malnutrition cause defective ovarian function, compromised oocyte and early embryo metabolism and survival, abnormal embryo cellular differentiation, fetal growth, and long-term outcomes such as metabolic syndrome, cardiovascular disease and infertility in offspring.

IV- PERSPECTIVES

Other environmental effects

Not only nutrition has detrimental impact on fetal programming. It is long established that *in utero* tobacco exposure affects fetal growth and neuronal development [123, 124]. Tobacco exposure during pregnancy may also affect offspring's fertility. Indeed, maternal smoking disturbs endocrine equilibrium of the fetus with potential consequences on gonadal development and further fertility [125-127]. Alcohol consumption during pregnancy affects fetus development and lead to long term cognitive, neuropsychological and behavioral issues [128, 129]. Maternal alcohol consumption during pregnancy affects Sertoli cells and is associated with diminished semen quality [130].

Bisphenol A is an endocrine disruptor highly detected in the environment (for example, alimentary plastic). It is known to affect reproductive axis, but it seems also have effect in fetal programming. Indeed, prenatal exposure to Bisphenol A leads to increased body weight later in life [131]. Further studies would be necessary to link Bisphenol A prenatal exposure to fertility later in life.

Paternally Transgenerational Effects

Whereas many studies about maternal imprinting have been published, paternal imprinting investigation is only emerging. The effect of father's unbalanced nutrition can be transmitted to the offspring through sperm epigenetic alterations, and merits further investigation. In conjunction with recent human epidemiological data, animals studies showed that offspring of males fed with a low-protein diet had a modified hepatic expression of many genes involved in lipid and cholesterol metabolism, relative to controls, with numerous ($\approx$20%) changes in cytosine methylation depending on paternal diet, including reproducible changes in methylation over a likely enhancer for the key lipid regulator PPARα [132].

In another study, paternal high-fat-diet exposure was shown to program β-cell 'dysfunction' in rat female offspring, with increased body weight, adiposity, impaired glucose tolerance and insulin sensitivity [133].

Epigenetic modifications in the sperm contribute to the developmental program of the future embryo [134]. Consequently, paternal nutrition may interfere with epigenetic marks of mature sperm and play a critical role in long-term health of the offspring including infertility issues.

Furthermore, epidemiological studies have suggested that exposure of paternal grandfathers to famine influences obesity and cardiovascular disease in subsequent generations [135, 136].

V- CONCLUSION

Adult lifestyle is an important factor affecting the fertility of men and women, and can also impact health of their children. Maternal high fat nutrition, diminished calorie intake and imbalanced micronutrient intakes impacts on offspring reproductive maturation resulting in impaired fertility. Both over and undernutrition can lead to fetal growth restriction (the thrifty phenotype) due to placental insufficiency. Nevertheless, birth weight alone is not a sufficient criterion to predict further fertility, because it does not take into account the alternative fetus mechanisms. Indeed, it is difficult to distinguish each mechanism. Maternal effects are difficult to separate from direct effects of *in utero* environmental exposure on offspring. Knowledge of the processes through which maternal nutrition affects reproductive function in the offspring reminds very limited but multifactorial mechanisms such as hormonal influence, oxidative stress and epigenetic conditions should be involved in the programming process. Each stages of gamete, fetus, or neonate development, are concerned by maternal nutrition. Nevertheless, numerous factors are still unknown. Complexity of the search for underlying mechanism of human fetal programming leads to use simplified animal models. Consequently to this simplistic view, some of the results should not be extrapolated to human condition. The key question is the prevention of such effects possible by changes in diet and lifestyle?

REFERENCES

[1]   Barker DJ, Eriksson JG, Forsen T, Osmond C. Fetal origins of adult disease: strength of effects and biological basis. Int J Epidemiol 2002; 31(6): 1235-9.
[2]   Silveira PP, Portella AK, Goldani MZ, Barbieri MA. Developmental origins of health and disease (DOHaD). J Pediatr (Rio J) 2000; 83(6): 494-504.
[3]   Sharpe RM, Franks S. Environment, lifestyle and infertility--an inter-generational issue. Nat Cell Biol 2002; 4 (Suppl): s33-40.
[4]   Chavatte-Palmer P, Al Gubory K, Picone O, Heyman Y. Maternal nutrition: effects on offspring fertility and importance of the periconceptional period on long-term development. Gynecol Obstet Fertil 2008; 36(9): 920-9.

[5]   Mandon-Pepin B, Oustry-Vaiman A, Vigier B, Piumi F, Cribiu E, Cotinot C. Expression profiles and chromosomal localization of genes controlling meiosis and follicular development in the sheep ovary. Biol Reprod 2003; 68(3): 985-95.

[6]   Rhind SM. Effects of maternal nutrition on fetal and neonatal reproductive development and function. Anim Reprod Sci 2004; 82-83: 169-81.

[7]   Sibley CP, Brownbill P, Dilworth M, Glazier JD. Review: Adaptation in placental nutrient supply to meet fetal growth demand: implications for programming. Placenta 2010; 31 (Suppl): S70-4.

[8]   Gatford KL, Simmons RA, De Blasio MJ, Robinson JS, Owens JA. Review: Placental programming of postnatal diabetes and impaired insulin action after IUGR. Placenta 2010; 31 (Suppl): S60-5.

[9]   Thornburg KL, O'Tierney PF, Louey S. Review: The placenta is a programming agent for cardiovascular disease. Placenta 2010; 31 (Suppl): S54-9.

[10]   Thornburg KL, Shannon J, Thuillier P, Turker MS. *In utero* life and epigenetic predisposition for disease. Adv Genet 2010; 71: 57-78.

[11]   Sharpe RM, McKinnell C, Kivlin C, Fisher JS. Proliferation and functional maturation of Sertoli cells, and their relevance to disorders of testis function in adulthood. Reproduction 2003; 125(6): 769-84.

[12]   O'Shaughnessy PJ, Fowler PA. Endocrinology of the mammalian fetal testis. Reproduction 2011; 141(1): 37-46.

[13]   Gluckman PD, Hanson MA, Bateson P, *et al.* Towards a new developmental synthesis: adaptive developmental plasticity and human disease. Lancet 2009; 373(9675): 1654-7.

[14]   Uller T. Developmental plasticity and the evolution of parental effects. Trends Ecol Evol 2008; 23(8): 432-8.

[15]   Rae MT, Palassio S, Kyle CE, *et al.* Effect of maternal undernutrition during pregnancy on early ovarian development and subsequent follicular development in sheep fetuses. Reproduction 2001; 122(6): 915-22.

[16]   Sankaran S, Kyle PM. Aetiology and pathogenesis of IUGR. Best Pract Res Clin Obstet Gynaecol 2009 Dec; 23(6): 765-77.

[17]   Lumey LH. Compensatory placental growth after restricted maternal nutrition in early pregnancy. Placenta 1998; 19(1): 105-11.

[18]   de Bruin JP, Dorland M, Bruinse HW, Spliet W, Nikkels PG, Te Velde ER. Fetal growth retardation as a cause of impaired ovarian development. Early Hum Dev 1998; 51(1): 39-46.

[19]   Ibanez L, Potau N, Ferrer A, Rodriguez-Hierro F, Marcos MV, de Zegher F. Reduced ovulation rate in adolescent girls born small for gestational age. J Clin Endocrinol Metab 2002; 87(7): 3391-3.

[20]   Ibanez L, de Zegher F. Puberty and prenatal growth. Mol Cell Endocrinol 2006; 254-255: 22-5.

[21]   Ibanez L, Valls C, Ong K, Dunger DB, de Zegher F. Metformin therapy during puberty delays menarche, prolongs pubertal growth, and augments adult height: a randomized study in low-birth-weight girls with early-normal onset of puberty. J Clin Endocrinol Metab 2006; 91(6): 2068-73.

[22]   Sloboda DM, Hickey M, Hart R. Reproduction in females: the role of the early life environment. Hum Reprod Update 2011; 17(2): 210-27.

[23]   Verkauskiene R, Beltrand J, Claris O, *et al.* Impact of fetal growth restriction on body composition and hormonal status at birth in infants of small and appropriate weight for gestational age. Eur J Endocrinol 2007 157(5): 605-12.

[24]   Ibanez L, Lopez-Bermejo A, Diaz M, Suarez L, de Zegher F. Low-birth weight children develop lower sex hormone binding globulin and higher dehydroepiandrosterone sulfate levels and aggravate their visceral adiposity and hypoadiponectinemia between six and eight years of age. J Clin Endocrinol Metab 2009; 94(10): 3696-9.

[25]   Nohr EA, Vaeth M, Rasmussen S, Ramlau-Hansen CH, Olsen J. Waiting time to pregnancy according to maternal birthweight and prepregnancy BMI. Hum Reprod 2009; 24(1): 226-32.

[26]   Cicognani A, Alessandroni R, Pasini A, *et al.* Low birth weight for gestational age and subsequent male gonadal function. J Pediatr 2002; 141(3): 376-9.

[27]   Boisen KA, Main KM, Rajpert-De Meyts E, Skakkebaek NE. Are male reproductive disorders a common entity? The testicular dysgenesis syndrome. Ann NY Acad Sci 2001; 948: 90-9.

[28]   Ramlau-Hansen CH, Hansen M, Jensen CR, Olsen J, Bonde JP, Thulstrup AM. Semen quality and reproductive hormones according to birthweight and body mass index in childhood and adult life: two decades of follow-up. Fertil Steril 2010; 94(2): 610-8.

[29]   Waterland RA, Michels KB. Epigenetic epidemiology of the developmental origins hypothesis. Annu Rev Nutr 2007; 27: 363-88.

[30]   Heijmans BT, Tobi EW, Stein AD, *et al.* Persistent epigenetic differences associated with prenatal exposure to famine in humans. Proc Natl Acad Sci USA 2008; 105(44): 17046-9.

[31]   ESHRE. Nutrition and reproduction in women. Hum Reprod Update 2006; 12(3): 193-207.

[32]   Meikle D, Westberg M. Maternal nutrition and reproduction of daughters in wild house mice (Mus musculus). Reproduction 2001; 122(3): 437-42.

[33]   Rhind SM, McNeilly AS. Effects of level of food intake on ovarian follicle number, size and steroidogenic capacity in the ewe. Anim Reprod Sci 1998; 52(2): 131-8.

[34] Rae MT, Kyle CE, Miller DW, Hammond AJ, Brooks AN, Rhind SM. The effects of undernutrition, *in utero*, on reproductive function in adult male and female sheep. Anim Reprod Sci 2002; 72(1-2): 63-71.

[35] Bernal AB, Vickers MH, Hampton MB, Poynton RA, Sloboda DM. Maternal undernutrition significantly impacts ovarian follicle number and increases ovarian oxidative stress in adult rat offspring. PLoS One 2010; 5(12): e15558.

[36] Lumey LH, Stein AD. *In utero* exposure to famine and subsequent fertility: The Dutch Famine Birth Cohort Study. Am J Public Health 1997; 87(12): 1962-6.

[37] Painter RC, Osmond C, Gluckman P, Hanson M, Phillips DI, Roseboom TJ. Transgenerational effects of prenatal exposure to the Dutch famine on neonatal adiposity and health in later life. BJOG 2008; 115(10): 1243-9.

[38] Kotsampasi B, Balaskas C, Papadomichelakis G, Chadio SE. Reduced Sertoli cell number and altered pituitary responsiveness in male lambs undernourished *in utero*. Anim Reprod Sci 2009; 114(1-3): 135-47.

[39] Alejandro B, Perez R, Pedrana G, *et al.* Low maternal nutrition during pregnancy reduces the number of Sertoli cells in the newborn lamb. Reprod Fertil Dev 2002; 14(5-6): 333-7.

[40] Genovese P, Nunez ME, Pombo C, Bielli A. Undernutrition during fetal and post-natal life affects testicular structure and reduces the number of Sertoli cells in the adult rat. Reprod Domest Anim 2010; 45(2): 233-6.

[41] Foreyt JP, Poston WS, 2nd. Obesity: a never-ending cycle? Int J Fertil Womens Med 1998; 43(2): 111-6.

[42] Keim SA, Branum AM, Klebanoff MA, Zemel BS. Maternal body mass index and daughters' age at menarche. Epidemiology 2009; 20(5): 677-81.

[43] Scaramuzzi RJ, Campbell BK, Downing JA, *et al.* A review of the effects of supplementary nutrition in the ewe on the concentrations of reproductive and metabolic hormones and the mechanisms that regulate folliculogenesis and ovulation rate. Reprod Nutr Dev 2006; 46(4): 339-54.

[44] Fouladi-Nashta AA, Gutierrez CG, Gong JG, Garnsworthy PC, Webb R. Impact of dietary fatty acids on oocyte quality and development in lactating dairy cows. Biol Reprod 2007; 77(1): 9-17.

[45] Wakefield SL, Lane M, Schulz SJ, Hebart ML, Thompson JG, Mitchell M. Maternal supply of omega-3 polyunsaturated fatty acids alter mechanisms involved in oocyte and early embryo development in the mouse. Am J Physiol Endocrinol Metab 2008; 294(2): E425-34.

[46] Wallace JM, Aitken RP, Cheyne MA. Nutrient partitioning and fetal growth in rapidly growing adolescent ewes. J Reprod Fertil 1996 ; 107(2): 183-90.

[47] Da Silva P, Aitken RP, Rhind SM, Racey PA, Wallace JM. Influence of placentally mediated fetal growth restriction on the onset of puberty in male and female lambs. Reproduction 2001; 122(3): 375-83.

[48] Da Silva P, Aitken RP, Rhind SM, Racey PA, Wallace JM. Impact of maternal nutrition during pregnancy on pituitary gonadotrophin gene expression and ovarian development in growth-restricted and normally grown late gestation sheep fetuses. Reproduction 2002; 123(6): 769-77.

[49] Sloboda DM, Howie GJ, Pleasants A, Gluckman PD, Vickers MH. Pre- and postnatal nutritional histories influence reproductive maturation and ovarian function in the rat. PLoS One 2009; 4(8): e6744.

[50] Nguyen RH, Wilcox AJ, Skjaerven R, Baird DD. Men's body mass index and infertility. Hum Reprod 2007; 22(9): 2488-93.

[51] Ramlau-Hansen CH, Nohr EA, Thulstrup AM, Bonde JP, Storgaard L, Olsen J. Is maternal obesity related to semen quality in the male offspring? A pilot study. Hum Reprod 2007; 22(10): 2758-62.

[52] Sallmen M, Sandler DP, Hoppin JA, Blair A, Baird DD. Reduced fertility among overweight and obese men. Epidemiology 2006; 17(5): 520-3.

[53] Chavarro JE, Toth TL, Wright DL, Meeker JD, Hauser R. Body mass index in relation to semen quality, sperm DNA integrity, and serum reproductive hormone levels among men attending an infertility clinic. Fertil Steril 2010; 93(7): 2222-31.

[54] Kort HI, Massey JB, Elsner CW, *et al.* Impact of body mass index values on sperm quantity and quality. J Androl 2006; 27(3): 450-2.

[55] Da Silva P, Aitken RP, Rhind SM, Racey PA, Wallace JM. Effect of maternal overnutrition during pregnancy on pituitary gonadotrophin gene expression and gonadal morphology in female and male fetal sheep at day 103 of gestation. Placenta 2003; 24(2-3): 248-57.

[56] Cetin I, Berti C, Calabrese S. Role of micronutrients in the periconceptional period. Hum Reprod Update 2010; 16(1): 80-95.

[57] Ashworth CJ, Antipatis C. Micronutrient programming of development throughout gestation. Reproduction. 2001 Oct; 122(4): 527-35.

[58] Zhang S, Rattanatray L, McMillen IC, Suter CM, Morrison JL. Periconceptional nutrition and the early programming of a life of obesity or adversity. Prog Biophys Mol Biol 2011; 106(1): 307-14.

[59] Sinclair KD, Allegrucci C, Singh R, *et al.* DNA methylation, insulin resistance, and blood pressure in offspring determined by maternal periconceptional B vitamin and methionine status. Proc Natl Acad Sci USA 2007; 104(49): 19351-6.

[60]   Steegers-Theunissen RP, Obermann-Borst SA, Kremer D, *et al.* Periconceptional maternal folic acid use of 400 microg per day is related to increased methylation of the IGF2 gene in the very young child. PLoS One 2009; 4(11): e7845.

[61]   Ly A, Lee H, Chen J, *et al.* Effect of maternal and postweaning folic Acid supplementation on mammary tumor risk in the offspring. Cancer Res 2011 1; 71(3): 988-97.

[62]   Watanabe T, Ebara S, Kimura S, *et al.* Maternal vitamin B12 deficiency affects spermatogenesis at the embryonic and immature stages in rats. Congenit Anom (Kyoto) 2007; 47(1): 9-15.

[63]   Fleming TP, Kwong WY, Porter R, *et al.* The embryo and its future. Biol Reprod 2004; 71(4): 1046-54.

[64]   Petrie L, Duthie SJ, Rees WD, McConnell JM. Serum concentrations of homocysteine are elevated during early pregnancy in rodent models of fetal programming. Br J Nutr 2002; 88(5): 471-7.

[65]   Cooney CA, Dave AA, Wolff GL. Maternal methyl supplements in mice affect epigenetic variation and DNA methylation of offspring. J Nutr 2002; 132(8 Suppl): 2393S-400S.

[66]   Aris A, Leblanc S, Ouellet A, Moutquin JM. Detrimental effects of high levels of antioxidant vitamins C and E on placental function: considerations for the vitamins in preeclampsia (VIP) trial. J Obstet Gynaecol Res 2008; 34(4): 504-11.

[67]   Church MW, Jen KL, Anumba JI, Jackson DA, Adams BR, Hotra JW. Excess omega-3 fatty acid consumption by mothers during pregnancy and lactation caused shorter life span and abnormal ABRs in old adult offspring. Neurotoxicol Teratol 2010; 32(2): 171-81.

[68]   Long NM, Nijland MJ, Nathanielsz PW, Ford SP. The effect of early to mid-gestational nutrient restriction on female offspring fertility and hypothalamic-pituitary-adrenal axis response to stress. J Anim Sci 2010; 88(6): 2029-37.

[69]   Agarwal A, Gupta S, Sikka S. The role of free radicals and antioxidants in reproduction. Curr Opin Obstet Gynecol 2006; 18(3): 325-32.

[70]   Martin KR, Barrett JC. Reactive oxygen species as double-edged swords in cellular processes: low-dose cell signaling versus high-dose toxicity. Hum Exp Toxicol 2002; 21(2): 71-5.

[71]   Fujii J, Iuchi Y, Okada F. Fundamental roles of reactive oxygen species and protective mechanisms in the female reproductive system. Reprod Biol Endocrinol 2005; 3: 43.

[72]   Heijmans BT, Tobi EW, Lumey LH, Slagboom PE. The epigenome: archive of the prenatal environment. Epigenetics 2009; 4(8): 526-31.

[73]   Szyf M. The early life environment and the epigenome. Biochim Biophys Acta 2009; 1790(9): 878-85.

[74]   Bettegowda A, Lee KB, Smith GW. Cytoplasmic and nuclear determinants of the maternal-to-embryonic transition. Reprod Fertil Dev 2008; 20(1): 45-53.

[75]   Bromfield J, Messamore W, Albertini DF. Epigenetic regulation during mammalian oogenesis. Reprod Fertil Dev 2008; 20(1): 74-80.

[76]   Dean W, Santos F, Reik W. Epigenetic reprogramming in early mammalian development and following somatic nuclear transfer. Semin Cell Dev Biol 2003; 14(1): 93-100.

[77]   Buckley AJ, Jaquiery AL, Harding JE. Nutritional programming of adult disease. Cell Tissue Res 2005; 322(1): 73-9.

[78]   Hanson MA, Gluckman PD. Developmental origins of health and disease: new insights. Basic Clin Pharmacol Toxicol 2008; 102(2): 90-3.

[79]   Kind KL, Moore VM, Davies MJ. Diet around conception and during pregnancy--effects on fetal and neonatal outcomes. Reprod Biomed Online 2006; 12(5): 532-41.

[80]   McMillen IC, MacLaughlin SM, Muhlhausler BS, Gentili S, Duffield JL, Morrison JL. Developmental origins of adult health and disease: the role of periconceptional and fetal nutrition. Basic Clin Pharmacol Toxicol 2008; 102(2): 82-9.

[81]   Doherty AS, Schultz RM. Culture of preimplantation mouse embryos. Methods Mol Biol 2000; 135: 47-52.

[82]   Fernandez-Gonzalez R, Moreira P, Bilbao A, *et al.* Long-term effect of *in vitro* culture of mouse embryos with serum on mRNA expression of imprinting genes, development, and behavior. Proc Natl Acad Sci USA 2004; 101(16): 5880-5.

[83]   Sinclair KD, Singh R. Modelling the developmental origins of health and disease in the early embryo. Theriogenology 2007; 67(1): 43-53.

[84]   Young LE, Fernandes K, McEvoy TG, *et al.* Epigenetic change in IGF2R is associated with fetal overgrowth after sheep embryo culture. Nat Genet 2001; 27(2): 153-4.

[85]   Kwong WY, Miller DJ, Ursell E, *et al.* Imprinted gene expression in the rat embryo-fetal axis is altered in response to periconceptional maternal low protein diet. Reproduction 2006; 132(2): 265-77.

[86]   Mann MR, Lee SS, Doherty AS, *et al.* Selective loss of imprinting in the placenta following preimplantation development in culture. Development 2004; 131(15): 3727-35.

[87]   Morgan HD, Jin XL, Li A, Whitelaw E, O'Neill C. The culture of zygotes to the blastocyst stage changes the postnatal expression of an epigenetically labile allele, agouti viable yellow, in mice. Biol Reprod 2008; 79(4): 618-23.

[88] Rivera RM, Stein P, Weaver JR, Mager J, Schultz RM, Bartolomei MS. Manipulations of mouse embryos prior to implantation result in aberrant expression of imprinted genes on day 9.5 of development. Hum Mol Genet 2008 ; 17(1): 1-14.

[89] Hajkova P, Erhardt S, Lane N, et al. Epigenetic reprogramming in mouse primordial germ cells. Mech Dev 2002; 117(1-2): 15-23.

[90] Walsh CP, Chaillet JR, Bestor TH. Transcription of IAP endogenous retroviruses is constrained by cytosine methylation. Nat Genet 1998; 20(2): 116-7.

[91] Tadros W, Lipshitz HD. The maternal-to-zygotic transition: a play in two acts. Development 2009; 136(18): 3033-42.

[92] Waterland RA. Do maternal methyl supplements in mice affect DNA methylation of offspring? J Nutr 2003; 133(1): 238; author reply 9.

[93] Raychaudhuri N, Raychaudhuri S, Thamotharan M, Devaskar SU. Histone code modifications repress glucose transporter 4 expression in the intrauterine growth-restricted offspring. J Biol Chem 2008; 283(20): 13611-26.

[94] Park JH, Stoffers DA, Nicholls RD, Simmons RA. Development of type 2 diabetes following intrauterine growth retardation in rats is associated with progressive epigenetic silencing of Pdx1. J Clin Invest 2008; 118(6): 2316-24.

[95] Brasacchio D, Okabe J, Tikellis C, et al. Hyperglycemia induces a dynamic cooperativity of histone methylase and demethylase enzymes associated with gene-activating epigenetic marks that coexist on the lysine tail. Diabetes 2009; 58(5): 1229-36.

[96] Miao F, Wu X, Zhang L, Riggs AD, Natarajan R. Histone methylation patterns are cell-type specific in human monocytes and lymphocytes and well maintained at core genes. J Immunol 2008; 180(4): 2264-9.

[97] Einstein F, Thompson RF, Bhagat TD, et al. Cytosine methylation dysregulation in neonates following intrauterine growth restriction. PLoS One 2010; 5(1): e8887.

[98] Fraga MF, Ballestar E, Paz MF, et al. Epigenetic differences arise during the lifetime of monozygotic twins. Proc Natl Acad Sci USA 2005; 102(30): 10604-9.

[99] Kaminsky ZA, Tang T, Wang SC, et al. DNA methylation profiles in monozygotic and dizygotic twins. Nat Genet 2009; 41(2): 240-5.

[100] Skinner MK, Manikkam M, Guerrero-Bosagna C. Epigenetic transgenerational actions of environmental factors in disease etiology. Trends Endocrinol Metab 2010; 21(4): 214-22.

[101] Attig L, Gabory A, Junien C. Early nutrition and epigenetic programming: chasing shadows. Curr Opin Clin Nutr Metab Care 2010; 13(3): 284-93

[102] Jungheim ES, Schoeller EL, Marquard KL, Louden ED, Schaffer JE, Moley KH. Diet-induced obesity model: abnormal oocytes and persistent growth abnormalities in the offspring. Endocrinology 2010; 151(8): 4039-46.

[103] Robker RL, Akison LK, Bennett BD, et al. Obese women exhibit differences in ovarian metabolites, hormones, and gene expression compared with moderate-weight women. J Clin Endocrinol Metab 2009; 94(5): 1533-40.

[104] Pisani LF, Antonini S, Pocar P, et al. Effects of pre-mating nutrition on mRNA levels of developmentally relevant genes in sheep oocytes and granulosa cells. Reproduction 2008; 136(3): 303-12.

[105] Igosheva N, Abramov AY, Poston L, et al. Maternal diet-induced obesity alters mitochondrial activity and redox status in mouse oocytes and zygotes. PLoS One 2010; 5(4): e10074.

[106] Wilms L, Larsen J, Pedersen PL, Kvetny J. Evidence of mitochondrial dysfunction in obese adolescents. Acta Paediatr 2010; 99(6): 906-11.

[107] Leese HJ, Hugentobler SA, Gray SM, et al. Female reproductive tract fluids: composition, mechanism of formation and potential role in the developmental origins of health and disease. Reprod Fertil Dev 2008; 20(1): 1-8.

[108] Mitchell M, Schulz SL, Armstrong DT, Lane M. Metabolic and mitochondrial dysfunction in early mouse embryos following maternal dietary protein intervention. Biol Reprod 2009; 80(4): 622-30.

[109] Kwong WY, Wild AE, Roberts P, Willis AC, Fleming TP. Maternal undernutrition during the preimplantation period of rat development causes blastocyst abnormalities and programming of postnatal hypertension. Development. 2000; 127(19): 4195-202.

[110] Kwong WY, Miller DJ, Wilkins AP, et al. Maternal low protein diet restricted to the preimplantation period induces a gender-specific change on hepatic gene expression in rat fetuses. Mol Reprod Dev 2007; 74(1): 48-56.

[111] Watkins AJ, Platt D, Papenbrock T, et al. Mouse embryo culture induces changes in postnatal phenotype including raised systolic blood pressure. Proc Natl Acad Sci USA 2007; 104(13): 5449-54.

[112] Watkins AJ, Wilkins A, Cunningham C, et al. Low protein diet fed exclusively during mouse oocyte maturation leads to behavioural and cardiovascular abnormalities in offspring. J Physiol 2008; 586(8): 2231-44.

[113] Brannian JD, Furman GM, Diggins M. Declining fertility in the lethal yellow mouse is related to progressive hyperleptinemia and leptin resistance. Reprod Nutr Dev 2005; 45(2): 143-50.

[114] Picone O, Laigre P, Fortun-Lamothe L, et al. Hyperlipidic hypercholesterolemic diet in prepubertal rabbits affects gene expression in the embryo, restricts fetal growth and increases offspring susceptibility to obesity. Theriogenology 2011; 75(2): 287-99.

[115] Farley D, Tejero ME, Comuzzie AG, et al. Feto-placental adaptations to maternal obesity in the baboon. Placenta 2009; 30(9): 752-60.

[116] Sjoblom C, Roberts CT, Wikland M, Robertson SA. Granulocyte-macrophage colony-stimulating factor alleviates adverse consequences of embryo culture on fetal growth trajectory and placental morphogenesis. Endocrinology. 2005; 146(5): 2142-53.

[117] Lucifero D, Chaillet JR, Trasler JM. Potential significance of genomic imprinting defects for reproduction and assisted reproductive technology. Hum Reprod Update 2004; 10(1): 3-18.

[118] Gallaher BW, Breier BH, Keven CL, Harding JE, Gluckman PD. Fetal programming of insulin-like growth factor (IGF)-I and IGF-binding protein-3: evidence for an altered response to undernutrition in late gestation following exposure to periconceptual undernutrition in the sheep. J Endocrinol 1998; 159(3): 501-8.

[119] Lea RG, Andrade LP, Rae MT, *et al.* Effects of maternal undernutrition during early pregnancy on apoptosis regulators in the ovine fetal ovary. Reproduction 2006; 131(1): 113-24.

[120] Rhind SM, Rae MT, Brooks AN. Environmental influences on the fetus and neonate--timing, mechanisms of action and effects on subsequent adult function. Domest Anim Endocrinol 2003; 25(1): 3-11.

[121] Murdoch WJ. Metaplastic potential of p53 down-regulation in ovarian surface epithelial cells affected by ovulation. Cancer Lett 2003; 191(1): 75-81.

[122] Rae MT, Rhind SM, Fowler PA, Miller DW, Kyle CE, Brooks AN. Effect of maternal undernutrition on fetal testicular steroidogenesis during the CNS androgen-responsive period in male sheep fetuses. Reproduction 2002 ; 124(1): 33-9.

[123] Swanson JM, Entringer S, Buss C, Wadhwa PD. Developmental origins of health and disease: environmental exposures. Semin Reprod Med 2009; 27(5): 391-402.

[124] Cornelius MD, Day NL. Developmental consequences of prenatal tobacco exposure. Curr Opin Neurol 2009; 22(2): 121-5.

[125] Mamsen LS, Lutterodt MC, Andersen EW, *et al.* Cigarette smoking during early pregnancy reduces the number of embryonic germ and somatic cells. Hum Reprod 2010; 25(11): 2755-61.

[126] Varvarigou AA, Liatsis SG, Vassilakos P, Decavalas G, Beratis NG. Effect of maternal smoking on cord blood estriol, placental lactogen, chorionic gonadotropin, FSH, LH, and cortisol. J Perinat Med 2009; 37(4): 364-9.

[127] Ratcliffe JM, Gladen BC, Wilcox AJ, Herbst AL. Does early exposure to maternal smoking affect future fertility in adult males? Reprod Toxicol. 1992; 6(4): 297-307.

[128] Hellemans KG, Sliwowska JH, Verma P, Weinberg J. Prenatal alcohol exposure: fetal programming and later life vulnerability to stress, depression and anxiety disorders. Neurosci Biobehav Rev 2010; 34(6): 791-807.

[129] Ornoy A, Ergaz Z. Alcohol abuse in pregnant women: effects on the fetus and newborn, mode of action and maternal treatment. Int J Environ Res Public Health 2010; 7(2): 364-79.

[130] Ramlau-Hansen CH, Toft G, Jensen MS, Strandberg-Larsen K, Hansen ML, Olsen J. Maternal alcohol consumption during pregnancy and semen quality in the male offspring: two decades of follow-up. Hum Reprod 2010; 25(9): 2340-5.

[131] Rubin BS, Soto AM. Bisphenol A: Perinatal exposure and body weight. Mol Cell Endocrinol 2009; 304(1-2): 55-62.

[132] Carone BR, Fauquier L, Habib N, *et al.* Paternally induced transgenerational environmental reprogramming of metabolic gene expression in mammals. Cell 2010; 143(7): 1084-96.

[133] Ng SF, Lin RC, Laybutt DR, Barres R, Owens JA, Morris MJ. Chronic high-fat diet in fathers programs beta-cell dysfunction in female rat offspring. Nature 2010; 467(7318): 963-6.

[134] Jenkins TG, Carrell DT. The paternal epigenome and embryogenesis: poising mechanisms for development. Asian J Androl 2011; 13(1): 76-80.

[135] Kaati G, Bygren LO, Edvinsson S. Cardiovascular and diabetes mortality determined by nutrition during parents' and grandparents' slow growth period. Eur J Hum Genet 2002; 10(11): 682-8.

[136] Kaati G, Bygren LO, Pembrey M, Sjostrom M. Transgenerational response to nutrition, early life circumstances and longevity. Eur J Hum Genet 2007; 15(7): 784-90.

CHAPTER 3

Fetal Programming of Hypothalamic-Pituitary-Adrenal Axis by Synthetic Glucocorticoids

Marion Tegethoff[1] and Gunther Meinlschmidt[2,3*]

[1] Division of Clinical Psychology and Psychiatry, Department of Psychology, University of Basel, Switzerland;
[2]Division of Clinical Psychology and Epidemiology, Department of Psychology, University of Basel, Switzerland and [3] National Centre of Competence in Research "Swiss Etiological Study of Adjustment and Mental Health (sesam)", Switzerland

Abstract: Major physiological systems, such as the hypothalamic-pituitary-adrenal (hpa) axis, are susceptible to certain intrauterine exposures of the fetus. These exposures may lead to long-term programming, with potential consequences for the individual throughout life. One such exposure is the administration of synthetic glucocorticoids that are commonly used in different medical fields. This chapter focuses on fetal programming of hpa axis by synthetic glucocorticoids. It introduces the pharmacological and physiological background of this topic, summarizes major findings from human and animal studies, and addresses potential biological mechanisms and the clinical relevance of such programming. In humans, exposure to synthetic glucocorticoids *in utero* reduces fetal and, in some cases, postnatal hpa activity under basal conditions, and following stress. Data from animal studies indicate that lifelong hpa axis dysregulation, rather than either static *hypo*activity or *hyper*activity of hpa axis, is a common consequence of early exposure to synthetic glucocorticoids. The mechanisms of glucocorticoid-induced changes in hpa axis function are complex, including possible alterations at subcortical and cortical levels of the brain. Emerging evidence indicates that early dysregulation of hpa axis is adverse, possibly leading to compromised development and health in the short term. It is as yet unclear as to whether long-term health disturbances are to be expected. More randomized human follow-up studies are needed to better understand the short- and long-term effects of intrauterine exposure to synthetic glucocorticoids on hpa axis and potential short- and long-term consequences on health and development.

Keywords: Hypothalamic-pituitary-adrenal axis, fetal programming, synthetic glucocorticoids, intrauterine exposures, preterm delivery, asthma.

INTRODUCTION

Several medical conditions, such as risk for preterm delivery or asthma may lead to the decision to treat a pregnant woman with synthetic glucocorticoids [1-3]. In obstetric practice, different types of synthetic glucocorticoids are used, for example betamethasone and dexamethasone. Synthetic glucocorticoids, agonists of the glucocorticoid receptor (GR, the symbol approved by the Human Genome Organisation Nomenclature Committee is NR3C1), predominantly act *via* genomic effects mediated by the GR, a nuclear transcription factor (for detailed description, see [4, 5]). With its marked GR expression, the fetal lung is one of the primary targets of synthetic glucocorticoids administered during fetal development. The short-term effects of synthetic glucocorticoids on the fetal and neonatal lung and other organ systems with high GR expression, including kidney and brain, have been described elsewhere [*e.g.* 1, 6-11]. Moreover, the clinical outcomes that are potentially related to structural and functional changes in the brain after intrauterine exposure to synthetic glucocorticoids, including cognitive, psychological or behavioral development, have been brought together in previous works [12, 13]. This chapter deals with the effects of prenatal exposure to synthetic glucocorticoids on hypothalamic-pituitary-adrenal (hpa) axis function.

What is the clinical use of synthetic glucocorticoids during pregnancy? On the one hand glucocorticoids may be applied to alleviate medical conditions in the mother, such as the administration of glucocorticoid containing inhalants in case of asthma [3]. On the other hand, glucocorticoids may be applied to target the fetus. Indeed, one major indication is their application to women with risk of preterm delivery. Glucocorticoids accelerate fetal lung

Address correspondence to Gunther Meinlschmidt: Faculty of Psychology, University of Basel, Missionsstrasse 60/62, CH-4055 Basel, Switzerland, Tel: ++41 61 267 02 75; Fax: ++41 61 267 06 59; E-mail: gunther.meinlschmidt@unibas.ch

Bashir M. Matata and Maqsood M. Elahi (Eds.)

maturation, thereby successfully reducing morbidity and mortality in preterm infants [2, 14, 15]. However, major concerns exist concerning the safety of such therapy, as there is evidence that prenatal exposure to synthetic glucocorticoids may compromise health and development [12, 13, 16, 17].

BACKGROUND

Medical Indications for the Application of Synthetic Glucocorticoids During Pregnancy

Glucocorticoids are important regulators of a wide range of physiological processes. For example, they influence lipid, protein, and carbohydrate metabolism, and regulate cardiovascular, neurobiological, and immunological function. One major function of glucocorticoids is to maintain homeostasis and to enable coping with and adaptation to stressful events [18]. Synthetic analogues of glucocorticoids are broadly used in clinical practice to treat a large variety of pathologies, which is due to the crucial role of endogenous glucocorticoids in the regulation of physiological processes.

During fetal development, glucocorticoids stimulate surfactant production and influence structural changes, growth factors, lung fluid metabolism, antioxidant enzymes, and adrenergic receptors, in the maturing fetal lung. In late gestation, feto-maternal cortisol secretion increases to complete pulmonary maturation, and prepare the fetal lungs for postnatal life [1, 19]. Consequently, preterm infants are at risk of pulmonary immaturity predisposing them to respiratory distress syndrome (RDS). Indeed, preterm birth is associated with an increased risk of neonatal complications, including RDS. Due to their potency in maturing fetal organ systems, synthetic glucocorticoids are commonly used to treat cases of high-risk preterm delivery to accelerate fetal lung maturation. Seven to ten percent of all pregnancies in North America are endangered by preterm birth [20]. In addition, during gestation, synthetic glucocorticoids are given for several other pathologies of the mother or the fetus, including asthma and congenital adrenal hyperplasia (CAH).

The use of synthetic glucocorticoids in reproductive medicine to prevent RDS originated in the work of Liggins in the late 1960s, who was the first to demonstrate in lambs the lung maturational properties of glucocorticoids [21]. Based on numerous subsequent studies replicating the initial findings [2, 22], in 1994, the National Institutes of Health (NIH) Consensus Developmental Conference on the Effects of Corticosteroids for Fetal Maturation on Perinatal Outcomes concluded that all fetuses between 24 and 34 weeks of gestation at risk of preterm delivery are potential candidates for prenatal treatment with glucocorticoids [20].

Today, antenatal glucocorticoid use in fetuses at risk of preterm delivery is common practice to prevent postnatal RDS, even though treatment protocols remain inconsistent across institutions and physicians. If women continue pregnancy after a single course of glucocorticoid treatment, in some cases further subsequent courses of synthetic glucocorticoids are administered. However, due to insufficient scientific data, in 2001 the NIH Consensus Developmental Panel recommended that repeated courses should not be used routinely until insightful findings are available [23].

Taken together, synthetic glucocorticoids are now used broadly in reproductive medicine to treat fetuses at risk of preterm birth in order to prevent RDS.

Besides this, synthetic glucocorticoids are also administered to pregnant women due to maternal medical conditions, including asthma, or due to fetal needs, other than lung maturation, such as CAH [24]. In contrast to preparation for preterm birth, treatment in the latter cases often begins early in pregnancy and lasts throughout gestation.

Determinants of Fetal Drug Exposure

Synthetic glucocorticoids differ from their endogenous equivalents in chemical structure [25], having stronger potency at the GR and reduced activity at the mineralocorticoid receptor (MR, the symbol approved by the HUGO Nomenclature Committee is NR3C2) [5]. Moreover, different types of synthetic glucocorticoids vary with regard to their pharmacokinetic and pharmacodynamic properties (in the mother and the fetoplacental unit), such as protein binding, drug absorption, distribution throughout fluids and tissues, metabolism, and elimination [26]. These properties are major determinants of fetal exposure to the administered synthetic glucocorticoids.

Pharmacokinetic Properties of Synthetic Glucocorticoids during Pregnancy

The pharmacokinetic and pharmacodynamic properties of synthetic glucocorticoids have mostly been investigated in non-pregnant women. However, changes in the renal, gastrointestinal, cardiovascular, and immune system, which occur during pregnancy [27], lead to pharmacokinetic changes [26-30]. For example, it has been shown that clearance of betamethasone and volume of distribution are higher in pregnant than in non-pregnant women, whereas half-life remained unchanged [31]. Moreover, pharmacokinetic properties were different between pregnancies, for example varying with the plurality of birth [32], and half-life of betamethasone was significantly shorter in twin than in singleton pregnancies. Moreover, it was shown in ewes that pharmacokinetic characteristics of betamethasone differ between mother and fetus: after injection into maternal muscle tissue, as is common practice in obstetrics, betamethasone half-life is longer in fetal than in maternal circulation, suggesting that the fetus is exposed stronger than would be anticipated from maternal pharmacokinetic data [33].

During pregnancy, maternal plasma volume progressively expands. Subsequently, concentration of albulim decreases, leading to a reduced protein-binding capacity despite elevated albumin synthesis [34, 35]. Synthetic glucocorticoids such as betamethasone and dexamethasone bind specifically to albumin. Therefore, the unbound, biologically active fraction of these glucocorticoids subsequently increases. Interestingly, only this unbound fraction passes the placenta. Therefore, as pregnancy proceeds, the fetus is exposed to a greater amount of synthetic glucocorticoids, with potential clinical consequences. The fetus, however increasingly compensates this process: During gestation, fetal albumin concentrations gradually increase, equaling [36] or even exceeding [37] maternal albumin concentrations at term. Subsequently, fetal plasma binds more and more glucocorticoids, reducing the biological activity of the glucocorticoids in the fetus. Additionally, the fetus may already have a moderate capacity to metabolize drugs itself [26].

How Synthetic Glucocorticoids Get from Mother to Fetus

Diverse factors determine transplacental drug/substance permeation, these being drug properties, placental characteristics, and additional maternal and fetal influencing factors [38]. One key enzyme which selectively regulates the transplacental passage of glucocorticoids is placental hydroxysteroid (11 beta) dehydrogenase 2 (11beta-HSD2, the symbol approved by the HUGO Nomenclature Committee is HSD11B2) [17]. 11beta-HSD2 is located in placental syncytiotrophoblast [39], and catalyzes the rapid inactivation of cortisol and corticosterone, thereby representing an effective but incomplete barrier [40]. Normally, the fetus has much lower concentrations than the mother, even though endogenous glucocorticoids are highly lipophilic and rapidly cross the placenta [41, 42]. Transplacental passage differs noticeably between endogenous and synthetic glucocorticoids [43]. In cells transfected with 11beta-HSD2, more than 95 percent of corticosterone, 63 percent of cortisol, but only 17 percent of dexamethasone had been metabolized after a one-hour incubation [39]. Furthermore, in contrast to endogenous glucocorticoids, betamethasone and dexamethasone show decreased local inactivation; while conversely, reduction by 11beta-HSD2 is increased in prednisolone [25]. Accordingly, it has been shown previously *in vitro* that 67 percent of cortisol and 52 percent of prednisolone, but only 2 percent of dexamethasone and 7 percent of betamethasone, were converted by 11beta-HSD2 to their inactive metabolites in human placental tissue [44]. When examining cord and maternal blood, some authors demonstrated ten-fold lower prednisolone [45] but only three-fold lower betamethasone [28, 46] concentrations in fetal as compared to maternal plasma. In the human placenta, betamethasone was more rapidly metabolized than dexamethasone and prednisolone, with their inactive metabolites being first observed after 60, 120, and 240 minutes, respectively [47]. With regard to the rates of inactivation by 11beta-HSD2, metabolism of both betamethasone and prednisolone was significantly greater than that of dexamethasone [47]. It is of note that synthetic glucocorticoids have been shown to up-regulate placental 11beta-HSD2 activity [48-50], which provides evidence that they themselves amplify the placental barrier.

Besides 11beta-HSD2, other mechanisms seem to be involved in creating the placental glucocorticoid barrier, reducing fetal exposure to elevated levels of glucocorticoids, with the ATP-binding cassette, sub-family B (MDR/TAP), member 1 (also known as P-glycoprotein [P-gp], the symbol approved by the HUGO Nomenclature Committee is Abcb1) being a prominent candidate [51-55]. Interestingly, P-gp activity seems to decrease in the placenta in late gestation, potentially reducing the ability of the placenta to exclude synthetic glucocorticoids from the fetus at the end of pregnancy [54-59].

Taken together, during pregnancy, synthetic glucocorticoids can cross the placental barrier and become active in the fetus, potentially affecting the developing systems that express GRs (see below), for example the fetal brain and hpa axis.

Fetal HPA Axis Development

The fetal hpa axis differs from the postnatal hpa axis that has been described in detail elsewhere [60]. Fetal hpa axis controls intrauterine homeostasis, the growth and maturation of fetal organ systems, and establishes the estrogenic milieu of pregnancy. It is critical that the fetal adrenocortical system and structures involved in its regulation develop and function properly to ensure fetal maturation. The major physiological role of the postnatal adrenocortical system is to synthesize and secrete glucocorticoids for the maintenance of metabolic homeostasis and the stress response and mineralocorticoids for the maintenance of fluid and electrolyte balance [61]. One reason for the functional differences of the pre- and postnatal hpa axis is that hypothalamus, pituitary, and adrenal gland are subject to dynamic morphological and/or functional changes *in utero*, attaining adult shape and function soon after birth. Furthermore, fetal hpa axis is considerably regulated by the placenta (for details see below). The present knowledge about the developmental biology of the human and nonhuman primate fetal hypothalamus, pituitary, and adrenal cortex has previously been reviewed extensively [61-64]. Based on these reviews, we here briefly summarize function, anatomy and development of the embryonic and fetal hpa axis.

Anatomy and Function

By the seventh week of gestation, the human fetal hypothalamus is detectable [63], and CRH-positive fibres exist by the 16th gestational week [65]. The portal system for the transport of hypothalamic releasing factors to the pituitary gland is detectable at 11.5 weeks of gestation, allowing the hypothalamus to exert control over pituitary corticotropes around midgestation [66]. A rudimentary adenohypophysis in the pituitary gland can be identified by six weeks of gestation, which matures within the subsequent eight weeks [63]. The presence of corticotropes has been demonstrated by immunohistochemical studies at seven weeks of gestation [67]. Accordingly, ACTH secretion has been shown to occur at eight weeks of gestation [68]. By eight weeks, the embryonic adrenal cortex is clearly defined with its characteristic zonal partitioning, while the anlage of the adrenal cortex is detectable already at four weeks of gestation [61]. The fetal adrenal cortex of the primate consists of three compartments that are morphologically and functionally different, and distinguishable on the basis of the expression of specific steroidogenic enzymes: the fetal, the definitive, and the transitional zone [61]. The former comprises the major portion of the fetal adrenal cortex, and represents the primary site of growth and steroidogenesis. The fetal zone produces dehydroepiandrosterone sulfate (DHEA-S), the principle steroid product of the primate fetal adrenal gland throughout gestation. Mineralocorticoids are produced in the definitive zone in late gestation, while the smaller transitional zone is the site of glucocorticoid production and thus the precursor of the adult zona fasciculata [61]. The fetal adrenal cortex, especially the fetal zone, begins to grow rapidly from ten weeks of gestation until term, and by midgestation, the fetal zone forms the major part of the adrenal. Size and weight of the fetal adrenals double between 20 and 30 weeks, achieving a relative size 10- to 20-times that of the adult adrenal, further doubling until term [61]. By the 30th week of gestation, the fetal adrenal cells begin to take on a rudimentary appearance of the adult adrenal cortex through remodeling [69]. During early gestation, the adrenals take up steroidogenic activity. After eight to ten weeks of gestation, low levels of estriol, indicative of DHEA-S production in the fetal adrenals [70], can first be detected in the maternal circulation. Within the subsequent month, estriol concentrations in the maternal circulation increase rapidly up to 100-fold. Activity of the fetal zone subsequently continues to increase during the second and third trimester, producing around 200 mg DHEA-S/day at term [61]. Cortisol production begins between ten and twenty weeks of gestation, with progesterone being a possible precursor [61, 71, 72]. However, *de novo* synthesis of cortisol from cholesterol starts rather late in gestation. This leads to a large increase of cortisol concentrations in the third trimester [61]. In summary, hpa axis structures are detectable early during pregnancy. They show rapid growth and start steroidogenic activity by about eight to ten weeks of gestation.

Regulation

Stimulators of the fetal hpa axis are acute hypoxia, systemic hypotension, hemorrhage, psychological stress, noxious stimuli and neuropeptides, while the fetal hpa axis can be inhibited by glucocorticoids and vagal stimulation [64]. The human fetus can mount hormonal stress responses to invasive stimuli, with rises in beta-endorphin, cortisol and noradrenaline [73, 74], wich are independent of maternal hormonal reactions to invasive procedures [75]. Ng and coworkers [64] have illustrated the neuroendocrine interaction between the fetal hpa axis and the placenta. ACTH secreted from the fetal pituitary is the major regulator of the human fetal adrenal cortex. However, the fetal adrenals are also influenced by growth factors, transcription factors, and placental factors including CRH [61, 76]. For example, the production of proopiomelanocortin (POMC) and ACTH in the fetal pituitary is stimulated by placental CRH [77, 78], which thereby regulates growth and function of pituitary corticotrope cells and adrenal cortex [61, 64]. Given that placental and hypothalamic CRH are identical in immunoreactivity, bioactivity, and structure, it is possible that both fetal hypothalamic and placental CRH stimulate fetal pituitary. However, circulating CRH seems to be largely of placental origin, as umbilical venous were higher than arterial CRH concentrations [79]. Fetal ACTH enhances adrenal secretion of cortisol, which in turn reduces the axis' activity *via* negative feedback mechanisms [64, 80]. Most importantly, fetal ACTH stimulates synthesis of DHEA-S [64], which itself is a substrate for placental estrogen synthesis [70]. In the baboon, placental estrogens were shown to inactivate cortisol by its conversion to cortisone in the placenta. By reducing fetal exposure to maternal cortisol, this inactivation decreases inhibition of the fetal hpa axis *via* negative feedback by maternal cortisol, thereby maintaining the concentrations of fetal ACTH, cortisol and DHEA-S synthesis. This mechanism may underlie the rapid adrenal cortex growth around midgestation [81, 82]. Moreover, fetal adrenal glucocorticoids stimulate placental CRH production *via* a positive feedback circuit, resulting in constantly increasing CRH, ACTH, and cortisol concentrations at the end of gestation [64]. Taken together, the fetal neuroendocrine system is subject to a complex pattern of regulation *via* negative and positive feedback mechanisms.

Adaptation to Extrauterine Life

The fetal zone of the adrenal cortex degenerates immediately after birth and the zona fasciculata matures within three weeks [83]. Despite the remodeling of the adrenal cortex, there is no evidence of adrenocortical insufficiency in term infants during this critical period [61]. In contrast, serum levels of cortisol were even shown to gradually increase after birth in term infants [84]. Even infants born preterm showed an increase in cortisol concentrations within the first day postpartum, with values decreasing again up to age four weeks, but they did not fall below concentrations observed around birth [85]. However, other investigators reported a rapid decrease in ACTH, cortisol and cortisone precursors in term and preterm infants immediately after birth, with a nadir approximately two months postpartum [62]. This has to be clarified in future studies.

Interestingly, premature infants maintain fetal patterns of hormonal regulation until remodeling of adrenals is complete. Therefore, it is not surprising that different patterns of hormonal activity have been reported in premature infants as compared to term infants and that these patterns are amongst others linked to gestational age [62-64].

Taking into consideration everything else hpa axis activity starts early in embryonic life, passing through dynamic changes throughout gestation and the neonatal period up to adult life. Adequate maturation of the hypothalamus, pituitary, adrenal cortex, and systems involved in the regulation of the hpa axis serves appropriate ontogeny. Disturbances of this complex maturational process may thus result in a dysfunctional endocrine system later on.

Development of Glucocorticoid Receptors

Synthetic glucocorticoids act *via* the intracellular GR that binds cortisol with low affinity and synthetic glucocorticoids with high affinity. GRs are expressed in most organ systems, including the brain, where high GR expression occurs in the amygdala [86], hippocampus [87, 88], and the paraventricular nucleus of the hypothalamus (PVNh) [87, 89]. High levels of GR are also expressed in the pituitary gland [90, 91]. Thus, GR expression is high in those regions involved in regulation of corticotropin releasing hormone (CRH) and adrenocorticotropic hormone (ACTH) synthesis and release, thereby being a major modulator of the hpa axis, which is the major source of endogenous glucocorticoid hormones.

The stage of maturation of GR expression in the fetal hpa axis or those regions involved in its regulation determines whether synthetic glucocorticoids administered during gestation can exert effects on fetal hpa axis [92, 93]. In mice, more GR messenger RNA (mRNA) is expressed in the fetal zone of the placenta than in the decidual zone from around midgestation [94], suggesting that synthetic glucocorticoids may become active at the placental level early during gestation. In humans, GR mRNA expression in the fetal hippocampus was detected at 24 weeks of gestation, meaning that the receptor is present in the fetal brain around the time when synthetic glucocorticoids are given to the mother to accelerate fetal lung maturation [95]. The ontogeny of GR in the fetal PVNh or pituitary in humans is as yet unknown. Interestingly in sheep, high levels of GR mRNA are present in the fetal cerebral cortex, hippocampus, and PVNh in mid-late gestation [96]. Sheep have a pattern of prenatal brain development similar to humans, and have a high degree of neurological maturity at birth [97]. In the mouse fetus, GR gene expression in hypothalamus and pituitary was detected around midgestation with salient increases in the pituitary towards the end of gestation, when glucocorticoid production rises. In contrast, in the mouse fetus adrenals, GR mRNA expression remains low throughout gestation [94]. In the common marmoset (*Callithrix jacchus*), GR expression in the neonate hippocampus and PVNh is similar to that of adults, indicating that brain GR expression is already mature at birth, and implying that fetal GR expression will also be substantial in those species that give birth to relatively mature offspring [98].

Taken together, there is evidence that brain GRs will be substantially activated in the fetus following glucocorticoid treatment, given the early presence of GRs in the fetal brain and given the evidence that synthetic GR agonists administered to the mother can enter the fetal brain. Consequently, offspring hpa axis function could be acutely or chronically influenced [99].

FETAL PROGRAMMING OF HPA AXIS BY SYNTHETIC GLUCOCORTICOIDS: EVIDENCE FROM HUMAN AND ANIMAL STUDIES

Human Studies

The effects of intrauterine exposure to synthetic glucocorticoids on hpa axis have been systematically reviewed in detail [100]. We here summarize the major findings regarding (a) basal hpa function, (b) hpa reactivity, (c) glucocorticoid dose and time between treatment and sample collection, and (d) an integrating model of altered hpa function due to intrauterine exposure to synthetic glucocorticoids.

Basal HPA Function

Basal fetal pituitary-adrenal function was assessed by measuring markers of fetal hpa activity, including ACTH, cortisol, and DHEA-S, in cord blood and amniotic fluid during gestation and at birth. Concentrations were lower in fetuses exposed to synthetic glucocorticoids *in utero* compared to unexposed fetuses.

Evidence from multiple studies [see 100] suggests that during the first postnatal days, plasma cortisol concentrations are reduced in infants exposed to glucocorticoids, compared to unexposed infants. Subsequently, cortisol levels seem to increase to normal until not later than 2 weeks postpartum. However, some studies did not confirm this picture. Interestingly, at the same time, hpa axis secretagogues other than cortisol, such as ACTH, 17-OHP and 11-deoxycortisol, were in the normal range. This suggests that pituitary function and adrenal steroidogenesis normalizes earlier than cortisol synthesis and secretion, in infants exposed to synthetic glucocorticoids *in utero* compared to unexposed infants.

In summary, the available literature suggests an overall time course pattern of basal hpa function related to intrauterine exposure to glucocorticoid exposure, consisting of a short period of reduced activity, followed by recovery to normal levels by approximately two weeks postpartum.

HPA Reactivity

To investigate the reactivity of neonatal and infant hpa axis, pharmacological challenges with substances such as ACTH or ACTH agonists, metyrapone, and human CRH were applied, and reactions to painful stressors were measured.

Pharmacological Challenge

Available evidence suggests that within the first six weeks postpartum, adrenocortical reactivity to a standard dose of ACTH is unaltered in infants exposed to synthetic glucocorticoids *in utero*. This may seem to some extent counter-intuitive in light of substantial evidence for suppressed basal hpa function after intrauterine exposure to synthetic glucocorticoids. However, the evidence would be consistent with a situation in which the level of hpa axis inhibition leading to reduced basal cortisol concentrations would be located at the hypothalamus or pituitary rather than the adrenocortex [100]. Indeed, evidence from metyrapone stimulation confirmed studies using stimulation by ACTH, both indicating an intact adrenocortical activity in infants exposed to synthetic glucocorticoids *in utero*, while demonstrating an uncompromised pituitary reserve and feedback [101].

There was only weak evidence for suppressed cortisol reaction to hCRH administration in infants exposed to dexamethasone *in utero*. Moreover, no significant influence of dexamethasone exposure on post-hCRH ACTH concentrations has been reported.

In conclusion, at present, the available evidence does not suggest suppression of hpa reaction to pharmacological stimulation in infants exposed to glucocorticoids *in utero* (except for limited evidence of mild inhibition of the cortisol response to hCRH administration seven days postpartum).

Painful Stressors

Most studies assessing changes in hpa axis *reactivity* in relation to glucocorticoid exposure *in utero* reported on hpa reactivity after moderate pain by pinprick or following discomfort triggered by a medical examination or intervention between the first days and 12 months after birth [102-108]. Most of these studies found evidence for reduced pain-related hpa axis reactivity in neonates and infants exposed to glucocorticoids *in utero*. The observation that hpa axis responses to pain-related stress are reduced within the first postnatal week in glucocorticoid exposed infants is in line with evidence for reduced basal hpa function shortly after birth, suggesting a rather general dampening of hpa axis function that is not restricted to reduced basal activity immediately after birth but also affects reactivity to painful stimulation. However, there is some evidence that glucocorticoid-exposure related reduced basal hpa activity and reduced hpa reactivity to pain-related stress de-couple after the first two weeks of life, with the former recovering and the latter persisting until four months of life.

Pharmacological Challenge Versus Painful Stressors

Interestingly, in infants exposed to synthetic glucocorticoids *in utero* compared to controls, pharmacological challenge revealed at best only slightly blunted cortisol reactivity shortly after birth, while pain-related stressors revealed sustained blunting of cortisol reactivity up to four months of age. A potential explanation of this putative discrepancy may be that hpa reactions to the applied pharmacological challenges do not reflect processes that occur at supra-hypothalamic levels. Hence, blunted hpa axis reactions to painful, but not to pharmacological, stimulation may reflect reduced hypothalamic input from higher levels (*e.g.* limbic system, cortical structures) [100].

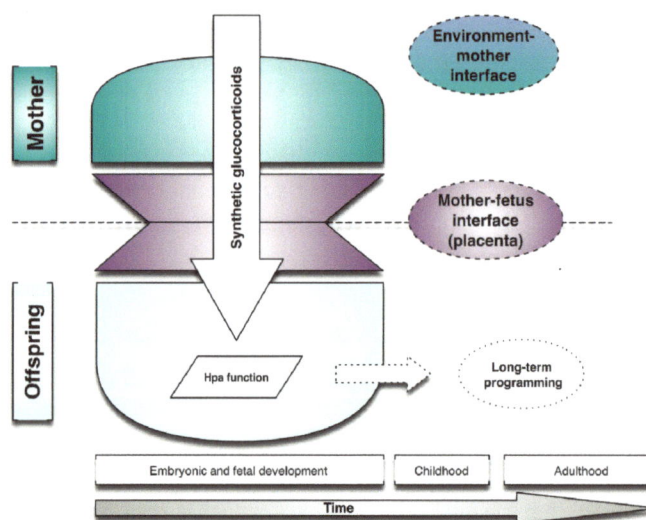

Figrue 1: Model of hpa Axis Programming by Synthetic Glucocorticoids *In Utero* (Figure is Reproduced and Adapted, with Permission, from Tegethoff, 2009. Copyright 2009 by Cuvillier).

Integrative Model of HPA Function Alterations Following Exposure to Synthetic Glucocorticoids in Utero

Current data provide the basis for the following model [100] (Fig. **1**): Exposure to synthetic glucocorticoids *in utero* leads 1) to a blunted fetal hpa activity at different levels, as indicated by substances assessed in cord blood and amniotic fluid; 2) to a subsequent normalization within the first week postpartum of basal hpa activity at the level of the pituitary, indicated by normalized ACTH levels, but an ongoing reduction of basal adrenocortical activity; 3) to a subsequent recovery of basal hpa activity at the level of the adrenocortex, as indicated by normalized basal concentrations of indicators of cortisol synthesis or secretion by the end of the second week post-partum, and 4) to ongoing reduced hpa reactivity during the first months of life that probably originates from changes at supra-pituitary levels, as suggested by evidence from pharmacological and psychological challenge.

The validity of this model is challenged by some methodological issues that complicate the interpretation of the available studies, such as the use of quasi-experimental study designs and potential confounding by treatment indication or small sample sizes, as well as risk of publication bias.

HPA, HYPOTHALMIC-PITUITARY-ADRENAL

Animal Studies

Some of the above-mentioned methodological limitations of human studies, especially the use of a quasi-experimental study design, due to the ethical barriers to experimentally manipulate exposure to glucocorticoids in humans, can be overcome in animal studies.

A study with rodents showed that exposure to synthetic glucocorticoids early in life can blunt basal hpa activity as well as hpa reactivity to stress during the neonatal period and in later life [*e.g.* 110, 111, 112]. In contrast to that, in an ample amount of studies, early exposure to synthetic glucocorticoids was related to increased hpa activity at different life stages in various species, including nonhuman primates [113-117]. If everything else is taken into consideration, the findings from animal studies suggest that long-term hpa dysregulation, rather than either static hpa *hypo*activity or *hyper*activity, is the overarching consequence of exposure to synthetic glucocorticoids early in life [12, 13, 16, 118-120]. There is a big need for a detailed and systematic comparison between findings from human and animal studies, taking into account potential heterogeneity between species in which the hpa axis primarily matures postnatally (such as rats, rabbits, and mice) and species in which the hpa axis primarily matures prenatally (such as primates, sheep, and guinea pigs) [97]. Such comparison of findings from animal and human studies may foster our understanding and interpretation of results from human studies, with a special emphasis on revealing the mechanisms underlying the observed effects of synthetic glucocorticoids on hpa axis.

POTENTIAL BIOLOGICAL MECHANISMS MEDIATING HPA AXIS PROGRAMMING BY GLUCOCORTICOIDS

Several biological mechanisms may mediate the hpa related consequences of intrauterine exposure to synthethic glucocorticoids. The blunting of fetal and newborn hpa activity may be a direct consequence of the suppressing effects of the synthetic glucocorticoids administered to the mother, while they are in the circulation. This is supported by several studies that assessed the effects of synthetic glucocorticoids close to their administration before they could have been cleared from blood. However, a range of studies assessed hpa reactivity at more than 72 hours after birth, which is at a time when synthetic glucocorticoids are most likely virtually cleared from blood [121, 122]. Such a lasting adrenal suppression beyond the clearance of the administered synthetic glucocorticoids [*e.g.* 102, 103-105, 123-126] indicates that changes in hpa activity become independent from current exogenous influence, suggesting the development of changes in structure or function of hpa axis or brain regions involved in hpa regulation, establishing a sustained dampening of hpa activity. For example, different alterations of hpa axis, such as primary or secondary adrenal insufficiency or (compensatory) down-regulation of receptors at higher hpa axis levels, may underlie the hypocortisolemic phenotype that was observed after exposure to synthetic glucocorticoids *in utero* [100]. Findings from animal studies suggest that functional hpa axis changes following intrauterine exposure to synthetic glucocorticoids are associated with (i) changes at higher brain levels, including alterations in diverse brain structures involved in hpa axis regulation, particularly the hippocampus, (ii) changes in GR expression and (iii) variations in other neuroendocrine and neurotransmitter systems [12, 16, 118]. In summary, while inducing a short-term hypercortisolemic state in the fetus due to their direct glucocorticoid properties, synthetic glucocorticoids concomittantly reduce hpa function. This blunting of hpa activity might be due to various biological mechanisms [for a detailed discussion, see 100].

CLINICAL RELEVANCE OF HPA HYPOACTIVITY IN INFANCY

A blunted hpa activity in infancy following exposure to glucocorticoids *in utero* may be of clinical relevance. Reduced fetal and infant hpa function will affect the tissue exposure to endogenous glucocorticoids, and may result in altered rate of development and/or health impairment. To the best of our knowledge, this question has, not yet been comprehensively addressed in humans. However, the broad physiological functions of endogenous glucocorticoids [18] and several experimental and clinical observations suggest that changes in endocrine activity at an early stage of life are likely to be of clinical relevance.

For example, the hypothesis that reduced hpa activity early in life may affect development is supported by several studies on the long-term consequences of early *postnatal* glucocorticoid therapy due to respiratory distress. Indeed, this treatment has repeatedly been linked to blunting of hpa function [*e.g.* 127, 128-132]. Infants postnatally treated with dexamethasone for respiratory distress show reduced behavioral and cognitive performance and compromised neuromotor and psychomotor development [*e.g.* 133, 134-136]. Notably, as yet we have no clear evidence that the observed suppression of hpa function in infants postnatally exposed to synthetic glucocorticoids mediates the reported developmental consequences of the treatment. Besides this, valid extrapolations from postnatal glucocorticoid treatment to make assumptions about prenatal glucocorticoid treatment may be limited as for example postnatal glucocorticoid therapy usually lasts longer than prenatal therapy, therefore leading to stronger changes.

Further evidence comes from a series of studies revealing an association between atopic diseases and attenuated cortisol stress responses in children [137, 138] and adults [139].

If everything is considered, the results from experimental and clinical studies suggest that blunted hpa activity early in life may impair development and health in the short and in the long term. More studies are highly warranted to evaluate the clinical implications of altered tissue exposure to endogenous glucocorticoids in fetuses and newborns following exposure to synthetic glucocorticoids *in utero*.

THE HPA AXIS AS PUTATIVE LINK BETWEEN INTRAUTERINE EXPOSURE TO GLUCOCORTICOIDS AND COMPROMISED HEALTH

Intrauterine exposure to synthetic glucocorticoids has been associated with impaired fetal growth [140], modulated fetal immune function [141], compromised cognitive [142, 143], neurological [144], and psychological function [145], as well as increased blood pressure [146] into adolescence [12, 13]. The question arises whether this association may be mediated (at least in part) by blunted hpa activity, as suggested by the above mentioned evidence that in humans (i) exposure to synthetic glucocorticoids *in utero* is blunting fetal and infant hpa activity and (ii) blunted hpa activity during infancy is associated with developmental and health impairment [141, 147-150]. However, there are other alternative mechanisms potentially underlying the link between intrauterine exposure to synthetic glucocorticoids and impaired developmental and health, such as changes in brain regions with GR expression that are not involved in regulation of the hpa axis, or changes in other organ systems that express GR. Further studies are needed to scrutinize the clinical relevance of changes in hpa axis activity following intrauterine exposure to synthetic glucocorticoids.

BENEFICIAL EFFECTS OF FUNCTIONAL HYPOCORTISOLISM: AN EVOLUTIONARY PERSPECTIVE

According to the thrifty phenotype hypothesis originally proposed by Hales and Barker, the observed changes of hpa function in infants exposed to synthetic glucocorticoids *in utero* may be advantageous from an evolutionary perspective [151]. Their hypothesis says that the fetus responds to an adverse prenatal environment by making developmental changes that are appropriate in the short run and that may also be adequate in the long run provided that the anticipated postnatal environment is as adverse as the prenatal environment [151]. Only if the postnatal environment is not as adverse as anticipated, the adaptive changes might be disadvantageous in the long run. Consequently, by decreasing hpa function, fetuses exposed to synthetic glucocorticoids, which simulate a stressful environment, compensate for the large amount of exogenous glucocorticoids that reach their body. By settling down at roughly normal total (exogenous plus endogenous) glucocorticoid concentrations, the prenatal adaptive changes appear to be appropriate. Apart from this immediate benefit, sustained hpa suppression into postnatal life would only be beneficial in the long run if fetuses were indeed born into the expected stressful environment. For instance, functional hypocortisolism may protect chronically stressed subjects against harmful effects of high allostatic load and be beneficial in terms of adaptation [147, 152]. However, as synthetic glucocorticoids are no longer given after birth in most cases, low endogenous cortisol production in the infant would be inappropriate under less stressful conditions, thereby possibly triggering diverse pathologies, as has been described above.

The thrifty phenotype hypothesis may not only illuminate the evolutionary perspective on the whole purpose of reduced hpa function in infants antenatally exposed to synthetic glucocorticoids. It may further explain why some studies detected hpa hyperactivity while others reported hpa hypoactivity in animals treated with synthetic glucocorticoids *in utero*, or why Miller and coworkers demonstrated an unstable endocrine system at baseline and following pain-related stress in humans, with an inverse relationship between cortisol concentrations at two months and cortisol levels at four months, those with increased cortisol concentrations at two months having decreased cortisol concentrations at four months, and vice versa [106]: In expectation of a stressful environment, it may not only be advantageous to reduce hpa activity, but to evolve an endocrine system that is able to flexibly change according to requirements.

Taken together, the observed patterns of fetal and newborn endocrine activity after antenatal treatment with synthetic glucocorticoids may, from an evolutionary perspective, reflect adaptive changes that are appropriate in the short run and may also be advantageous in the long run, provided that the fetus is born into the expected environment. Otherwise, the mal-adaptation may trigger adverse developmental and health outcomes, as has been described above.

CONCLUSION AND OUTLOOK

Synthetic glucocorticoids serve as common pharmacological treatment of numerous medical conditions. There is considerable evidence that exposure to synthetic glucocorticoids *in utero* is blunting fetal and, in some cases, newborn and infant hpa activity under basal conditions, and following pain-related stress. While the available data suggest that baseline hpa function recovers during the first two weeks postpartum, there is some evidence that reduced hpa axis reactivity to pain-related stressors persists throughout the first four months postpartum. More studies are needed to scrutinize whether exposure to synthetic glucocorticoids *in utero* profoundly influences hpa function beyond the first months into adult life. While, there is some data suggesting that early hpa dysregulation following exposure to synthetic glucocorticoids can be adverse, compromising development and health in the short term, more studies are needed to determine whether long-term health disturbances are to be expected. Potential mechanisms underlying changes in hpa axis activity following exposure to glucocorticoids *in utero* include alterations at subcortical and cortical levels of the brain. Further randomized follow-up studies are highly warranted to unravel the short- and long-term effects of intrauterine exposure to synthetic glucocorticoids on the offspring's hpa axis, and their consequences for development and health throughout life.

ACKNOWLEDGEMENTS

This work has been funded by the German National Academic Foundation and the Research Foundation of the University of Basel (to MT), and the Swiss National Science Foundation (to GM). We thank Dr. Christopher Pryce for critical reading of a previous version of this chapter.

REFERENCES

[1]   Bolt RJ, van Weissenbruch MM, Lafeber HN, Delemarre-van de Waal HA. Glucocorticoids and lung development in the fetus and preterm infant. Pediatr Pulmonol 2001;32(1):76-91.

[2]   Roberts D, Dalziel S. Antenatal corticosteroids for accelerating fetal lung maturation for women at risk of preterm birth. Cochrane Database Syst Rev 2006;3:CD004454.

[3]   National Heart Lung and Blood Institute, National Asthma Education and Prevention Program Asthma and Pregnancy Working Group. NAEPP expert panel report. Managing asthma during pregnancy: recommendations for pharmacologic treatment-2004 update. The J Allergy Clinl Immunol 2005;115(1):34-46.

[4]   Bamberger CM, Schulte HM, Chrousos GP. Molecular determinants of glucocorticoid receptor function and tissue sensitivity to glucocorticoids. Endocr Rev 1996;17(3):245-61.

[5]   Grossmann C, Scholz T, Rochel M, *et al.* Transactivation *via* the human glucocorticoid and mineralocorticoid receptor by therapeutically used steroids in CV-1 cells: a comparison of their glucocorticoid and mineralocorticoid properties. Eur J Endocrinol 2004;151(3):397-406.

[6]   Grier DG, Halliday HL. Effects of glucocorticoids on fetal and neonatal lung development. Treat Respir Med 2004;3(5):295-306.

[7]   Cintra A, Bhatnagar M, Chadi G, *et al.* Glial and neuronal glucocorticoid receptor immunoreactive cell populations in developing, adult, and aging brain. Ann NY Acad Sci 1994;746:42-61; discussion -3.

[8]   Condon J, Gosden C, Gardener D, *et al.* Expression of type 2 11beta-hydroxysteroid dehydrogenase and corticosteroid hormone receptors in early human fetal life. J Clin Endocrinol Metab 1998;83(12):4490-7.

[9]   Cattarelli D, Chirico G, Simeoni U. Renal effects of antenatally or postnatally administered steroids. Pediatr Med Chir 2002;24(2):157-62.

[10]   Jahnukainen T, Chen M, Berg U, Celsi G. Antenatal glucocorticoids and renal function after birth. Semin Neonatol 2001;6(4):351-5.

[11]   O'Shea TM, Doyle LW. Perinatal glucocorticoid therapy and neurodevelopmental outcome: an epidemiologic perspective. Semin Neonatol 2001;6(4):293-307.

[12]   Owen D, Andrews MH, Matthews SG. Maternal adversity, glucocorticoids and programming of neuroendocrine function and behaviour. Neurosci Biobehav Rev 2005;29(2):209-26.

[13]   Sloboda DM, Challis JR, Moss TJ, Newnham JP. Synthetic glucocorticoids: antenatal administration and long-term implications. Curr Pharm Des 2005;11(11):1459-72.

[14]   Crowley P. Prophylactic corticosteroids for preterm birth. Cochrane Database Syst Rev 2000(2):CD000065.

[15]   Lee BH, Stoll BJ, McDonald SA, Higgins RD. Adverse neonatal outcomes associated with antenatal dexamethasone versus antenatal betamethasone. Pediatrics 2006;117(5):1503-10.

[16]   Matthews SG. Antenatal glucocorticoids and programming of the developing CNS. Pediatr Res 2000;47(3):291-300.

[17]   Seckl JR. Prenatal glucocorticoids and long-term programming. Eur J Endocrinol 2004;151 (Suppl 3):U49-62.

[18]   Sapolsky RM, Romero LM, Munck AU. How do glucocorticoids influence stress responses? Integrating permissive, suppressive, stimulatory, and preparative actions. Endocr Rev 2000;21(1):55-89.

[19]   Lindsay JR, Nieman LK. The hypothalamic-pituitary-adrenal axis in pregnancy: challenges in disease detection and treatment. Endocr Rev 2005;26(6):775-99.

[20]   National Institutes of Health Consensus Development Panel. Effect of corticosteroids for fetal maturation on perinatal outcomes. NIH Consens Statement 1994;12(2):1-24.

[21]   Liggins GC. Premature delivery of foetal lambs infused with glucocorticoids. J Endocrinol 1969;45(4):515-23.

[22]   Crowley PA. Antenatal corticosteroid therapy: a meta-analysis of the randomized trials, 1972 to 1994. Am J Obstet Gynecol 1995;173(1):322-35.

[23]   National Institutes of Health Consensus Development Panel. Antenatal corticosteroids revisited: repeat courses - National Institutes of Health Consensus Development Conference Statement, August 17-18, 2000. Obstet Gynecol 2001;98(1):144-50.

[24]   Dorr HG, Sippell WG. Prenatal dexamethasone treatment in pregnancies at risk for congenital adrenal hyperplasia due to 21-hydroxylase deficiency: effect on midgestational amniotic fluid steroid levels. J Clin Endocrinol Metab 1993;76(1):117-20.

[25]   Diederich S, Eigendorff E, Burkhardt P, *et al.* 11beta-hydroxysteroid dehydrogenase types 1 and 2: an important pharmacokinetic determinant for the activity of synthetic mineralo- and glucocorticoids. J Clin Endocrinol Metab 2002;87(12):5695-701.

[26]   Loebstein R, Koren G. Clinical relevance of therapeutic drug monitoring during pregnancy. Ther Drug Monit 2002;24(1):15-22.

[27]   Pacheco LD, Ghulmiyyah LM, Snodgrass WR, Hankins GD. Pharmacokinetics of corticosteroids during pregnancy. Am J Perinatol 2007;24(2):79-82.

[28]   Anderson GD. Pregnancy-induced changes in pharmacokinetics: a mechanistic-based approach. Clin Pharmacokinet 2005;44(10):989-1008.

[29]   Dawes M, Chowienczyk PJ. Drugs in pregnancy. Pharmacokinetics in pregnancy. Best Pract Res Clin Obstet Gynaecol 2001;15(6):819-26.

[30]   Little BB. Pharmacokinetics during pregnancy: evidence-based maternal dose formulation. Obstet Gynecol 1999;93(5 Pt 2):858-68.

[31]   Petersen MC, Collier CB, Ashley JJ, McBride WG, Nation RL. Disposition of betamethasone in parturient women after intravenous administration. Eur J Clin Pharmacol 1983;25(6):803-10.

[32]   Ballabh P, Lo ES, Kumari J, et al. Pharmacokinetics of betamethasone in twin and singleton pregnancy. Clin Pharmacol Ther 2002;71(1):39-45.

[33]   Moss TJ, Doherty DA, Nitsos I, Harding R, Newnham JP. Pharmacokinetics of betamethasone after maternal or fetal intramuscular administration. Am J Obstet Gynecol 2003;189(6):1751-7.

[34]   Olufemi OS, Whittaker PG, Halliday D, Lind T. Albumin metabolism in fasted subjects during late pregnancy. Clin Sci (Lond) 1991;81(2):161-8.

[35]   Whittaker PG, Lind T. The intravascular mass of albumin during human pregnancy: a serial study in normal and diabetic women. Br J Obstet Gynaecol 1993;100(6):587-92.

[36]   Benassayag C, Souski I, Mignot TM, et al. Corticosteroid-binding globulin status at the fetomaternal interface during human term pregnancy. Biol Reprod 2001;64(3):812-21.

[37]   Krauer B, Dayer P, Anner R. Changes in serum albumin and alpha 1-acid glycoprotein concentrations during pregnancy: an analysis of fetal-maternal pairs. Br J Obstet Gynaecol 1984;91(9):875-81.

[38]   Audus KL. Controlling drug delivery across the placenta. Eur J Pharm Sci 1999;8(3):161-5.

[39]   Brown RW, Chapman KE, Kotelevtsev Y, et al. Cloning and production of antisera to human placental 11 beta-hydroxysteroid dehydrogenase type 2. Biochem J 1996;313 (Pt 3):1007-17.

[40]   Benediktsson R, Calder AA, Edwards CR, Seckl JR. Placental 11 beta-hydroxysteroid dehydrogenase: a key regulator of fetal glucocorticoid exposure. Clin Endocrinol (Oxf) 1997;46(2):161-6.

[41]   Klemcke HG. Placental metabolism of cortisol at mid- and late gestation in swine. Biol Reprod 1995;53(6):1293-301.

[42]   Osathanondh R, Tulchinsky D, Kamali H, Fencl M, Taeusch HW, Jr. Dexamethasone levels in treated pregnant women and newborn infants. J Pediatr 1977;90(4):617-20.

[43]   van Runnard Heimel PJ, Franx A, Schobben AF, Huisjes AJ, Derks JB, Bruinse HW. Corticosteroids, pregnancy, and HELLP syndrome: a review. Obstet Gynecol Surv 2005;60(1):57-70; quiz 3-4.

[44]   Blanford AT, Murphy BE. In vitro metabolism of prednisolone, dexamethasone, betamethasone, and cortisol by the human placenta. Am J Obstet Gynecol 1977;127(3):264-7.

[45]   van Runnard Heimel PJ, Schobben AF, Huisjes AJ, Franx A, Bruinse HW. The transplacental passage of prednisolone in pregnancies complicated by early-onset HELLP syndrome. Placenta 2005;26(10):842-5.

[46]   Ballard PL, Granberg P, Ballard RA. Glucocorticoid levels in maternal and cord serum after prenatal betamethasone therapy to prevent respiratory distress syndrome. J Clin Invest 1975;56(6):1548-54.

[47]   Murphy VE, Fittock RJ, Zarzycki PK, Delahunty MM, Smith R, Clifton VL. Metabolism of synthetic steroids by the human placenta. Placenta 2007;28(1):39-46.

[48]   Clifton VL, Rennie N, Murphy VE. Effect of inhaled glucocorticoid treatment on placental 11beta-hydroxysteroid dehydrogenase type 2 activity and neonatal birthweight in pregnancies complicated by asthma. Aust N Z J Obstet Gynaecol 2006;46(2):136-40.

[49]   Kajantie E, Dunkel L, Turpeinen U, et al. Placental 11 beta-hydroxysteroid dehydrogenase-2 and fetal cortisol/cortisone shuttle in small preterm infants. J Clin Endocrinol Metab 2003;88(1):493-500.

[50]   Murphy VE, Gibson PG, Giles WB, et al. Maternal asthma is associated with reduced female fetal growth. Am J Respir Crit Care Med 2003;168(11):1317-23.

[51]   Mark PJ, Waddell BJ. P-glycoprotein restricts access of cortisol and dexamethasone to the glucocorticoid receptor in placental BeWo cells. Endocrinology 2006;147(11):5147-52.

[52]   Stein WD. Kinetics of the multidrug transporter (P-glycoprotein) and its reversal. Physiol Rev 1997;77(2):545-90.

[53]   Uhr M, Holsboer F, Muller MB. Penetration of endogenous steroid hormones corticosterone, cortisol, aldosterone and progesterone into the brain is enhanced in mice deficient for both mdr1a and mdr1b P-glycoproteins. J Neuroendocrinol 2002;14(9):753-9.

[54]   Kalabis GM, Kostaki A, Andrews MH, Petropoulos S, Gibb W, Matthews SG. Multidrug resistance phosphoglycoprotein (ABCB1) in the mouse placenta: fetal protection. Biol Reprod 2005;73(4):591-7.

[55]   Sun M, Kingdom J, Baczyk D, Lye SJ, Matthews SG, Gibb W. Expression of the multidrug resistance P-glycoprotein, (ABCB1 glycoprotein) in the human placenta decreases with advancing gestation. Placenta 2006;27(6-7):602-9.

[56]   Kalabis GM, Petropoulos S, Gibb W, Matthews SG. Breast cancer resistance protein (Bcrp1/Abcg2) in mouse placenta and yolk sac: ontogeny and its regulation by progesterone. Placenta 2007;28(10):1073-81.

[57]   Kapoor A, Petropoulos S, Matthews SG. Fetal programming of hypothalamic-pituitary-adrenal (HPA) axis function and behavior by synthetic glucocorticoids. Brain Res Rev 2008;57(2):586-95.

[58]   Mark PJ, Augustus S, Lewis JL, Hewitt DP, Waddell BJ. Changes in the Placental Glucocorticoid Barrier During Rat Pregnancy: Impact on Placental Corticosterone Levels and Regulation by Progesterone. Biol Reprod 2009;80(6):1209-15.

[59]   Petropoulos S, Kalabis GM, Gibb W, Matthews SG. Functional changes of mouse placental multidrug resistance phosphoglycoprotein (ABCB1) with advancing gestation and regulation by progesterone. Reprod Sci 2007;14(4):321-8.

[60]   Tsigos C, Chrousos GP. Hypothalamic-pituitary-adrenal axis, neuroendocrine factors and stress. J Psychosom Res 2002;53(4):865-71.

[61]   Mesiano S, Jaffe RB. Developmental and functional biology of the primate fetal adrenal cortex. Endocr Rev 1997;18(3):378-403.

[62]   Bolt RJ, van Weissenbruch MM, Lafeber HN, Delemarre-van de Waal HA. Development of the hypothalamic-pituitary-adrenal axis in the fetus and preterm infant. J Pediatr Endocrinol Metab 2002;15(6):759-69.

[63]   Brosnan PG. The hypothalamic pituitary axis in the fetus and newborn. Semin Perinatol 2001;25(6):371-84.

[64]   Ng PC. The fetal and neonatal hypothalamic-pituitary-adrenal axis. Arch Dis Child Fetal Neonatal Ed 2000;82(3):F250-4.

[65]   Bresson JL, Clavequin MC, Fellmann D, Bugnon C. Anatomical and ontogenetic studies of the human paraventriculo-infundibular corticoliberin system. Neuroscience 1985: 14(4):1077-90.

[66]   Thliveris JA, Currie RW. Observations on the hypothalamo-hypophyseal portal vasculature in the developing human fetus. Am J Anat 1980;157(4):441-4.

[67]   Baker BL, Jaffe RB. The genesis of cell types in the adenohypophysis of the human fetus as observed with immunocytochemistry. Am J Anat 1975;143(2):137-61.

[68]   Asa SL, Kovacs K, Laszlo FA, Domokos I, Ezrin C. Human fetal adenohypophysis. Histologic and immunocytochemical analysis. Neuroendocrinology 1986;43(3):308-16.

[69]   Sucheston ME, Cannon MS. Development of zonular patterns in the human adrenal gland. J Morphol 1968;126(4):477-91.

[70]   Baulieu EE, Dray F. Conversion of H3-Dehydroisoandrosterone (3beta-Hydroxy-Delta5-Androsten-17-One) Sulfate to H3-Estrogens in Normal Pregnant Women. J Clin Endocrinol Metab 1963;23:1298-301.

[71]   Macnaughton MC, Taylor T, McNally EM, Coutts JR. The effect of synthetic ACTH on the metabolism of [4-14C]-progesterone by the previable human fetus. J Steroid Biochem 1977;8(5):499-504.

[72]   Seron-Ferre M, Lawrence CC, Siiteri PK, Jaffe RB. Steroid production by definitive and fetal zones of the human fetal adrenal gland. J Clin Endocrinol Metab 1978;47(3):603-9.

[73]   Giannakoulopoulos X, Sepulveda W, Kourtis P, Glover V, Fisk NM. Fetal plasma cortisol and beta-endorphin response to intrauterine needling. Lancet 1994;344(8915):77-81.

[74]   Giannakoulopoulos X, Teixeira J, Fisk N, Glover V. Human fetal and maternal noradrenaline responses to invasive procedures. Pediatr Res 1999;45(4 Pt 1):494-9.

[75]   Gitau R, Fisk NM, Teixeira JM, Cameron A, Glover V. Fetal hypothalamic-pituitary-adrenal stress responses to invasive procedures are independent of maternal responses. J Clin Endocrinol Metab 2001;86(1):104-9.

[76]   Parker CR, Jr., Stankovic AM, Goland RS. Corticotropin-releasing hormone stimulates steroidogenesis in cultured human adrenal cells. Mol Cell Endocrinol 1999;155(1-2):19-25.

[77]   Blumenfeld Z, Jaffe RB. Hypophysiotropic and neuromodulatory regulation of adrenocorticotropin in the human fetal pituitary gland. J Clin Invest 1986;78(1):288-94.

[78]   Gibbs DM, Stewart RD, Vale W, Rivier J, Yen SS. Synthetic corticotropin-releasing factor stimulates secretion of immunoreactive beta-endorphin/beta-lipotropin and ACTH by human fetal pituitaries *in vitro*. Life Sci 1983;32(5):547-50.

[79]   Goland RS, Wardlaw SL, Stark RI, Brown LS, Jr., Frantz AG. High levels of corticotropin-releasing hormone immunoactivity in maternal and fetal plasma during pregnancy. J Clin Endocrinol Metab 1986;63(5):1199-203.

[80]   Reichardt HM, Schutz G. Feedback control of glucocorticoid production is established during fetal development. Mol Med 1996;2(6):735-44.

[81]   Pepe GJ, Albrecht ED. Actions of placental and fetal adrenal steroid hormones in primate pregnancy. Endocr Rev 1995 Oct;16(5):608-48.

[82]   Pepe GJ, Waddell BJ, Stahl SJ, Albrecht ED. The regulation of transplacental cortisol-cortisone metabolism by estrogen in pregnant baboons. Endocrinology 1988;122(1):78-83.

[83]   Keene MF. Observations on the Development of the Human Suprarenal Gland. J Anat 1927;61(Pt 3):302-24.

[84]   Nomura S. Immature adrenal steroidogenesis in preterm infants. Early Hum Dev 1997 Oct 10;49(3):225-33.

[85]   Banks BA, Stouffer N, Cnaan A, *et al.* Association of plasma cortisol and chronic lung disease in preterm infants. Pediatrics 2001;107(3):494-8.

[86]   Pryce CR. Postnatal ontogeny of expression of the corticosteroid receptor genes in mammalian brains: Inter-species and intra-species differences. Brain Res Rev 2008;57(2):596-605.

[87]   Patel PD, Lopez JF, Lyons DM, Burke S, Wallace M, Schatzberg AF. Glucocorticoid and mineralocorticoid receptor mRNA expression in squirrel monkey brain. J Psychiatr Res 2000;34(6):383-92.

[88]   Seckl JR, Dickson KL, Yates C, Fink G. Distribution of glucocorticoid and mineralocorticoid receptor messenger RNA expression in human postmortem hippocampus. Brain Res 1991;561(2):332-7.

[89]   Sanchez MM, Young LJ, Plotsky PM, Insel TR. Distribution of corticosteroid receptors in the rhesus brain: relative absence of glucocorticoid receptors in the hippocampal formation. J Neurosci 2000;20(12):4657-68.

[90]   Kononen J, Honkaniemi J, Gustafsson JA, Pelto-Huikko M. Glucocorticoid receptor colocalization with pituitary hormones in the rat pituitary gland. Mol Cell Endocrinol 1993;93(1):97-103.

[91]   Ozawa H, Ito T, Ochiai I, Kawata M. Cellular localization and distribution of glucocorticoid receptor immunoreactivity and the expression of glucocorticoid receptor messenger RNA in rat pituitary gland. A combined double immunohistochemistry study and in situ hybridization histochemical analysis. Cell Tissue Res 1999;295(2):207-14.

[92]   De Kloet ER, Vreugdenhil E, Oitzl MS, Joels M. Brain corticosteroid receptor balance in health and disease. Endocr Rev 1998;19(3):269-301.

[93]   Herman JP, Ostrander MM, Mueller NK, Figueiredo H. Limbic system mechanisms of stress regulation: hypothalamo-pituitary-adrenocortical axis. Prog Neuropsychopharmacol Biol Psychiatry 2005;29(8):1201-13.

[94]   Speirs HJ, Seckl JR, Brown RW. Ontogeny of glucocorticoid receptor and 11beta-hydroxysteroid dehydrogenase type-1 gene expression identifies potential critical periods of glucocorticoid susceptibility during development. J Endocrinol 2004;181(1):105-16.

[95]   Noorlander CW, De Graan PN, Middeldorp J, Van Beers JJ, Visser GH. Ontogeny of hippocampal corticosteroid receptors: effects of antenatal glucocorticoids in human and mouse. J Comp Neurol 2006;499(6):924-32.

[96]   Andrews MH, Matthews SG. Regulation of glucocorticoid receptor mRNA and heat shock protein 70 mRNA in the developing sheep brain. Brain Res 2000;878(1-2):174-82.

[97]   Dobbing J, Sands J. Comparative aspects of the brain growth spurt. Early Hum Dev 1979;3(1):79-83.

[98]   Pryce CR, Feldon J, Fuchs E, *et al.* Postnatal ontogeny of hippocampal expression of the mineralocorticoid and glucocorticoid receptors in the common marmoset monkey. Eur J Neurosci 2005;21(6):1521-35.

[99]   Bertram CE, Hanson MA. Prenatal programming of postnatal endocrine responses by glucocorticoids. Reproduction 2002;124(4):459-67.

[100] Tegethoff M, Pryce C, Meinlschmidt G. Effects of intrauterine exposure to synthetic glucocorticoids on fetal, newborn, and infant hypothalamic-pituitary-adrenal axis function in humans: a systematic review. Endocr Rev 2009;30(7):753-89.

[101] Fiad TM, Kirby JM, Cunningham SK, McKenna TJ. The overnight single-dose metyrapone test is a simple and reliable index of the hypothalamic-pituitary-adrenal axis. Clin Endocrinol (Oxf) 1994;40(5):603-9.

[102] Ashwood PJ, Crowther CA, Willson KJ, *et al.* Neonatal adrenal function after repeat dose prenatal corticosteroids: a randomized controlled trial. Am J Obstet Gynecol 2006;194(3):861-7.

[103] Davis EP, Townsend EL, Gunnar MR, *et al.* Effects of prenatal betamethasone exposure on regulation of stress physiology in healthy premature infants. Psychoneuroendocrinology 2004 Sep;29(8):1028-36.

[104] Davis EP, Townsend EL, Gunnar MR, Guiang SF, Lussky RC, Cifuentes RF, *et al.* Antenatal betamethasone treatment has a persisting influence on infant HPA axis regulation. J Perinatol 2006;26(3):147-53.

[105] Glover V, Miles R, Matta S, Modi N, Stevenson J. Glucocorticoid exposure in preterm babies predicts saliva cortisol response to immunization at 4 months. Pediatr Res 2005;58(6):1233-7.

[106] Miller NM, Williamson C, Fisk NM, Glover V. Infant cortisol response after prolonged antenatal prednisolone treatment. BJOG 2004;111(12):1471-4.

[107] Davis EP, Waffarn F, Sandman CA. Prenatal treatment with glucocorticoids sensitizes the hpa axis response to stress among full-term infants. Dev Psychobiol 2010 [Epub ahead of print]

[108] Schaffer L, Luzi F, Burkhardt T, Rauh M, Beinder E. Antenatal betamethasone administration alters stress physiology in healthy neonates. Obstet Gynecol [Controlled Clinical Trial] 2009;113(5):1082-8.

[109] Tegethoff M. Fetal origins of pediatric disease: Intrauterine programming by stress and glucocorticoids. Göttingen: Cuvillier 2009.

[110] Burlet G, Fernette B, Blanchard S, *et al.* Antenatal glucocorticoids blunt the functioning of the hypothalamic-pituitary-adrenal axis of neonates and disturb some behaviors in juveniles. Neuroscience 2005;133(1):221-30.

[111] Felszeghy K, Bagdy G, Nyakas C. Blunted pituitary-adrenocortical stress response in adult rats following neonatal dexamethasone treatment. J Neuroendocrinol 2000;12(10):1014-21.

[112] Kamphuis PJ, Bakker JM, Broekhoven MH, *et al.* Enhanced glucocorticoid feedback inhibition of hypothalamo-pituitary-adrenal responses to stress in adult rats neonatally treated with dexamethasone. Neuroendocrinology 2002;76(3):158-69.

[113] Barbazanges A, Piazza PV, Le Moal M, Maccari S. Maternal glucocorticoid secretion mediates long-term effects of prenatal stress. J Neurosci 1996;16(12):3943-9.

[114] Haussmann MF, Carroll JA, Weesner GD, Daniels MJ, Matteri RL, Lay DC, Jr. Administration of ACTH to restrained, pregnant sows alters their pigs' hypothalamic-pituitary-adrenal (HPA) axis. J Anim Sci 2000;78(9):2399-411.

[115] Levitt NS, Lindsay RS, Holmes MC, Seckl JR. Dexamethasone in the last week of pregnancy attenuates hippocampal glucocorticoid receptor gene expression and elevates blood pressure in the adult offspring in the rat. Neuroendocrinology 1996;64(6):412-8.

[116] Muneoka K, Mikuni M, Ogawa T, *et al.* Prenatal dexamethasone exposure alters brain monoamine metabolism and adrenocortical response in rat offspring. Am J Physiol 1997;273(5 Pt 2):R1669-75.

[117] Uno H, Eisele S, Sakai A, *et al.* Neurotoxicity of glucocorticoids in the primate brain. Horm Behav 1994;28(4):336-48.

[118] Kapoor A, Dunn E, Kostaki A, Andrews MH, Matthews SG. Fetal programming of hypothalamo-pituitary-adrenal function: prenatal stress and glucocorticoids. J Physiol 2006;572(Pt 1):31-44.

[119] Seckl JR, Meaney MJ. Glucocorticoid programming. Ann NY Acad Sci 2004;1032:63-84.

[120] Welberg LA, Seckl JR. Prenatal stress, glucocorticoids and the programming of the brain. J Neuroendocrinol 2001;13(2):113-28.

[121] Ballard PL, Gluckman PD, Liggins GC, Kaplan SL, Grumbach MM. Steroid and growth hormone levels in premature infants after prenatal betamethasone therapy to prevent respiratory distress syndrome. Pediatr Res 1980;14(2):122-7.

[122] Kajantie E, Raivio T, Janne OA, Hovi P, Dunkel L, Andersson S. Circulating glucocorticoid bioactivity in the preterm newborn after antenatal betamethasone treatment. J Clin Endocrinol Metab 2004;89(8):3999-4003.

[123] Ng PC, Lam CW, Lee CH, *et al.* Reference ranges and factors affecting the human corticotropin-releasing hormone test in preterm, very low birth weight infants. J Clin Endocrinol Metab 2002;87(10):4621-8.

[124] Ng PC, Lam CW, Lee CH, *et al.* Changes of leptin and metabolic hormones in preterm infants: a longitudinal study in early postnatal life. Clin Endocrinol (Oxf) 2001;54(5):673-80.

[125] Ng PC, Wong GW, Lam CW, *et al.* Effect of multiple courses of antenatal corticosteroids on pituitary-adrenal function in preterm infants. Arch Dis Child Fetal Neonatal Ed 1999;80(3):F213-6.

[126] Parker CR, Jr., Atkinson MW, Owen J, Andrews WW. Dynamics of the fetal adrenal, cholesterol, and apolipoprotein B responses to antenatal betamethasone therapy. Am J Obstet Gynecol 1996;174(2):562-5.

[127] Alkalay AL, Pomerance JJ, Puri AR, *et al.* Hypothalamic-pituitary-adrenal axis function in very low birth weight infants treated with dexamethasone. Pediatrics 1990;86(2):204-10.

[128] Bettendorf M, Albers N, Bauer J, Heinrich UE, Linderkamp O, Maser-Gluth C. Longitudinal evaluation of salivary cortisol levels in full-term and preterm neonates. Horm Res 1998;50(6):303-8.

[129] Cole CH, Shah B, Abbasi S, *et al.* Adrenal function in premature infants during inhaled beclomethasone therapy. J Pediatr 1999;135(1):65-70.

[130] Ford LR, Willi SM, Hollis BW, Wright NM. Suppression and recovery of the neonatal hypothalamic-pituitary-adrenal axis after prolonged dexamethasone therapy. J Pediatr 1997;131(5):722-6.

[131] Kari MA, Raivio KO, Stenman UH, Voutilainen R. Serum cortisol, dehydroepiandrosterone sulfate, and steroid-binding globulins in preterm neonates: effect of gestational age and dexamethasone therapy. Pediatr Res 1996;40(2):319-24.

[132] Rizvi ZB, Aniol HS, Myers TF, Zeller WP, Fisher SG, Anderson CL. Effects of dexamethasone on the hypothalamic-pituitary-adrenal axis in preterm infants. J Pediatr 1992;120(6):961-5.

[133] Karemaker R, Heijnen CJ, Veen S, *et al.* Differences in behavioral outcome and motor development at school age after neonatal treatment for chronic lung disease with dexamethasone versus hydrocortisone. Pediatr Res 2006;60(6):745-50.

[134] van der Heide-Jalving M, Kamphuis PJ, van der Laan MJ, *et al.* Short- and long-term effects of neonatal glucocorticoid therapy: is hydrocortisone an alternative to dexamethasone? Acta Paediatr 2003;92(7):827-35.

[135] Yeh TF, Lin YJ, Huang CC, *et al.* Early dexamethasone therapy in preterm infants: a follow-up study. Pediatrics 1998;101(5):E7.

[136] Yeh TF, Lin YJ, Lin HC, *et al.* Outcomes at school age after postnatal dexamethasone therapy for lung disease of prematurity. N Engl J Med 2004;350(13):1304-13.

[137] Buske-Kirschbaum A, Jobst S, Psych D, *et al.* Attenuated free cortisol response to psychosocial stress in children with atopic dermatitis. Psychosom Med 1997;59(4):419-26.

[138] Buske-Kirschbaum A, von Auer K, Krieger S, Weis S, Rauh W, Hellhammer D. Blunted cortisol responses to psychosocial stress in asthmatic children: a general feature of atopic disease? Psychosom Med 2003;65(5):806-10.

[139] Buske-Kirschbaum A, Geiben A, Hollig H, Morschhauser E, Hellhammer D. Altered responsiveness of the hypothalamus-pituitary-adrenal axis and the sympathetic adrenomedullary system to stress in patients with atopic dermatitis. J Clin Endocrinol Metab 2002;87(9):4245-51.

[140] Schatz M, Dombrowski MP, Wise R, *et al.* The relationship of asthma medication use to perinatal outcomes. J Allergy Clin Immunol 2004;113(6):1040-5.

[141] Kavelaars A, van der Pompe G, Bakker JM,, *et al.* Altered immune function in human newborns after prenatal administration of betamethasone: enhanced natural killer cell activity and decreased T cell proliferation in cord blood. Pediatr Res 1999;45(3):306-12.

[142] French NP, Hagan R, Evans SF, Godfrey M, Newnham JP. Repeated antenatal corticosteroids: size at birth and subsequent development. Am J Obstet Gynecol 1999;180(1 Pt 1):114-21.

[143] Modi N, Lewis H, Al-Naqeeb N, Ajayi-Obe M, Dore CJ, Rutherford M. The effects of repeated antenatal glucocorticoid therapy on the developing brain. Pediatr Res 2001;50(5):581-5.

[144] MacArthur BA, Howie RN, Dezoete JA, Elkins J. School progress and cognitive development of 6-year-old children whose mothers were treated antenatally with betamethasone. Pediatrics 1982;70(1):99-105.

[145] French NP, Hagan R, Evans SF, Mullan A, Newnham JP. Repeated antenatal corticosteroids: effects on cerebral palsy and childhood behavior. Am J Obstet Gynecol 2004;190(3):588-95.

[146] Doyle LW, Ford GW, Davis NM, Callanan C. Antenatal corticosteroid therapy and blood pressure at 14 years of age in preterm children. Clin Sci (Lond) 2000;98(2):137-42.

[147] Fries E, Hesse J, Hellhammer J, Hellhammer DH. A new view on hypocortisolism. Psychoneuroendocrinology 2005;30(10):1010-6.

[148] Heim C, Ehlert U, Hellhammer DH. The potential role of hypocortisolism in the pathophysiology of stress-related bodily disorders. Psychoneuroendocrinology 2000;25(1):1-35.

[149] White BP, Gunnar MR, Larson MC, Donzella B, Barr RG. Behavioral and physiological responsivity, sleep, and patterns of daily cortisol production in infants with and without colic. Child Dev 2000;71(4):862-77.

[150] Van Hoof E, De Becker P, Lapp C, Cluydts R, De Meirleir K. Defining the occurrence and influence of alpha-delta sleep in chronic fatigue syndrome. Am J Med Sci 2007;333(2):78-84.

[151] Hales CN, Barker DJ. Type 2 (non-insulin-dependent) diabetes mellitus: the thrifty phenotype hypothesis. Diabetologia 1992;35(7):595-601.

[152] Hellhammer J, Schlotz W, Stone AA, Pirke KM, Hellhammer D. Allostatic load, perceived stress, and health: a prospective study in two age groups. Ann NY Acad Sci 2004;1032:8-13.

CHAPTER 4

Epigenetic Developmental Origins Hypothesis and Oxidative Stress

Kaoru Nagai[*]

Department of Epigenetic Medicine, Interdisciplinary Graduate School of Medicine and Engineering, University of Yamanashi, Yamanashi, 409-3898, Japan

Abstract: Epigenetics is a heritable transcriptional regulation mechanism independent of DNA sequence. Epigenetic transcriptional control is achieved by regulation of chromatin conformation. The molecular mechanisms of epigenetics include post-translational modifications of histone and DNA methylation. Histone acetylation is the mostly studied epigenetic regulation. Histone deacetylase (HDAC) deacetylates histones and induce chromatin condensation, which prevent the approach of transcriptional regulating proteins. Methylated DNA is recognized by methyl-CpG binding protein (MBD) which recruits HDAC to the methylated region. Epigenetic status is known to be affected by oxidative stress condition via altering metabolic pathway associated with methylation reaction, and epigenetic abnormality on the developmental stage can influence brain and mental development. These suggest that oxidative stress condition affects brain and mental development via altering epigenetic regulation. In some mental retardation, such as Rett syndrome (RTT) and fetal alcohol syndrome (FAS), patients show microcephaly which may be caused by glial growth abnormality. The responsible gene of RTT is one of the MBDs, MeCP2. We discovered that knock down of MeCP2 in astrocytes reduced the growth rate, and DNA methyltransferase (DNMT) and HDAC inhibitors also did the same. Thus, epigenetic dysregulation induced mental disorder may be, at least partly, caused by abnormality of glial cells.

Keywords: Epigenetic transcriptional control, DNA methylation, histone deacetylase, methyl-CpG binding protein, Rett syndrome, fetal alcohol syndrome.

INTRODUCTION

Transcriptional Regulation by Epigenetics

Epigenetics is transcriptional regulating mechanisms independent of genomic DNA sequence. Epigenetics is heritable, but can be influenced by environment. Epigenetic transcriptional regulation is not encoded in the DNA sequence, but involves persistent changes in chromatin conformation. The molecular mechanisms of epigenetics include post-translational modification of histones and DNA methylation.

Post-translational histone modifications are precisely and reversibly regulated for epigenetic regulation. The modification includes acetylation, methylation, and phosphorylation. The acetylation is known as a transcription-activating modification, and mostly focused histone modification on epigenetics. The modification is achieved by the transfer of acetyl group from acetyl Coenzyme A to one or more lysine residues at the α-amino group by histone acetyltransferase (HAT). The acetylation neutralizes the positive charge of the lysine residues, and reduces overall positive charge of histones. Thus, it weakens the affinity of histones to negatively charged DNA.

The reduced histone-DNA interaction results in a decondensed (*i.e.* open) chromatin conformation which allows transcriptional activators to gain access to their recognition elements (Fig. **1**). Mainly three HAT families, p300/CBP family, GNAT family, and MYST family have been reported [1]. Deacetylation of the acetylated histone is also precisely regulated. Since acetylation of histone induces decondensed chromatin conformation, the deacetylation induces condensed (*i.e.* close) conformation (Fig. **1**).

The deacetylation is achieved by histone deacetylases (HDAC). In mammals, HDACs are divided into four major classes based on their homology. Class I HDACs include HDAC1, 2, 3, and 8. Class II HDACs include HDAC4, 5,

---

*Address correspondence to Kaoru Nagai: Department of Epigenetic Medicine, Interdisciplinary Graduate School of Medicine and Engineering, University of Yamanashi, 1110 Shimokato, Chuo-shi, Yamanashi, 409-3898, Japan; Tel: +81-55-273-9557; Fax: +81-55-273-9561; E-mail: kaoru@yamanashi.ac.jp

6, 7, 9, and 10. Class III HDACs include SIRT1-7, and are also known as sirtuin family. They are nicotinamide adenine dinucleotide (NAD^+) dependent enzymes, and focused on their important roles in longevity. Most recently identified HDAC11 is classified as class IV HDAC due to its distinct structure. HDAC I, II, and IV are zinc-dependent enzymes [2].

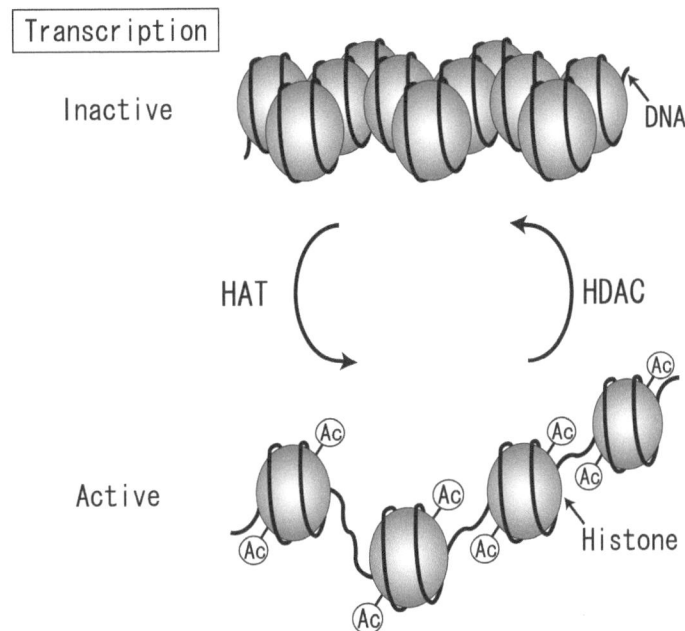

Figure 1: The Mechanisms of Histone Acetylation Dependent Transcriptional Regulation.

DNA methylation is generally known as a transcriptional repression signal. DNA methylation involves covalent modification at carbon-5 position of cytosine (C) residues of CG dinucleotide sequences (CpG) in DNA. The responsible enzyme is DNA methyltransferase (DNMT), which transfer methyl-group from S-adenosylmethionine (SAM) to C residues (Fig. **2**). The both strands of C in CpG are generally methylated.

During DNA replication, the parent strand remains methylated, but the daughter strand is not methylated. The unmethylated C residues in daughter strand are then methylated by maintenance DNMT, and the parental methylation patterns can be restored. There are two types of DNMTs. One is responsible for *de novo* methylation which establishes the methylation pattern, and the other is maintenance DNMT. In mammals, four DNMTs have been reported: DNMT1, 2, 3A, and 3B. DNMT3A and B are known as de novo DNMTs, while DNMT1 is maintenance DNMT [3].

DNA methylation dependent transcriptional repression is also achieved by condensation of chromatin conformation. Methylated DNA is recognized by methyl DNA binding proteins (MBD). MBD includes MeCP1, 2, and MBD1-4. MeCP2 has been studied in detail about transcriptional repression mechanisms. MeCP2 contains two functional domains, a methyl-CpG-binding domain (MBD) essential for binding to 5-methyl cytosine, and a transcriptional repression domain (TRD) which interacts with a corepressor complex (Fig. **2**).

The co-repressor complex contains HDAC and a transcriptional repressor Sin3a. When MeCP2 bind to methylated DNA via MBD, HDAC is recruited to the MeCP2 binding region, and deacetylates the histones. It results in condensed chromatin conformation which is the transcriptionally silenced state (Fig. **2**).

Oxidative Stress and Epigenetics

Redox state can affect methylation via SAM synthetic pathway. Methylation needs SAM as a donor substrate. SAM is synthesized by one-carbon metabolism which is consisted with interconnection between folate cycle and methionine cycle (Fig. **3**).

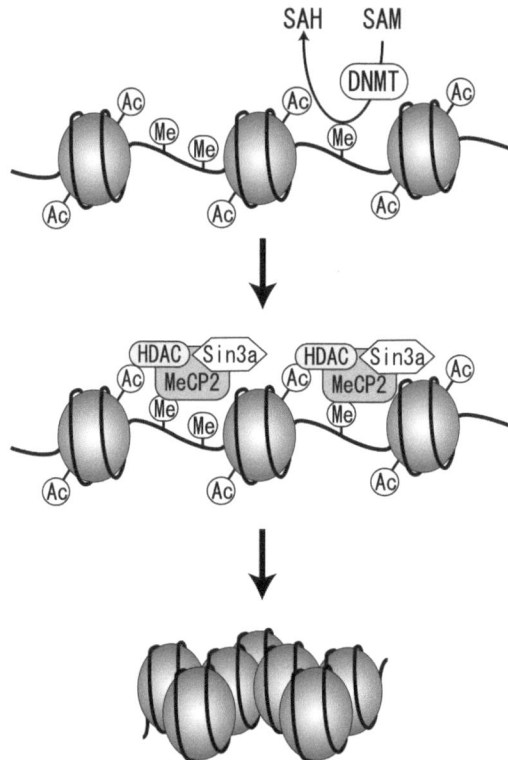

Figure 2: The Mechanisms of DNA Methylation Dependent Transcriptional Regulation. Ac: Acetyl Group, Me: Methyl Group.

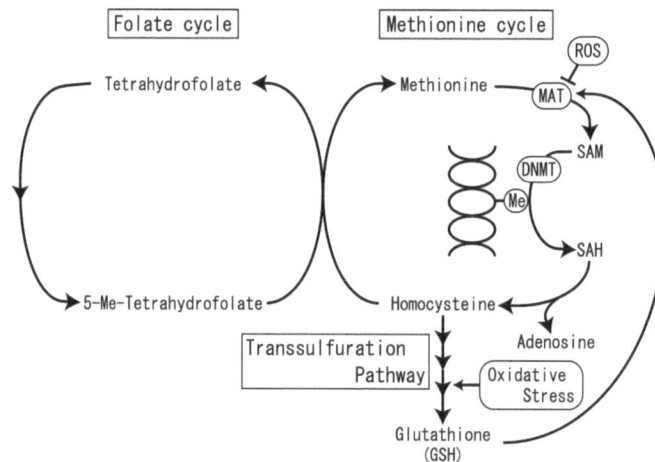

Figure 3: Effects of Oxidative Stress on One-Carbon Metabolic Pathway Associating with DNA Methylation.

It was reported that dietary folate influenced epigenetics by altering the synthesis of SAM [4], and mutations in genes of folate metabolism prior to the SAM synthesis disrupted DNA methylation [5]. During methylation reaction, the donor substrate SAM is changed to S-adenosylhomocysteine (SAH). SAH is then hydrolyzed to adenosine and homocysteine. The one-carbon metabolism includes trans-sulfuration pathway, which is a synthetic pathway of glutathione (GSH) from homocysteine. On the other hand, homocysteine is also utilized for resynthesis of SAM via methionine cycle. It indicates that SAM synthesis is competitive metabolic pathway to glutathione synthesis (Fig. **3**).

GSH is an important low-molecular weight thiol antioxidant. On the oxidative stress condition or in the case of development, increased production of GSH is required. It was reported that depleting GSH decreased the level of SAM, and led to genome-wide DNA hypomethylation [6]. It indicates that altering the level or synthesis of GSH can directly impact the level of DNA methylation by altering SAM pools. It suggests that the conditions changing the

GSH synthesis can affect the epigenetic patterns. In gametes or during developmental stage, glutathione synthesis changes to prevent reactive oxygen species (ROS)-induced damage. Therefore, we can speculate that oxidative stress condition or GSH synthesis during development mechanistically linked to epigenetic transcriptional regulation via synthesis of SAM.

The redox state of a cell can also affect the SAM synthesis by altering the activity of SAM synthase. SAM synthase, also known as methionine adenosyl transferase (MAT), catalyzes the conversion of methionine, in the presence of ATP, into SAM. In mammals, there are three forms of MAT, MAT I, MAT II, and MAT III. Since MAT has 10 cysteine residues per subunit, MAT activity may be sensitive to oxidation or nitrosylation. It was reported that hydrogen peroxide (H_2O_2) inactivate MAT via the modification of cysteine residues [7]. Nitric oxide (NO) can also inactivate MAT via S-nitrosylation of cysteine residue [8] (Fig. **3**). Regarding the GSH, increasing level of GSH enhances the MAT activity, and GSH / GSSG ratio influence the activity. High GSH / GSSG ratio maintains MAT in a reduced state, and allow the enzyme to achieve maximum activity (Fig. **3**). Therefore, oxidative stress and the GSH / GSSG ratio during development directly affects MAT activity, and in turn influence the epigenetic pattern by altering the level of SAM [9].

Oxidative stress leads to increased production of ROS. Generation of hydroxyl radical causes a wide range of DNA lesions including base modifications, deletions, strand breakage, and chromosomal rearrangements. Such DNA lesions have been shown to interfere with the ability of DNA to function as a substrate for DNMTs, resulting in hypomethylation. In CpG dinucleotides, the C residue is the base for DNA methylation, whereas the G residue is the site for oxidative damage. The guanine oxidative product, 8-oxoguanine (8-oxoG), is a major form of DNA damage, and 8-oxoG is used as a marker of oxidative damage. Conversion of G to 8-oxoG in methylated CpG dinucleotide diminishes MBP binding to DNA (Fig. **4**). In addition, the methyl group of 5-methylcytosine is susceptible to oxidation and generates 5-hydroxymethyl cytosine. Conversion of 5-methyl C to 5-hydroxymethyl C also diminishes MBP binding (Fig. **4**) [10]. Thus, these nucleotide modifications by ROS interferes with DNA methylation dependent transcriptional regulation, and results in epigenetic alterations.

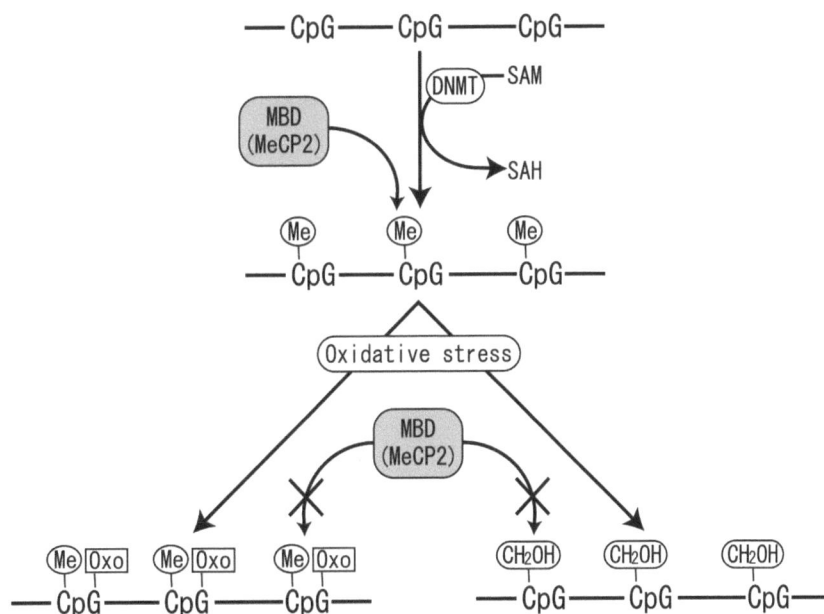

Figure 4: Modification of DNA by Oxidative Stress and its Effects on the Binding of MBD to DNA. CH_2OH: Hydroxymethyl Group, Me: Methyl Group, Oxo: 8-Oxo Group.

Epigenetic Alteration and Risk of Developmental Disorder

After the discovery of MeCP2 as a responsible gene of heritable autistic disease Rett syndrome (RTT) [11], the importance of epigenetics on development has been noticed. Recently, it has been reported that perinatal environment which affects epigenetic status has important impacts on not only mental development but also health trajectories later in life [12].

RTT is an X-linked disorder which primarily affects females. Classic RTT is characterized by apparently normal early development for the first 6 to 18 months of life followed by a period of regression and loss of acquired skills that results in intellectual disability, loss of speech and purposeful hand movements, ataxia, seizures, and respiratory abnormalities. About 96% of classic RTT cases are associated with MeCP2 mutations.

Significant phenotypic variability exists in classic RTT, even among individuals with the same MeCP2 mutation. The variability has been explained by skewed X-chromosome inactivation (XCI) pattern [13]. Although much progress has been made in understanding the functions of MeCP2, it is still unclear exactly how MeCP2 mutations contribute to the pathogenesis of RTT. Synapse formation and maturation requires activity-dependent gene expression. MeCP2 has been reported to control the expression of some of them, such as BDNF, and MeCP2 mutations dysregulate the expression of them [13]. This is thought to be an underlying cause of RTT.

Antiepileptic drug valproate (VPA), which is also known as HDAC inhibitor, is used to control various types of convulsive disorder or as mood stabilizer. However, VPA is known to be teratogenic. When it is used by pregnant mother, the risk of congenital abnormalities in the embryo and fetus is increased [14]. One of the major symptoms is autistic spectrum disorder (ASD), and prenatal exposure of VPA in rodents is used as autistic model [15].

The abnormality induced by VPA was reported to interfere with folic acid [14] which can contribute to the synthesis of methyl donor SAM. VPA was reported to change gene expressions via its HDAC inhibition activity. These suggest that VPA shows teratogenicity including autistic symptom via dysregulation of epigenetics.

The long-term effects of maternal behavior in the rat on the stress responsivity of the offspring during adulthood were reported [16]. The adult offspring of mothers which exhibit high levels of pup licking / grooming (*i.e.*, high LG mothers) over the first week of life show increased hippocampal GR expression compared to rats reared by low LG mothers. Cross fostering studies suggest that maternal care affects both GR gene expression and stress responsivity. It raises the possibility that maternal care influences epigenetic regulation. Actually, differences in DNA methylation and histone acetylation state in the regulatory region of GR gene were observed in the hippocampus of the offspring between high and low LG mothers. It suggests that epigenetic patterns, which are elaborated early in life in response to maternal behavior, remain stable into adulthood.

As described above, epigenetics closely associates with mental development. Recently, not only mental development but also the risk of metabolic syndrome or diabetes associates perinatal epigenetic change [12]. Therefore, epigenetics will be a target for broad range of health.

Epigenetic Dysregulation and Glial Growth Abnormality

In the brain, there are mainly two classes of cells, neuron and glia. Neuron is information processing cells by organizing neuronal circuit. Glia includes three types of cells, astrocytes, oligodendrocytes, and microglia.

Astrocytes have been thought to be just supporting cells for neurons. Recent finding demonstrated that astrocytes regulate neuronal information process more directly. Therefore, astrocyte abnormality induced by epigenetic dysregulation can influence brain development.

Some mental developmental disorder, such as RTT and fetal alcohol syndrome (FAS), show microcephaly [17]. FAS is a disease that prenatal alcohol exposure leads abnormality, including mental retardation and microcephaly. Brain growth is achieved not only by neuronal maturation and circuit formation but also glial proliferation and maturation.

In FAS, ethanol induced growth retardation of astrocytes was reported. In addition, ethanol was reported to affect epigenetic regulation. Thus, we studied if epigenetic dysregulation associates growth retardation of astrocytes. The responsible gene for RTT is MeCP2, which is known as an epigenetic transcriptional regulator as described above. In the past, MeCP2 was thought to be exclusively expressed in neurons [20], mainly studied in postnatal brain. Whereas, it is known that RTT shows microcephaly [17].

From this observation, we speculated the possibility that MeCP2 is expressed in glial cells, including astrocytes, at least on developmental stage, and affects growth rate of astrocytes. We prepared primary cultured glial cells from embryonic day 18 (E18) mouse cortex, and studied if astrocytes express MeCP2 [21]. After passage for removing neurons, the cells were immunostained against MeCP2 and astrocyte marker GFAP. In this condition, we observed the presence of the cells which expressed both MeCP2 and GFAP (Fig. **5**).

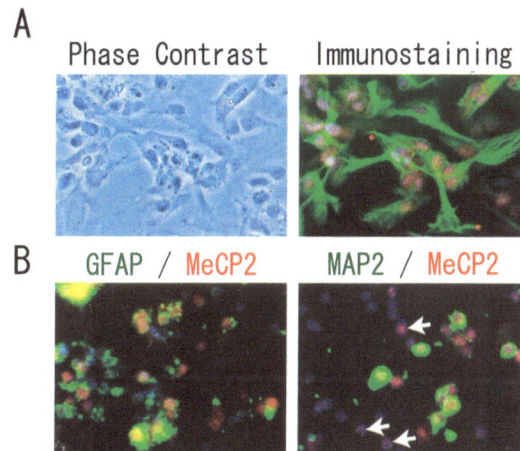

Figure 5: Expression of MeCP2 in Glial Cells. Primary Cultured Glial Cells (A) Or Acutely Dissociated Cortical Cells from E18 Mice were Subjected to Immunocytochemical Staining. (A) The Glial Cells were Stained with Mecp2 (Red) and GFAP (Green) Antibodies. (B) The Brain Cells were Stained with Mecp2 (Red) and GFAP (Green in Left Panel) or MAP2 (Green N Right Panel). The Nuclei were Stained with hoechst33342.

The evidence strongly suggests that embryonic astrocytes express MeCP2. However, it raises the possibility that MeCP2 is upregulated during culture *in vitro*. Thus, we stained the primary cultured cells which are acutely prepared. In the acutely prepared cortical cells, we could observe MeCP2 and GFAP double positive cells and MeCP2 positive cells without neuronal marker MAP2 (Fig. **5**). Next, we studied if MeCP2 regulates growth of astrocytes. To achieve a knockdown on astrocyte's MeCP2 we transfected siRNA against MeCP2. The siRNA transfected astrocytes showed reduced growth rate comparing to non-treated and control siRNA transfected astrocytes (Fig. **6**).

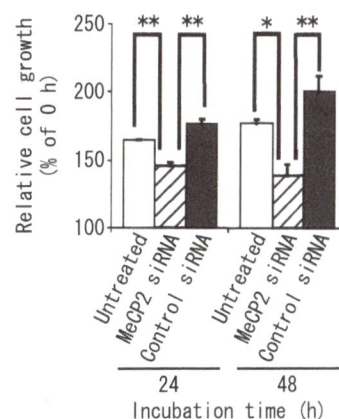

Figure 6: The Effect of Mecp2 Knock Down on Glial Cell Growth. Mecp2 and Control Sirna were Transfected to Glial Cells. After Incubation 24 and 48 H, the Cell Numbers were Evaluated by MTT Assay.

It suggests that MeCP2 dysfunction reduced embryonic glial growth rate, and then caused a disorder associated with dysfunctional brain development like FAS. Recently, another group reported that MeCP2 is expressed in astrocytes and MeCP2 null astrocytes showed reduced neurotogenic activity [22].

Since there are some reports that MeCP2 can bind unmethylated DNA [23], we studied whether DNA methylation and / or histone modification actually reduce astrocytic growth rate [24]. Primary cultured astrocytes were treated with DNMT inhibitor 5-aza-deoxycytidine (5adC) or HDAC inhibitor VPA. Both of the inhibitor reduced the cell number and the reduction was abolished in the DNA polymerase inhibitor aphidicolin (Fig. **7**).

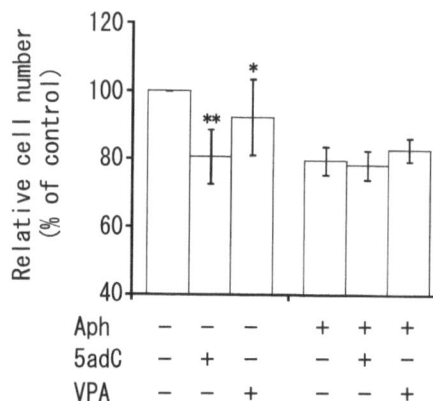

Figure 7: Effects of DMNT Inhibitor 5adc and HDAC Inhibitor VPA on Glial Cell Growth. E18 Mouse Cortical Glial Cells were Treated With 10μm 5adc or 100μm VPA in the Presence or Absence of DNA Polymerase Inhibitor Aphidicolin (Aph).

It indicates that epigenetic dysregulation in astrocytes reduced the cell growth rate, but not induced cell death. Regarding the effects *in vivo*, we treated VPA to fetal mice by intraperitoneal injection of VPA to pregnant mother on E12. Prenatal VPA exposed mice is used as an autistic model [25], but it has not been reported whether this model mouse showed microcephaly. Thus, we made the autistic model mice and brain and body weight on postnatal days 0, 5, 10. The brain / body ratio was significantly lower in the VPA exposed autistic model (Fig. **8**).

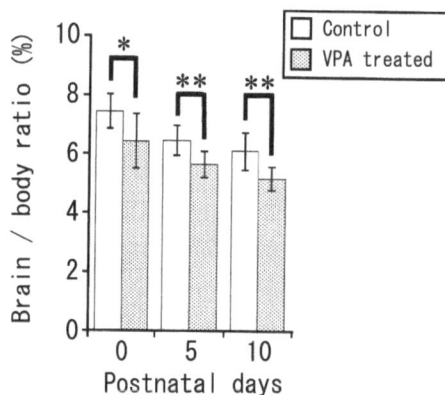

Figure 8: Prenatal VPA Treatment Induced Microcephaly in Neonatal Mice. Brain and Body Weights Were Measured in VPA Treated Autistic Model Mice.

CONCLUSION

Our observations suggest that epigenetic dysregulation in astrocytes cause growth retardation of the astrocytes and microcephaly, that might associates with disorders in mental development. From these observations, epigenetic regulation on glial growth is suggested to be crucial for mental development. Therefore, epigenetic regulation in glial cells will be a target for treating mental disorder. In addition, oxidative stress can alter epigenetic regulation as described above. Some epigenetic abnormality induced mental disorder might be caused by oxidative stress.

ACKNOWLEDGEMENT

This work was supported by Television Yamanashi Welfare and Culture Foundation.

CONFLICT OF INTEREST

The author declares no conflict of interest.

REFERENCES

[1]   Selvi BR, Cassel JC, Kundu TK, Boutillier AL. Tuning acetylation levels with HAT activators: therapeutic strategy in neurodegenerative diseases. Biochim Biopys Acta 2010; 1799:840-53.

[2]   Lane AA, Chabner BA. Histone deacetylase inhibitors in cancer therapy. J Clin Oncol 2009; 27: 5459-68.

[3]   Cheng X, Blumenthal RM. Mammalian DNA methyltransferases: a structural perspective. Structure 2008; 16: 341-50.

[4]   Kronenberg G, Colla M, Endres M. Folic acid, neurodegenerative and neuropsychiatric disease. Curr Mol Med 2009; 9: 315-23.

[5]   Lawrance AK, Deng L, Brody LC, Finnell RH, Shane B, Rozen R. Genetic and nutritional deficiencies in folate metabolism influence tumorigenicity in Apcmin/+ mice. J Nutr Biochem 2007; 18: 305-12.

[6]   Lee DH, Jacobs DR Jr, Porta M. Hypothesis: a unifying mechanism for nutrition and chemicals as lifelong modulators of DNA hypomethylation. Environ Health Perspect 2009; 117: 1799-802.

[7]   Sánchez-Góngora E, Ruiz F, Mingorance J, An W, Corrales FJ, Mato JM. Interaction of liver methionine adenosyltransferase with hydroxyl radical. FASEB J 1997; 11: 1013-9.

[8]   Ruiz F, Corrales FJ, Miqueo C, Mato JM. Nitric oxide inactivates rat hepatic methionine adenosyltransferase *In vivo* by S-nitrosylation. Hepatology 1998; 28(4): 1051-7.

[9]   Hitchler MJ, Domann FE. An epigenetic perspective on the free radical theory of development. Free Radic Biol Med 2007; 43: 1023-36.

[10]   Donkena KV, Young CY, Tindall DJ. Oxidative stress and DNA methylation in prostate cancer. Obstet Gynecol Int 2010;2010:302051.

[11]   Amir RE, Van den Veyver IB, Wan M, Tran CQ, Francke U, Zoghbi HY. Rett syndrome is caused by mutations in X-linked MECP2, encoding methyl-CpG-binding protein 2. Nat Genet 1999; 23:185-8.

[12]   Choudhuri S, Cui Y, Klaassen CD. Molecular targets of epigenetic regulation and effectors of environmental influences. Toxicol Appl Pharmacol 2010; 245: 378-93.

[13]   Gonzales ML, LaSalle JM. The role of MeCP2 in brain development and neurodevelopmental disorders. Curr Psychiatry Rep 2010; 12: 127-34.

[14]   Ornoy A. Valproic acid in pregnancy: how much are we endangering the embryo and fetus. Reprod Toxicol 2009; 28: 1-10.

[15]   Sadamatsu M, Kanai H, Xu X, Liu Y, Kato N. Review of animal models for autism: implication of thyroid hormone. Congenit Anom 2006; 46: 1-9.

[16]   Weaver IC, Cervoni N, Champagne FA, *et al.* Epigenetic programming by maternal behavior. Nat Neurosci 2004; 7: 847-54.

[17]   Zoll B, Huppke P, Wessel A, Bartels I, Laccone F. Fetal alcohol syndrome in association with Rett syndrome. Genet Couns 2004; 15: 207-12.

[18]   Costa LG, Vitalone A, Guizzetti M. Signal transduction mechanisms involved in the antiproliferative effects of ethanol in glial cells. Toxicol Lett 2004; 149: 67-73.

[19]   Haycock PC. Fetal alcohol spectrum disorders: the epigenetic perspective. Biol Reprod 2009; 81(4): 607-17.

[20]   Kishi N, Macklis JD. Dissecting MECP2 function in the central nervous system. J Child Neurol 2005; 20: 753-9.

[21]   Nagai K, Miyake K, Kubota T. A transcriptional repressor MeCP2 causing Rett syndrome is expressed in embryonic non-neuronal cells and controls their growth. Dev Brain Res 2005; 157: 103-6.

[22]   Ballas N, Lioy DT, Grunseich C, Mandel G. Non-cell autonomous influence of MeCP2-deficient glia on neuronal dendritic morphology. Nat Neurosci 2009; 12: 311-7.

[23]   Hansen JC, Ghosh RP, Woodcock CL. Binding of the Rett syndrome protein, MeCP2, to methylated and unmethylated DNA and chromatin. IUBMB Life 2010; 62: 732-8.

[24]   Nagai K, Natori T, Nishino T, Kodaira F. Epigenetic disregulation induces cell growth retardation in primary cultured glial cells. J Biosci Bioeng 2008; 105: 470-5.

[25]   Wagner GC, Reuhl KR, Cheh M, McRae P, Halladay AK. A new neurobehavioral model of autism in mice: pre- and postnatal exposure to sodium valproate. J Autism Dev Disord 2006; 36(6): 779-93.

CHAPTER 5

Endothelial Dysfunction during Cardiac Development: A Heart to Heart Discussion of the Significance of the Nitrosative-Oxidative Disequilibrium Hypothesis

Maqsood M. Elahi[1] and Bashir M. Matata[2,*]

[1]Department of Cardiothoracic Surgery, Prince of Wales and Sydney Children Hospital, Randwick, NSW, Australia and [2]Liverpool Heart & Chest Hospital NHS Foundation Trust, Thomas Drive, Liverpool, United Kingdom

Abstract: Endothelial dysfunction as a consequence of a variety of common cardiovascular disease risk factors is thought to be associated with increased reactive oxygen species (ROS) and the subsequent decrease in vascular bioavailability of nitric oxide (NO). In this article we give a detailed discussion of evidence of the impact of oxidative-nitrosative stress during maternal pregnancy on fetal development in animal models and also the association with the onset of cardiovascular conditions in adult humans. We highlighted specifically the presence of ROS in circulating blood as the key intermediary related to vascular injury and organ dysfunction. In addition, the evidence that red blood cells regulate the arteriolar microcirculation, coupling oxygen delivery with blood flow, highlighting their role in NO bioavailability. The unique natures of relationship between cell-signalling, transcriptional mechanisms and oxidative-nitrosative stress in the progression of coronary heart disease have also been discussed in greater detail. We have also discussed the emerging concepts that pharmacological prevention of cardiovascular events in the future might consists of the control of classical risk factors with specific interventions targeting oxidative stress while simultaneously improving NO production.

Keywords: Oxidative stress, cardiac development, developmental programming.

INTRODUCTION

Experimental studies have so far reported the significance of the vascular endothelium in the regulation of homeostasis and myocardial wellbeing [1-9] through the participation of different metabolic, synthetic, and regulatory pathways within our body. We now know that a normal endothelial function is needed to maintain the control of antithrombotic and thrombolytic activity, vascular architecture and permeability, leukocyte interactions with the vessel wall, and regulation of vascular tone. In this context we and others have suggested the particular importance of endothelium derived nitric oxide (NO) bioavailability within blood [10-14]. In addition, the modulation of the bioavailability of NO and its precursors plays a key role in the oxidative-nitrosative disequilibrium phenomenon and that this may be related to the development of atherosclerotic lesions [15].

NO is a free radical species (been investigated extensively over the years) that diffuses and concentrates in the hydrophobic core of low-density lipoprotein (LDL) to serve as a potent antioxidant [16,17]. Peroxynitrite (ONOO⁻), the product of the diffusion-limited reaction between NO and superoxide anion, as well as lipoxygenase, represent relevant mediators of oxidative modifications in LDL. Previously we have suggested the interactions between NO, peroxynitrite and lipoxygenase during LDL oxidation, are relevant in the development of early steps of myocardial remodelling in the disease phase as well as progression of atherosclerosis [18,19]. We have suggested at length in our recent review the role of NO in redirecting peroxynitrite reactivity in LDL, the lipophilic antioxidant sparing actions of NO and the effects of novel potential pharmacological strategies against such process [20]. Thus the knowledge of reduced NO bioavailability in human circulation is of prime interest to comprehend fascinating issues regarding cardiovascular disease process and heart-failure pathophysiology. Attempting to understand these issues requires insight into the pharmacologic and biologic underpinnings of mechanisms that enhance NO availability.

Here we summarize the present understanding of NO metabolism in blood and its availability towards signalling mechanism responsible for heart-endothelial cells interaction in maintaining homeostasis. We also discuss in detail

Address correspondence to Bashir M. Matata: Head of Clinical Trials Unit, Liverpool Heart & Chest Hospital NHS Foundation Trust, Liverpool, L14 3PE, UK; Tel: +44 151 600 1380; Fax: +44 151 600 1647; E-mail: matata_bashir@hotmail.com

Bashir M. Matata and Maqsood M. Elahi (Eds.)

the emerging concepts that pharmacological prevention of cardiovascular events in the future might consists of the control of classical risk factors with specific interventions targeting oxidative stress while simultaneously improving NO production.

BIOMECHANICS OF NO

NO is a ubiquitous signalling molecule that influences cardiovascular functioning by modifying post-translational effectors of cysteine residues [21]. This process is called *S*-nitrosylation that regulates key processes in both the heart and the vascular tree, and thus, can affect both cardiac performance and vascular tone [22, 23].

This is a highly versatile signalling mechanism, facilitated by superoxide (O_2^-) in dual faceted moieties in a concentration dependent manner [21]. Excess O_2^- also reacts directly with NO, disrupting its physiologic signalling and potentially leading to the production of other toxic and reactive molecules, notably $ONOO^-$ [22, 23].

Thus, a central pathophysiological consequence of oxidative stress is the disruption of NO signalling causing nitrosative oxidative redox imbalance in the myocardium. In medium-to-large size conductance vessels, NO acts as the prototypical endothelium-derived relaxing factor by activating guanylyl cyclase to produce cyclic guanosine monophosphate.

Finally, in the microcirculation, NO carried by *S*-nitrosohemoglobin (SNOHb) regulates blood flow [24,25]. It is important to note that NO is not produced by endothelial cells in the microcirculation but, rather, is carried there by hemoglobin itself [26-28]. Thus, to help guide the reader through these various reactions, it is useful to elaborate reactive indices of NO bioavailability that contribute to cardiovascular disruptive signaling.

NITROSATION CHEMISTRY AND NITROSATIVE-OXIDATIVE DISEQUILIBRIUM *IN VIVO*

A better knowledge of the fate of NO is an important prerequisite for a proper understanding of its physiology in blood. It is well opinionated that a continuous production and release of endothelial NO plays an important role in vascular homeostasis and cardiac function [29,30]. The supposedly rapid conversion of NO to biologically inactive metabolites in human blood formed the rationale for utilisation of inhaled NO therapy, where the rationale is that the short half-life of NO should confine its effect to the pulmonary circulation [31]. To address this issue, we recently studied the impact of inspired NO gas on physiological function and markers of inflammation-oxidative stress for coronary artery bypass graft patients. Outcomes from subjects that received 5 ppm and 20 ppm of inspired NO were compared to those not given NO gas.

Breath-to-breath measurement commenced at the start of intubation and continued up to 4 hours later. Indices of cardiovascular function, alveolar-capillary gas exchange and haematological parameters were not significantly different in outcomes for the inspired NO groups as compared with control. We observed a reduction in mean systemic arterial pressure in all subjects at 30 minutes and 4 hours after bypass when compared with pre bypass values. Markers of systemic inflammatory response and oxidative stress increased during CPB particularly at 4 hours and 24 hours after the initiation of bypass. In contrast, we observed a reduction in expired NO, at 24 hours after surgery in the groups given inspired NO. In addition, there was also a significant reduction in oxidative stress markers in blood at 24 hours after surgery for the groups given inspired NO as compared with the control group. In contrast, cytokines response remained similar in all the three groups at all time points. The results suggested that inspired NO gas has an antioxidant property that reduces the levels of cell death, and is not associated with significantly worse-off physiological outcomes [19].

In circulation, red blood cells (RBCs) are believed to be a major sink for NO by virtue of the rapid co-oxidation reaction of NO with oxyhemoglobin to form methemoglobin (metHb) and nitrate [32,33]. Alternatively, NO may react with hemoglobin (Hb) to form either nitrosylhemoglobin (NOHb) or SNOHb as discussed above. In addition to its reaction with RBCs, NO has to interact at some stage with plasma constituents, especially in view of the existence of an RBC-free zone close to the vessel wall. Recently, we provided evidence that how ROS in blood augment the cell signalling processes involved in the pathogenesis of coronary heart disease [9-11, 15, 20]. In particular, ROS is an important component of the cross-talk between blood and elements of the vasculature during the initial and latter stages of vascular injury and development of atherosclerotic lesions [9,10]. Currently, the thinking prevails although inflammatory processes may be prompted by different etiological factors from that of coronary heart disease, the presence of ROS in circulating blood is the key intermediary related to vascular injury and organ dysfunction. We reviewed, the clinical and experimental data of the mechanisms involved, and evaluated the wider implications of this concept (results discussed in the next section).

In an elegant series of experiments carried out by Jonathan Stamler's group [34] and recently confirmed by others, red cells were shown to regulate the arteriolar microcirculation, coupling oxygen delivery with blood flow [35-40]. A disruption in nitrosative-oxidative redox signalling clearly has the potential to contribute to events related to myocardial injury. At an enzymatic level, oxidant-producing enzymes are up-regulated and the level or spatial location of nitric oxide–producing enzymes - nitric oxide synthases are altered within cells [41]. In addition, a deficiency of NO- synthase actually increases the activity of oxidases, since NO may be a physiologic down-regulator of superoxide production [22].

On the other hand, levels of specific vascular NADPH oxidases have been reported to increase in the failing circulatory system, at least partly in response to increased levels of angiotensin II. This suggests a link between neurohormonal activation and a nitrosative-oxidative imbalance [42]. Along with this, the levels and activity of xanthine oxidase produced in myocardium, circulates *via* the blood throughout the cardiovascular system and contributes to vasoconstriction and depressed myocardial function [25,41,43]. Datta and colleagues recently demonstrated that the delivery of *S*-nitrosohemoglobin is impaired in the presence of both myocardial failure and one of the major risk factors for myocardial failure, diabetes [44]. Disruption of nitric oxide delivery to the microcirculation almost certainly contributes to the vasoconstriction and uncoupling of oxygen delivery in skeletal muscle that are characteristic of myocardial failure. Thus, although the sources of oxidative stress may differ and several different enzymatic and biochemical mechanisms can disrupt NO signalling, a central problem in the failing myocardial circulation appears to be a shift in the nitrosative-oxidative imbalance away from physiologic *S*-nitrosylation to one of oxidative stress [45-48].

Cellular damage in this situation is often potentiated due to the stimuli leading to formation of iNOS capable of up-regulating oxidases, elevation in NO and concomitant the formation of peroxynitrite with the help of superoxide. A prolonged nitrosative-oxidative imbalance thus leads to the consequences more traditionally ascribed to oxidative stress-cell damage as a result of the oxidation of nucleic acids and proteins, cell loss owing to apoptosis, and phenotypic alteration as a result of the activation of abnormal gene programs (the fetal gene program and resultant cardiac hypertrophy are a prime example of this phenomenon) [49]. The results of upcoming work from our laboratory and others have shown regimens with the potential to restore such imbalance that leads to myocardial remodelling [49-51].

ENHANCED S-NITROSO-ALBUMIN FORMATION DURING ISCHEMIA/REPERFUSION STATE

In relation to NO reaction with heme groups, for rapid clearance of NO from blood, NO also reacts with the thiol of cysteine-93 on the hemoglobin chain thus forming SNO-Hb within red blood cells and allows blood to function as an important transport system [51]. In addition, potent nitrosating and nitrosylating reactions can occur in the presence of plasma constituents that could yield NO-carrying molecules which include the *S*-nitrosothiols (RSNOs) [52,53]. Moreover, RSNOs including low molecular weight *S*-nitrosocysteine (CysNO), *S*-nitrosoglutathione (GSNO), and high molecular weight *S*-nitroso-albumin (SNO-Alb) have been detected in plasma with the latter molecule being the dominant circulating pool of NO in plasma [34]. However, despite the endogenous existence of these molecules, there remains considerable debate regarding physiological effects of these compounds on the myocardium and endothelium. The variation in levels detected by different groups of researchers is likely due to the analytical techniques used. Moreover, the link between inhaled NO and SNO-Alb formation is tenuous.

Interestingly, we observed that the use of inhaled NO gas alone at different concentrations elicited no significant change in the level of NO and SNO-Alb in circulating blood [19]. Since, NO is detectable in the exhaled gas, its quantification as a measure of intrinsic metabolism has attracted much attention in recent years. Various clinical and experimental models have investigated the role of endogenous NO production in the pulmonary vasculature and bronchial systems and have reported that inhaled NO improves lung function in same settings [54]. However, we have shown that inspired NO gas has significant effect on the alveolar-capillary gaseous exchange rate. However, whether endogenous NO plays any part in the development of reperfusion injury and pulmonary endothelial dysfunction remains unclear. Evidence suggests that endogenous NO production decreases during reperfusion after brief episodes of ischemia in the pulmonary extremities, myocardial and skeletal muscles [54]. This may be due to a temporary endothelial cell dysfunction resulting in the inability to produce sufficient NO during early reperfusion [54].

In 1992, Stamler and colleagues [52] proposed that NO undergoes S-nitrosylation with protein-bound thiol groups, forming stable *S*-nitrosoproteins, including SNO-Alb. This molecule could conceivably stabilize NO, thereby establishing an NO delivery system *in vivo*. Since that time, it has been demonstrated that multiple biochemical pathways exist *in vitro* that cause the formation of RSNOs from NO and thiol-containing plasma proteins. Unfortunately, much less evidence exists that these biochemical pathways and their end products play any role as either homeostatic regulators of myocardial function or as mediators of pathophysiology *in vivo*. Studies have so far elucidated the link between oxidation of plasma proteins [55] and the secretion of proinflammatory factors by tissue cells [56], a hypothesis supported by evidence obtained from our studies on blood from ischemic heart disease (IHD) patients, which demonstrated that scavenging of peroxynitrite and inhibiting nitric oxide synthase activity significantly reduced IL-6, IL-8 and TNF-alpha production [57]. This may be explained by the reported observations that levels of reactive oxygen species (ROS) already present in IHD blood completely overwhelms antioxidant capacity and probably alter the function of enzymes such as SOD, glutathione peroxidase and catalase [58]. This thesis is supported by the fact that during neutrophils respiratory burst, up to 17% of the glutathione (GSH) can become protein-bound. This potentially decreases the level of glutathione; hence, reducing potential for the glutathione disulfide-glutathione couple (GSSG/2GSH) half-cell. Moreover, the efflux of GSSG-59 to maintain the redox status during oxidative stress will result in the loss of glutathione from the cell, thereby decreasing the reducing capacity [58]. Both oxidative and reductive stresses may trigger redox cascades that bring about changes in the thiol status of the cell [59]. Changes in the cellular redox environment consequently can alter signal transduction, DNA and RNA synthesis, protein synthesis, enzyme activation, and even regulation of the cell cycle, thus determining the survival of the cell [59].

Whether this may be a reflection of an existing pro-oxidant state symbolized by an upregulation of genes for enzymes responsible for increased production of ROS is yet to be investigated. Indeed, this supposition has a bearing on the observed contrasting roles of NADPH oxidase isoforms in pressure-overload versus angiotensin II-induced cardiac hypertrophy that differentially activate the enzyme gp91phox involved in the NADH/NADPH pathway of superoxide production [60]. Overall, findings from the studies discussed here suggest that there is a differential response to stress by blood, which may directly reflect upon the induction of a proinflammatory state. This mechanism may involve the early activation of neutrophils the most likely source of free radicals during the initial stages. We therefore, propose that the cardiovascular disease process is associated with a phenotypic alteration in cells of the endothelium that increases their capacity to produce ROS in endothelium, characterized by an increased superoxide production *via* an elevated NAD(P)H oxidase activity [61]. More recent work has also demonstrated that oxidative inactivation of tetrahydrobiopterin (H_4B) may cause uncoupling of eNOS to initiate increased production of superoxide [62]. Though these *in vivo* studies did not address the mechanisms of action of NO transport, herein, we hypothesized that SNO-Alb may be one transporter in this situation.

The mechanism of RSNO formation *in vivo* is unclear at this time but likely involves multiple reaction pathways. The S-nitrosylation of thiols by the NO autoxidation intermediate dinitrogen trioxide (N_2O_3) is well documented, but increased oxidative stress during ischemia reperfusion could also induce an increase in one electron oxidation intermediates of thiols, which may provide an important source of thiol radicals (RS·) available for direct radical-radical combination with NO to form RSNOs [63]. An important alternative pathway is the reaction of thiols with peroxynitrite ($ONOO^-$/ $ONOOH$), the diffusion-limited reaction product of NO with O_2^- [64]. Several investigators reported that a number of molecules (albumin, uric acid, and glutathione) present in blood could combine with $ONOO^-$ to generate NO donor compounds [65]. Ischemia reperfusion would be an extremely conducive environment for the latter reaction of cardiac developmental physiology to take place in as much as this pathology is associated with a burst of O_2^- formation and a reduction in antioxidants such as glutathione peroxidase [45].

Because this antioxidant has been shown to reduce S-nitrosylation by ONOO, a reduction of glutathione peroxidase would potentially enhance these reactions. The elevated levels of SNO-Alb in arterial blood suggest that this molecule was made before reaching the myocardium [45]. Moreover, reports have suggested that tissues can release

NO from stored RSNOs [47-48], though O_2^- has never been tested for its ability to induce the release of NO from RSNOs in tissues. Sources of O_2^- in the myocardium after ischemia reperfusion would include activated neutrophils and macrophages, as well as perhaps circulating xanthine oxidase [48]. Consistent with this hypothesis is the observation that during ischemia reperfusion of various peripheral tissues, a dramatic increase in neutrophil recruitment into lungs occurs [66]. The possibility therefore exists that oxidative stress stimulates the release of NO from RSNOs in tissues by either circulating xanthine oxidase and/or inflammatory leukocytes in the pulmonary circulation. Finally, it should be noted that HbNO directly or *via* a SNO-Hb intermediate was stabilized and transported in blood peripherally to modulate blood flow. Finally, one can envisage both NO carrying molecules in plasma (SNO-Alb) and in RBCs transporting NO from lung to periphery in a cooperative manner [67]. Clearly, examination of the RBC compartment in our model system is warranted.

BIOLOGICAL IMPLICATIONS OF NITROSATION CHEMISTRY IN ADULTS WITH CARDIAC DISEASE

Nitrosative stress modulated factors are suggested to be elevated in the aging heart (unstable angina and heart failure). However whether such an increase is sufficient to elicit a biological response and whether these findings can be extrapolated to the *in vivo* situation in blood with RBCs being present as a potentially important intravascular sink for NO remains unclear. Keeping this in view, we carried out prospectively designed experiments where blood and myocardial biopsies (right atrium and left ventricular) were obtained from 3 groups of patients (n=20/ group) undergoing elective coronary artery bypass graft surgery before the surgical correction: The groups are (i) stable angina (SA), (ii) unstable angina (UA), (iii) and stable angina with severely impaired left ventricular function (ILVF), EF ≤30% (Table **1** and **2**).

Table 1: Preoperative Clinical Characteristics, Results Presented as Mean ± SE Mean

	Stable angina	**Unstable angina**	**Impaired LV function**
Number of patients	20	20	20
Age (years)	62.0±1.8	65.0±1.6	62.8±2.9
Male: female	16:4	17:3	18:2
Diseased vessels (3:2:1)	9:3:8	10:2:8	8:4:8
Angina class (CCS)	2.2±0.2	3.4±0.1*	2.6±0.3
Dyspnoea class (NYHA)	1.6±0.2	2.4±0.1*	2.2±0.3*
LV ejection fraction (%)	48.0±2.9	50.0±3.9	16.5±1.4 *
Hypertension	9	10	8
Hypercholesterolemia	9	7	8
Previous MI	5	3	12*
Atrial fibrillation	0	1	1
Active smokers	1	2	2
Plasma TNF-α (pg/mL)	20±3	12±2*	11±3*
SolubleTNF-R1 (ng/mL)	1.5±0.1	1.8±0.2*	1.8±0.3*
Infections	0	0	0
CRP (mg/dL)	1.6±0.2	10.3±1.4*	8.2±3.4*

Table 2: Preoperative Medication and Peripheral Blood Mononuclear Cell Subsets

	Stable angina (n=20)	Unstable angina (n=20)	Impaired LV Function (n=20)
Medical treatment			
Beta-blockers	17	16	13
Organic nitrates	9	12	9

Ca2+ antagonists	7	8	8
ACE inhibitors	11	14	12
Aspirin	17	16	14
Statins	15	13	13
CD3 (x 106) cells	17.3±5.6	18.0±1.2	18.4±6.1
CD14 (x 106) cells	5.9±0.9	8.7±0.8*	4.9±0.9
CD19 x 106) cells	1.8±0.4*	4.0±0.5	3.6±1.1

* $P<0.05$ compared with the other group(s).

Our results demonstrated that peripheral blood mononuclear cells subsets CD14-positive cells were significantly greater in UA patients as compared with SA, and these cells produced significantly greater superoxide in UA and ILVF patients (see Fig. **1**).

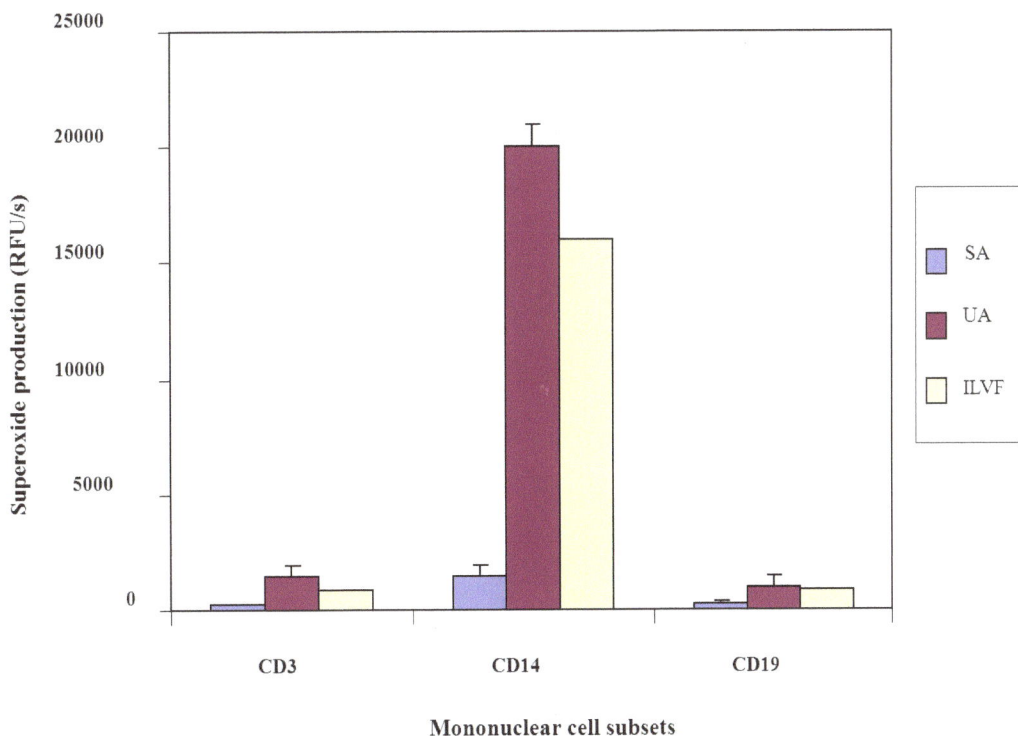

Figure 1: Superoxide production of peripheral blood mononuclear cells (PMBC) subsets. This demonstrates that PMBC subsets CD14-positive cells were significantly greater in UA patients as compared with SA, and these cells produced significantly greater superoxide in UA and ILVF patients.

ELISA assays demonstrated soluble TNF-alpha in circulation to be greatest for SA patients, whereas in contrast tissue TNF-alpha was greatest in myocardial extracts for UA and ILVF groups. Immunohistochemical staining for protein 3-nitrotyrosine, NF-κB subunit p65, and iNOS was greater in the myocardium from UA and ILVF patients, and staining for CD45 followed an identical pattern. Interestingly, apoptosis in the right atrium (Fig. **2**) and left ventricle (Fig. **3**) biopsies of the ILVF group was significantly greater compared with the SA group, but the greatest values were observed in the UA group.

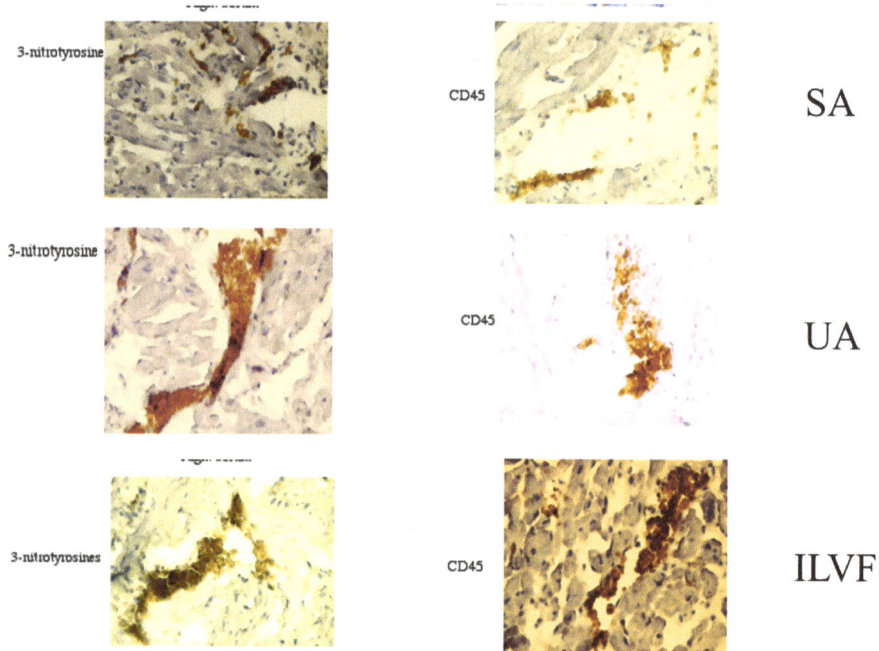

Figure 2: Immunohistochemical staining for protein 3-nitrotyrosine, NF-κB subunit p65, and iNOS was greater in the myocardium from UA and ILVF patients, and staining for CD45 followed an identical pattern. Interestingly, apoptosis in the right atrium biopsies of the ILVF group was significantly greater compared with the SA group, but the greatest values were observed in the UA group (p<0.001).

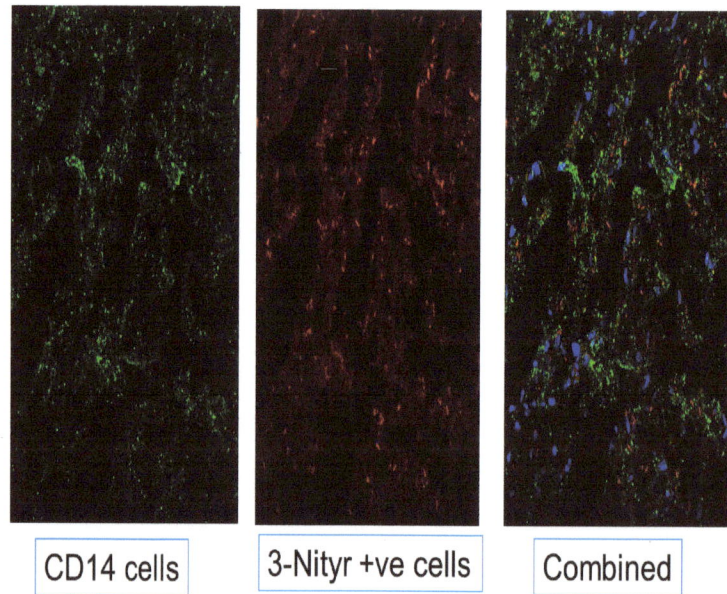

Figure 3: Co-localization of CD14 and 3-nitrotyrosine positive cells in unstable angina ventricular myocardium.

Protein nitration and lipid hydroperoxides were significantly (P<0.05) elevated in mononuclear lysates and plasma from UA and ILVF when compared with the myocardial extracts. Immunoblots and citrulline-conversion assays also showed that the iNOS content and activities were greater in mononuclear cell extracts than in the myocardium of UA and ILVF groups. Furthermore, NF-κB activities were significantly greater in the UA and ILVF groups than in the SA group in both myocardial tissue and mononuclear cell extracts. The results of our this work clearly proposed that excessive oxidative/nitrosative stress induced by activated circulating leukocytes may be responsible for the elevated transcriptional activities and the induction of apoptosis observed in the myocardium of patients with unstable angina and severely impaired LV function, a process that may involve an increase in iNOS activity.

In the present study, we demonstrate for the first time that release of NO *via* iNOS activity exerts systemic hemodynamic effects as judged by NF-κB activity found to be greater in UA and ILVF groups than in the SA group in both myocardial tissue and mononuclear cell extracts. In a separate set of experiments, we reported the mechanism of release of proinflammatory cytokines by blood granulocytes *via* NO-dependent pathways and modulation of nitrosation bioavailability [68]. Taken together, these results provide unequivocal evidence for the occurrence of nitrosation chemistry in the human myocardium and possible hemodynamic consequences.

CROSS TALK BETWEEN NO BIOAVAILABILITY, OXIDATIVE STRESS AND CARDIAC DEVELOPMENTAL DYSFUNCTION

In view of the evidence discussed above, we believe that ROS are implicated in the initiation and progression of cardiovascular disease even at the fetal developmental stage. It has already been observed in several studies [69-73] that ROS can oxidize lipoproteins, limit the bioavailability of NO, and promote translational expression of cytokines and adhesion molecules in dying cardiomyocytes. In addition, Nox proteins of the NADPH oxidase family are prominent sources of this, and Nox protein-dependent ROS production has been linked to this pathophysiology [69-71]. Together with the phagocyte NADPH oxidase itself (NOX_2/gp91^{phox} gets upregulated at the mRNA and protein level [70,71]. In addition to NF-κB, activator protein 1 is an important transcription factor that may mediate pathogenic effects due to an increased proinflammatory state with direct effect on Forkhead O (FOXO) transcription factors as a direct target of phosphatidylinositol-3 kinase/Akt signalling in skeletal and smooth muscle and regulate the expression of the Cip/Kip family of cyclin kinase inhibitors in other cell types [72,73]. The desensitization of protein kinase B/Akt kinase activity and Akt-dependent phosphorylation may downregulate the translocation of p21 into the cytoplasm which in turn may lead to the promotion of Rho-kinases, a contributor to cardiomyocytes dysfunction [70-73]. This leads to increased muscle loss or increased load, with time, progressive ventricular dilatation, increasing interstitial fibrosis and arrhythmia, and a decline in ejection fraction [69-73].

Therefore, inhibition of ROS production, inhibition of NF-κB and inflammatory protein production, and improvement in NO bioactivity may have additive beneficial effects on endothelial function, and overall cardiovascular pathophysiology. To test this hypothesis we investigated using animal models, whether feeding dams with a high fat (HF) diet during pregnancy and/or lactation can result impaired cardiac development and hypertension in their offspring [74]. Our findings suggested that maternal hypercholesterolemia increases ROS-mediated inflammation and inhibits EPC differentiation, survival and function in the cardiomyocytes. It therefore affects key components of angiogenesis and endothelial repair in these offspring [75]. Interestingly, treatment of hypercholesterolemic dams with Statins improved the number of circulating EPC and reduced ROS levels in the adult offspring and may prevent the risk of later cardiovascular pathophysiology [76]. We further elucidated that the ability of maternal hypercholesterolemia to reduce EPC survival and differentiation may represent an important mechanism in the developmental origins of cardiovascular disease [77,78]. However, the impact of HF feeding during pregnancy and lactation on EPC biology and CRP levels in the offspring remains to be determined.

In recent years, immune-mediated mechanisms have also been shown to play important roles in the pathophysiology of cardiovascular diseases. These levels are reported to be increased with the severity of cardiomyopathy. However, it is not clear how individual complement pathways could be affected by ROS. We have also shown previously that complement activation in normal human serum and that there is a concentration-dependent modification of protein residues by ROS and that ROS plays an important role in regulating complement activation independently of the classical and mannan binding lectin (MBL) pathways and that increased activities of cardiomyocytes and endothelial dysfunction may be attributable to a direct effect on the alternate pathway [79].

OXIDATIVE STRESS HYPOTHESIS AND THE EVOLUTION OF CARDIAC DEVELOPMENTAL DYSFUNCTION

Cardiac developmental dysfunction characterised by progressive left ventricular (LV) systolic impairment is believed to be modulated by the ROS. Evidence of this comes from studies that have investigated the impact of excess free-radical generation from a variety of sources in animal and human models, such as vascular nicotinamide adenine dinucleotide oxidases, [80] xanthine oxidases, autooxidation of catecholamines, [81] nitric oxide synthase activation, [82,83] or mitochondrial leakage [84]. The evidence also suggested that besides excessive ROS generation, myocardial antioxidant defences are also impaired [85,86]. These observations have prompted the formulation of an oxidative stress hypothesis of cardiac dysfunction. We hypothesized that nitrosative oxidative disequilibrium is characterized by generalized and cardiac-specific oxidative stress, and that chronic oxidant injury contributes to impairment of myocardial function and ultimately clinical progression into heart failure state.

We now know that oxidative-nitrosative stress is a common feature of many commonly described risk factors of or conditions associated with adverse (poor or excessive) fetal growth and/or preterm birth, such as preeclampsia, diabetes, smoking, malnutrition or excessive nutrition, infection or inflammation [88-90]. Plausibly, oxidative stress may be the key link underlying this pathophysiology. Oxidative stress insults may directly link or accompany many genetic, nutritional and environmental risk factors in association with the elevated risks of adverse cardiac dysfunctional growth indirectly through increasing gestational morbidities such as gestational hypertension and gestational diabetes (Fig. **4**).

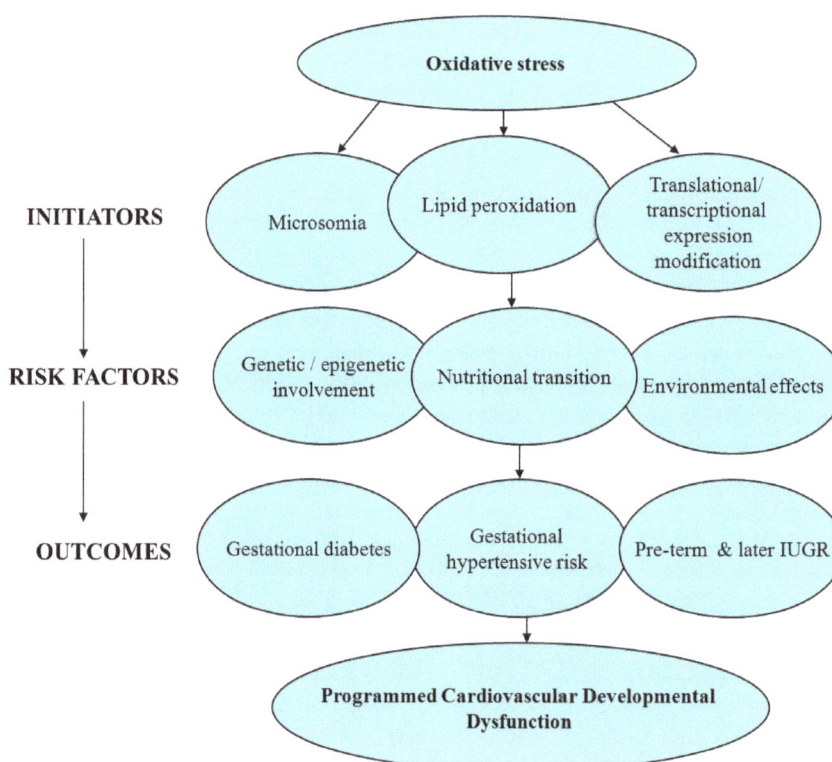

Figure 4: Modified from *Luo et al.*, 2006 [118]. Oxidative stress may be the key link between adverse insults and cardiovascular developmental programming through directly modulating gene expression and/or the indirect effects of oxidized lipids or other molecules. IUGR= Intrauterine growth retardation.

Oxidative stress programming may operate either directly through the modulation of gene expression or indirectly through the adverse effects of oxidized lipids or other molecules at critical developmental windows and therefore resetting/programming the susceptibility to the cardiovascular developmental disorders [91-92]. The susceptibility of biological systems due to oxidative insults is likely dependent on its resilience and maturity stage at the time of insult. There could be different critical time windows (prenatal or even postnatal) in ''programming'' different diseases. Plausibly, prenatal and early postnatal periods are the most critical ''windows'' for oxidative stress programming.

Many studies on cells and tissues have demonstrated the deleterious effects of oxidized LDL (oxLDL) contributing to cellular toxicity, inflammation, vascular apoptosis and endothelial cell dysfunction [93,94]. Some F2-isoprostanes, such as F2α-8-isoprostanes (8-iso-PGF2-α), are associated with potent vasoconstriction and the modulation of platelet functions (pro-aggregation) [95-97]. These or other yet unknown oxidized molecules may be involved in adverse programming by modulating tissue blood supply and growth through affecting vascular physiology or other mechanisms.

Although relatively little is known about the role of oxidative stress in cardiac growth, experimental studies have already demonstrated the role of redox imbalance in modulating gene expression and cell signal cascades [98,99]. ROS is capable of modifying the structure and functions of cellular proteins in defined ways (conformational changes by oxidation of cysteine residues to form disulfide and cyclic sulfonamide covalent bonds) to regulate signal transduction pathways and gene expression [100]. Recent studies in animal model observed that manipulating antioxidant-oxidant balance in pregnancy could alter blood pressure and vascular reactivity in rat offspring [101,102]. Furthermore, in mitochondria the cellular organelles responsible for regulating energy metabolism and monitoring of blood sugar, the DNA is much more vulnerable to ROS damage than nuclear DNAs [103] which may offer an additional venue of programming the risk of cardiovascular dysfunction as subtle damages which may be magnified with advancing age. It can be envisioned that the effects of oxidative insults on myocytes proliferation, function or energy metabolism at critical developmental windows in early life will have the maximal effects that will be further magnified or aggregated with additional oxidative insults in later life with the eventual manifestations of the heart failure.

CONCLUSION

Oxidative-nitrosative stress is an important therapeutic target as it represents a common mechanism associated with a multitude of cardiovascular disease risk factors and also during cardiac development. There is extensive evidence from *in vitro* research and from experimental *in vivo* animal models in support of the hypothesis that oxidative stress has a negative impact on cardiac development. *In vitro* experiments [104-109] have also demonstrated that excess ROS generation or impaired antioxidant function adversely affects several cardiac myocytes functions such as depression of myocardial contractility, myocardial tissue injury, and induction of myocytes apoptosis. *In vivo* animal models [110-115] have also demonstrated the significance of oxidative injury to cardiac function; the best-studied example is that of myocardial stunning and injury due to reperfusion after a period of ischemia thus confirming the role of oxidative stress. Moreover, myocardial oxidative stress through the targeting of redox sensitive proteins and enzymes is now known to be an important regulator of cardiac developmental dysfunction; and also a regulator of the extracellular matrix deposition and degradation that contributes to ventricular remodelling and LV dilatation. In agreement with others [116], we propose that the manipulation of ROS production and the simultaneous increase in NO production could be the basis for future novel therapeutic strategies for halting cardiovascular dysfunction particularly during fetal development.

REFERENCES

[1]   Boucher JL, Moali C, Tenu JP. Nitric oxide biosynthesis, nitric oxide synthase inhibitors and arginase competition for L-arginine utilization. Cell Mol Life Sci 1999; 55: 1015-28.

[2]   Cannon RO III, Schechter AN, Panza JA, *et al.* Effects of inhaled nitric oxide on regional blood flow are consistent with intravascular nitric oxide delivery. J Clin Invest 2001; 108 (2): 279-87.

[3]   Garlichs CD, Beyer J, Zhang H, *et al.* Decreased plasma concentrations of L-hydroxyarginine as a marker of reduced NO formation in patients with combined cardiovascular risk factors. J Lab Clin Med 2000; 135 (5): 419-25.

[4]   Gladwin MT, Ognibene FP, Pannell LK, *et al.* Relative role of heme nitrosylation and β-cysteine 93 nitrosation in the transport and metabolism of nitric oxide by hemoglobin in the human circulation. Proc Natl Acad Sci USA 2000; 97 (18): 9943-48.

[5]   Kelm M. Nitric oxide metabolism and breakdown. Biochim Biophys Acta 1999; 1411 (2): 273-89.

[6]   Lauer T, Preik M, Rassaf T, *et al.* Plasma nitrite rather than nitrate reflects regional endothelial nitric oxide synthase activity but lacks intrinsic vasodilator action. Proc Natl Acad Sci USA 2001; 98 (22): 12814-819.

[7]   Miyazaki H, Matsuoka H, Cooke JP, *et al.* Endogenous nitric oxide synthase inhibitor. A novel marker of atherosclerosis. Circulation 1999; 99 (9): 1141-46,

[8]   Moncada S, Higgs EA. Molecular mechanisms and therapeutic strategies related to nitric oxide. FASEB J 1995; 9 (13): 1319-30.

[9]   Elahi MM, Yii M, Matata BM Significance of oxidants and inflammatory mediators in blood of patients undergoing cardiac surgery. J Cardiothorac Vasc Anesth 2008; 22 (3):455-67.

[10]   Elahi MM, Kong YX, Matata BM. Oxidative stress as a mediator of cardiovascular disease. Oxid Med Cell Longev 2009; 2 (5): 259-69.

[11]   Elahi M, Asopa S, Matata B.NO-cGMP and TNF-alpha counter regulatory system in blood: understanding the mechanisms leading to myocardial dysfunction and failure. Biochim Biophys Acta 2007; 1772 (1): 5-14.

[12]   Bian K, Doursout MF, Murad F. Vascular system: role of nitric oxide in cardiovascular diseases. J Clin Hypertens 2008; 10 (4): 304-10.

[13]   Napoli C, Ignarro LJ. Nitric oxide and pathogenic mechanisms involved in the development of vascular diseases. Arch Pharm Res 2009; 32 (8):1103-8.

[14]   Crimi E, Ignarro LJ, Napoli C. Microcirculation and oxidative stress. Free Radic Res 2007; 41 (12):1364-75.

[15]   Elahi MM, Naseem KM, Matata BM. Nitric oxide in blood. The nitrosative-oxidative disequilibrium hypothesis on the pathogenesis of cardiovascular disease. FEBS J 2007; 274 (4): 906-23.

[16]   Baker PR, Schopfer FJ, O'Donnell VB, Freeman BA. Convergence of nitric oxide and lipid signaling: anti-inflammatory nitro-fatty acids. Free Radic Biol Med 2009; 46 (8): 989-1003.

[17]   Rubbo H, Trostchansky A, O'Donnell VB. Peroxynitrite-mediated lipid oxidation and nitration: mechanisms and consequences. Arch Biochem Biophys 2009; 484 (2): 167-72.

[18]   Rubbo H, O'Donnell V. Nitric oxide, peroxynitrite and lipoxygenase in atherogenesis: mechanistic insights. Toxicology 2008; 208 (2): 305-17.

[19]   Elahi MM, Worner M, Khan JS, Matata BM. Inspired nitric oxide and modulation of oxidative stress during cardiac surgery. Curr Drug Saf 2009; 4 (3): 188-98.

[20]   Elahi MM, Matata BM. Myocardial protection against ischemia-reperfusion injury: novel approaches in maintaining homeostatic stability in blood. Recent Pat Cardiovasc Drug Discov 2006; 1 (3): 291-305.

[21]   Stamler JS, Lamas S, Fang FC. Nitrosylation: the prototypic redox- based signaling mechanism. Cell 2001; 106 (6): 675-83.

[22.   Khan S, Lee KH, Minhas KM, *et al.* Neuronal nitric oxide synthase negatively regulates xanthine oxidoreductase inhibition of cardiac excitation-contraction coupling. Proc Natl Acad Sci USA 2004; 101 (45): 15944-48.

[23]   Xu L, Eu JP, Meissner G, Stamler JS. Activation of the cardiac calcium release channel (ryanodine receptor) by poly-S-nitrosylation. Science 1998; 279 (5348): 234-37.

[24]   Lima B, Forrester MT, Hess DT, *et al.* S-nitrosylation in cardiovascular signaling. Circ Res 2010; 106 (4): 633-46.

[25]   Berry CE, Hare JM. Xanthine oxidoreductase and cardiovascular disease: molecular mechanisms and pathophysiological implications. J Physiol 2004; 555 (3): 589-606.

[26]   Hare JM. Nitric oxide and excitation-contraction coupling. J Mol Cell Cardiol 2003; 35 (7):719-29.

[27]   Singel DJ, Stamler JS. S-Nitrosylation of cardiac ion channels Blood traffic control. Nature 2004; 430 (6997): 297.

[28]   Gonzalez DR, Treuer A, Sun QA, *et al.* S-Nitrosylation of cardiac ion channels. J Cardiovasc Pharmacol 2009; 54 (3): 188-95.

[29]   Heusch G, Post H, Michel MC, *et al.* Endogenous nitric oxide and myocardial adaptation to ischemia. Circ Res 2000; 87 (2): 146-52.

[30]   Bolli R. Cardioprotective function of inducible nitric oxide synthase and role of nitric oxide synthase and role of nitric oxide in myocardial ischemia and preconditioning: an overview of a decade of research. J Mol Cell Cardiol 2001; 33 (11):1897-918.

[31]   Rossaint R, Falke KJ, Lopez F, *et al.* Inhaled nitric oxide for the adult respiratory distress syndrome. N Engl J Med 1993; 328 (6): 399-405.

[32]   Cannon RO III, Schechter AN, Panza JA, *et al.* Effects of inhaled nitric oxide on regional blood flow are consistent with intravascular nitric oxide delivery. J Clin Invest 2001; 108 (2): 279-87.

[33]   Jia L, Bonaventura C, Bonaventura J, *et al.* S-nitrosohaemoglobin: a dynamic activity of blood involved in vascular control. Nature 1996; 380 (6571):221–26.

[34]   Stamler JS, Simon DI, Osborne JA, *et al.* S-nitrosylation of proteins with nitric oxide: synthesis and characterization of biologically active compounds. Proc Natl Acad Sci USA 1992; 89 (1): 444–48. 1992.

[35]   Adlam D, Bendall JK, De Bono JP, *et al.* Cardiovascular control: relationships between nitric oxide-mediated endothelial function, eNOS coupling and blood pressure revealed by eNOS-GTP cyclohydrolase 1 double transgenic mice. Exp Physiol 2007; 92: 119–26.

[36]   Landmesser U, Harrison DG, Drexler H: Oxidant stress: a major cause of reduced endothelial nitric oxide availability in cardiovascular disease. Eur J Clin Pharmacol 2006; 62 (1):13-9.

[37]   Geiszt M: NADPH oxidases: new kids on the block. Cardiovasc Res 2006; 71 (2):289 –99.

[38]   Harrison DG, Widder J, Grumbach I, *et al.* Endothelial: mechanotransduction, nitric oxide and vascular inflammation. J Intern Med 2006; 259 (4):351–63.

[39]   DeLano FA, Parks DA, Ruedi JM, *et al.* Microvascular display of xanthine oxidase and NADPH oxidase in the spontaneously hypertensive rat. Microcirculation 2006; 13 (7): 551–66.

[40]   Andrew PJ, Mayer B: Enzymatic function of nitric oxide synthases. Cardiovasc Res 1999; 43:521–31.

[41]   Cappola TP, Kass DA, Nelson GS, *et al.* Allopurinol improves myocardial efficiency in patients with idiopathic dilated cardiomyopathy. Circulation 2001; 104 (20): 2407-11.

[42]   Mollnau H, Wendt M, Szocs K, *et al.* Effects of angiotensin II infusion on the expression and function of NAD(P)H oxidase and components of nitric Oxide/cGMP signaling. Circ Res 2002; 90 (4): 58-65.

[43]   Landmesser U, Spiekermann S, Dikalov S, *et al.* Vascular oxidative stress and endothelial dysfunction in patients with chronic heart failure: role of xanthine-oxidase and extracellular superoxide dismutase. Circulation 2002; 106 (24): 3073-78.

[44]   Datta B, Tufnell-Barrett T, Bleasdale RA, *et al.* Red blood cell nitric oxide as an endocrine vasoregulator: a potential role in congestive heart failure. Circulation 2004; 109 (11): 1339-42.

[45]   Kuo WN, Kocis JM. Nitration/S-nitrosation of proteins by peroxynitritetreatment and subsequent modification by glutathione *S*-transferase and glutathione peroxidase. Mol Cell Biochem 2002; 233 (1-2): 57–63.

[46]   Rodriguez J, Maloney RE, Rassaf T, *et al.* Chemical nature of nitric oxide storage forms in rat vascular tissue. Proc Natl Acad Sci USA 2003; 100 (1): 336–41.

[47]   Feelisch M, Rassaf T, Mnaimneh S, *et al.* Concomitant *S*-, *N*-, and heme-nitros(yl)ation in biological tissues and fluids: implications for the fate of NO *in vivo.* FASEB J 2002; 16 (13): 1775–85.

[48]   Repine JE, Parsons PE. Oxidant-antioxidant balance in endotoxin induced oxidative injury and tolerance to oxidative injury. In: Brigham KL, Ed. Endotoxin and the Lungs. New York, NY: Marcel Dekker, Inc 1994; Vol. 77; pp. 207–27.

[49]   Matata BM, Elahi MM. Mechanisms of ROS formation In: Matata B, Elahi M, Eds. Oxidative Stress and Biomedical Implications. New York, NY: Nova Publishers, Inc 2007; pp. 23-38.

[50]   Circu M, Aw TY. Redox regulation of cell signalling In: Matata B, Elahi M, Eds. Oxidative Stress and Biomedical Implications. New York, NY: Nova Publishers, Inc 2007; pp. 103-132.

[51]   Taylor EL, Winyard PG. S-Nitrosothiols and disease mechanisms. In: Matata B, Elahi M, Eds. Oxidative Stress and Biomedical Implications. New York, NY: Nova Publishers, Inc. 2007; pp. 157-170.

[52]   Stamler JS, Jaraki O, Osborne J, *et al.* Nitric oxide circulates in mammalian plasma primarily as an S-nitroso adduct of serum albumin. Proc Natl Acad Sci USA1992; 89 (16): 7674–77.

[53]   Keaney JF, Simon DI, Stamler JS, *et al.* NO forms an adduct with serum albumin that has endothelium-derived relaxing factor-like properties. J Clin Invest 1993; 91 (4):1582–89.

[54]   Ishibe Y, Liu R, Ueda M, Mori K, Miura N. Role of inhaled nitric oxide in ischaemia-reperfusion injury in the perfused rabbit lung. Br J Anaesth 1999; 83 (3): 430-5.

[55]   Okusawa S, Yancey KB, van der Meer JW, *et al.* C5a stimulates secretion of tumour necrosis factor from human mononuclear cells *in vitro.* J Exp Med 1988; 168 (1): 443-48.

[56]   Pantke U, Volk T, Schmutzler M, Kox WJ, Sitte N, Grune T. Oxidised proteins as a marker of oxidative stress during coronary heart surgery. Free Radic Biol Med 1999; 27 (9-10): 1080-86.

[57]   Elahi M, Matata BM. The interaction between reactive oxygen species and proinflammatory cytokines in human blood during extracorporeal circulation. Filtration 1: 89-94. 2005.

[58]   Mezzetti A, Lapenna D, Pierdomenico SD, *et al.* Myocardial antioxidant defences during cardiopulmonary bypass. J Cardiac Surg 1993; 8 (2): 167- 71.

[59]   Schafer FQ, Buettner GR. Redox environment of the cell as viewed through the redox state of the glutathione disulfide/ glutathione couple. Free Radic Biol Med 2001; 30 (11): 1191-212.

[60]   Byrne JA, Grieve DJ, Bendall JK, *et al.* Contrasting roles of NADPH oxidase isoforms in pressure- overload versus angiotensin II-induced cardiac hypertrophy. Circ Res 2003; 93 (9): 802-5.

[61]   Guzik TJ, Sadowski J, Kapelak B, *et al.* Systemic regulation of vascular NAD(P)H oxidase activ- ity and nox isoform expression in human arteries and veins. Arterioscler Thromb Vasc Biol 2004; 24 (9): 1614-20.

[62]   Chalupsky K, Cai H. Endothelial dihydrofolate reductase: critical for nitric oxide bioavailability and role in angiotensin II uncoupling of endothelial nitric oxide synthase. Proc Natl Acad Sci USA 2005; 102 (25): 9056-61.

[63]   Jourd'heuil D, Jourd'heuil FL, Feelisch M. Oxidation and nitrosation of thiols at low micromolar exposure to nitric oxide: evidence for a free radical mechanism. J Biol Chem 2003; 278 (18): 15720–26.

[64]   van der Vliet A, Chr.'t Hoen PA, Wong PSY, *et al.* Formation of *S*-nitrosothiols *via* direct nucleophilic nitrosation of thiols by peroxynitrite with elimination of hydrogen peroxide. J Biol Chem 1998; 273 (46): 30255–62.

[65]   Ma XL, Gao F, Lopez BL, *et al.* Peroxynitrite, a two-edged sword in post-ischemic myocardial injury: dichotomy of action in crystalloid- versus blood-perfused hearts. J Pharmacol Exp Ther 2000; 292 (3): 912–20.

[66]   Koike K, Moore F, Moore EE, *et al.* Gut ischemia mediates lung injury by a xanthine oxidase-dependent neutrophil mechanism. J Surg Res 1993; 54 (5): 469–73.

[67]   Gow AJ, Luchsinger BP, Pawloski JR, Singel DJ, Stamler JS. The oxyhemoglobin reaction of nitric oxide. Proc Natl Acad Sci USA 1999; 96 (16): 9027–32.

[68]   Elahi M, Matata B. Nitric Oxide-dependent Pathway Regulates Granulocytes Cytokines Release in Cultured Human Leucocytes from Type-II Diabetes Mellitus. Proceedings of the 13th Biennial Congress of the International Society for Free Radical Research 2006; pp. 115-118 [SFRRI -XIII Congress]   .

[69]   Babior BM. NADPH oxidase. Curr Opin Immunol 2004; 16 (1):42– 47.

[70]   Chabrashvili T, Tojo A, Onozato ML, *et al.* Expression and cellular localization of classic NADPH oxidase subunits in the spontaneously hypertensive rat kidney. Hypertension 2002; 39 (2): 269 –74.

[71] Touyz RM, Yao G, Schiffrin EL. c-Src induces phosphorylation and translocation of p47phox: role in superoxide generation by angiotensin II in human vascular smooth muscle cells. Arterioscler Thromb Vasc Biol 2003; 23 (6):981–87.

[72] Bokoch GM, Zhao T. Regulation of the phagocyte NADPH oxidase by Rac GTPase. Antioxid Redox Signal 2006; 8 (9-10):1533– 48.

[73] Ambasta RK, Kumar P, Griendling KK, Schmidt HH, Busse R, Brandes RP. Direct interaction of the novel Nox proteins with p22phox is required for the formation of a functionally active NADPH oxidase. J Biol Chem 2004; 279 (44): 45935–41.

[74] Elahi MM, Cagampang FR, Mukhtar D, *et al.* Long-term maternal high-fat feeding from weaning through pregnancy and lactation predisposes offspring to hypertension, raised plasma lipids and fatty liver in mice. Br J Nutr 2009; 102 (4): 514-19.

[75] Elahi MM, Mukhtar D, Cagampang FR, *et al.* High Fat High Cholesterol diet consumption in Pregnancy Attenuates Bone Marrow- Derived Circulating Endothelial Progenitor Cells and Increases the Risk of Cardiovascular Disorders in the Offspring. Early Hum Develop 2007; 83 (Suppl-1): 5D-6, S74.

[76] Elahi MM, Cagampang FR, Anthony FW, Curzen N, Ohri SK, Hanson MA. Statin treatment in hypercholesterolemic pregnant mice reduces cardiovascular risk factors in their offspring. Hypertension 2008; 51 (4): 939-44.

[77] Elahi MM, Mukhtar D, Kahraman N, Cagampang FR, Ohri, SK, Hanson MA. Statin Therapy Improves Blood Pressure and Lipid Profiles in Hypercholesterolemic Mothers but not C-reactive proteins levels or Endothelial Progenitor Cell Expression. Early Hum Development 2007; 83: 6, S60.

[78] Elahi MM, Cagampang FR, Mukhtar D, Ohri SK, Hanson MA. Statin treatment in female mice has sex specific effects on cardiovascular risk factors and circulating endothelial progenitor cells in their offspring. Reprod Sci 2009; 16: 412.

[79] Elahi MM, Elahi M, Matata BM. Reactive Oxidant Species Augment Complement Function in Human Blood independently of Classical and MBL-Pathways. Int J Mol Med Adv Sci 2005; 1: 382-91.

[80] Rajagopalan S, Kurz S, Munzel T, *et al.* Angiotensin II mediated hypertension in the rat increases vascular superoxide production *via* membrane NADH/NADPH oxidase activation. J Clin Invest 1996; 97 (2): 1916–23.

[81] Singal PK, Beamish RE, Dhalla NS. Potential oxidative pathways of catecholamines in the formation of catecholamines in the formation of lipid peroxidation. Adv Exp Med Biol 1983; 161: 391–401.

[82] Habib FM, Springall DR, Davies GJ, *et al.* Tumour necrosis factor and inducible nitric oxide synthase in dilated cardiomyopathy. Lancet 1996; 347 (9009): 1151–55.

[83] Oyama J, Shimokawa H, Momii H, *et al.* Role of nitric oxide and peroxynitrite in the cytokine-induced sustained myocardial dysfunction in dogs *in vivo*. J Clin Invest 1998; 101 (10):2207– 14.

[84] Ozawa T, Tanaka M, Sugiyama S, *et al.* Multiple mitochondrial DNA deletions exist in cardiomyocytes of patients with hypertrophic or dilated cardiomyopathy. Biochem Biophys Res Commun 1990; 170 (2): 830–36.

[85] Dhalla AK, Hill MF, Singal PK. Role of oxidative stress in transition of hypertrophy to heart failure. J Am Coll Cardiol 1996; 28 (2):506–14.

[86] Hill MF, Singal PK. Right and left myocardial antioxidant responses during heart failure subsequent to myocardial infarction. Circulation 1997; 96 (7):2414-20.

[87] Roberts JM, Lain KY. Recent Insights into the pathogenesis of pre-eclampsia. Placenta 2002; 23 (5):359–72.

[88] Peuchant E, Brun JL, Rigalleau V, *et al.* Oxidative and antioxidative status in pregnant women with either gestational or type 1 diabetes. Clin Biochem 2004; 37 (4): 293–8.

[89] Block G, Dietrich M, Norkus EP, *et al.* Factors associated with oxidative stress in human populations. Am J Epidemiol 2002; 156 (3): 274–85.

[90] Higdon JV, Frei B. Obesity and oxidative stress: a direct link to CVD? Arterioscler Thromb Vasc Biol 2003; 23 (3): 365–7.

[91] Takano H, Zou Y, Hasegawa H, Akazawa H, Nagai T, Komuro I. Oxidative stress-induced signal transduction pathways in cardiac myocytes: involvement of ROS in heart diseases. Antioxid Redox Signal 2003; 5 (6): 789-94.

[92] Reed R, Potter B, Smith E, Jadhav R, Villalta P, Jo H, Rocic P. Redox-sensitive Akt and Src regulate coronary collateral growth in metabolic syndrome. Am J Physiol Heart Circ Physiol 2009; 296 (6): 1811-21.

[93] Frostegard J. Autoimmunity, oxidized LDL and cardiovascular disease. Autoimmun Rev 2002;1 (4): 233–7.

[94] Itabe H. Oxidized low-density lipoproteins: what is understood and what remains to be clarified. Biol Pharm Bull 2003; 26 (1): 1–9.

[95] Basu S. Isoprostanes: novel bioactive products of lipid peroxidation. Free Radic Res 2004; 38 (2):105–22.

[96] Morrow JD, Minton TA, Roberts LJ. The F2-isoprostane, 8-epi-prostaglandin F2 alpha, a potent agonist of the vascular thromboxane/endoperoxide receptor, is a platelet thromboxane/endoperoxide receptor antagonist. Prostaglandins 1992; 44 (2): 155–63.

[97] Pratico D, Smyth EM, Violi F, *et al.* Local amplification of platelet function by 8-Epi prostaglandin F2alpha is not mediated by thromboxane receptor isoforms. J Biol Chem 1996; 271 (25):14916–24.

[98] Turpaev KT. Reactive oxygen species and regulation of gene expression. Biochemistry (Mosc) 2002; 67 (3): 281–92.

[99]   Hancock JT, Desikan R, Neill SJ. Role of reactive oxygen species in cell signalling pathways. Biochem Soc Trans 2001; 29 (2): 345–50.

[100]   Barford D. The role of cysteine residues as redox-sensitive regulatory switches. Curr Opin Struct Biol 2004; 14 (6): 679–86.

[101]   Franco Mdo C, Dantas AP, Akamine EH, *et al*. Enhanced oxidative stress as a potential mechanism underlying the programming of hypertension *in utero*. J Cardiovasc Pharmacol 2002;40 (4): 501–9.

[102]   Racasan S, Braam B, van der Giezen DM, *et al*. Perinatal L-arginine and antioxidant supplements reduce adult blood pressure in spontaneously hypertensive rats. Hypertension 2004; 44 (1): 83–88.

[103]   Droge W. Free radicals in the physiological control of cell function. Physiol Rev 2002; 82 (1):47–95.

[104]   Dhalla AK, Hill MF, Singal PK. Role of oxidative stress in transition of hypertrophy to heart failure. J Am Coll Cardiol 1996; 28 (2): 506–14.

[105]   Hill MF, Singal PK. Right and left myocardial antioxidant responses during heart failure subsequent to myocardial infarction. Circulation 1997; 96 (7):2414–20.

[106]   Goldhaber JI, Ji S, Lamp ST, *et al*. Effects of exogenous free radicals on electromechanical function and metabolism in isolated rabbit and guinea pig ventricle. J Clin Invest 1989; 83 (6):1800–9.

[107]   Kim M, Akera T. O_2 free radicals: cause of ischemia reperfusion injury to cardiac Na-K-ATP'ase. Am J Physiol 1987; 252 (2): 252–57.

[108]   Kaneko M, Beamish RE, Dhalla NS. Depression of heart sarcolemmal Ca^{2+}-pump activity by oxygen free radicals. Am J Physiol 1989; 256 (2): 368–74.

[109]   Rowe GT, Manson NH, Caplan M, *et al*. Hydrogen peroxide and hydroxyl radical mediate leukocyte depression of cardiac sarcoplasmic reticulum: participation of the cyclooxygenase pathway. Circ Res 1983; 53 (5): 584–91.

[110]   Blaustein AS, Schine L, Brooks WW, *et al*. Influence of exogenously generated oxidant species on myocardial function. Am J Physiol 1986; 250 (4): 595–99.

[111]   Schrier GM, Hess ML. Quantitative identification of superoxide anion as a negative inotropic species. Am J Physiol 1988; 255: 138-43.

[112]   Burton KP, McCord JM, Ghai G. Myocardial alterations due to free-radical generation. Am J Physiol 1984; 246 (1): 776–83.

[113]   Gottlieb RA, Burleson KO, Kloner RA, *et al*. Reperfusion injury induces apoptosis in rabbit cardiomyocytes. J Clin Invest 1998; 94 (4):1621–28.

[114]   Bolli R, Zhu WX, Hartley CJ,, *et al*. Attenuation of dysfunction in the postischemic "stunned" myocardium by dimethylthiourea. Circulation 1987; 76 (2):458–68.

[115]   Bolli R, Zughaib M, Li XY, *et al*. Recurrent ischemia in the canine heart causes recurrent bursts of free radical production that have a cumulative effect on contractile function: a pathophysiological basis for chronic myocardial "stunning." J Clin Invest 1995; 96 (2):1066–84.

[116]   MunzelIT, Goril T, Bruno RM, Taddei S. Is oxidative stress a therapeutic target in cardiovascular disease? Eur Heart J 2010; 31 (22):2741–49.

[117]   Lauer T, Kleinbongard P, Kelm M. Indexes of NO bioavailability in human blood. News Physiol Sci 2002;17: 251-5.

CHAPTER 6

Fetal and Neonatal Programming in Current Practice

Tetyana H. Nesterenko and Hany Aly[*]

Department of Newborn Services, The George Washington University and the Children's National Medical Center, Washington, DC, USA

Abstract: Fetal and neonatal programming is a phenomenon produced by deviations from the normal development during prenatal or early postnatal life. These deviations can increase risk for different diseases later in life and are an example of phenotypic plasticity throughout the nature. For instance, infants born with low birth weight, as a marker of an unfavorable intrauterine environment, are programmed differently and face additional challenges in adulthood; thereby encountering more risks for coronary artery diseases, diabetes, hypertension, metabolic syndrome, imbalanced immune response, renal insufficiency, and suboptimal cognition. Advances in research in the last decade significantly improved the understanding of underlying mechanisms. Once these mechanisms are understood it is very tempting to implicate them into management. However, the risk and benefit of each new implication into clinical practice need to be considered carefully and evaluated by randomized controlled trials. This chapter will propose and discuss some of the possible clinical implications of fetal and neonatal programming which can lead to possible changes in current clinical management in reflection of latest knowledge on this topic.

Keywords: Neonatal programming, gestational age pregnancy, postnatal nutrition, neuro-developmental impairment, malnutrition.

CLINICAL APPLICABILITY OF FETAL-NEONATAL PROGRAMMING

"The theory without the practice is dead and practice without the theory is blind." Clinical applications of this new concept of fetal-neonatal programming may challenge some of the standard current practices. Looking at the umbrella-shaped model for programming [1] each of the five elements can be addressed clinically. Clinical changes in some of them such as gene expression and change in surface receptors belong rather to experimental medicine. Clinical changes in others, such as nutrients, immune system maturation and oxidative stress can be explored and implemented at the level of current knowledge and management. (Fig. **1**).

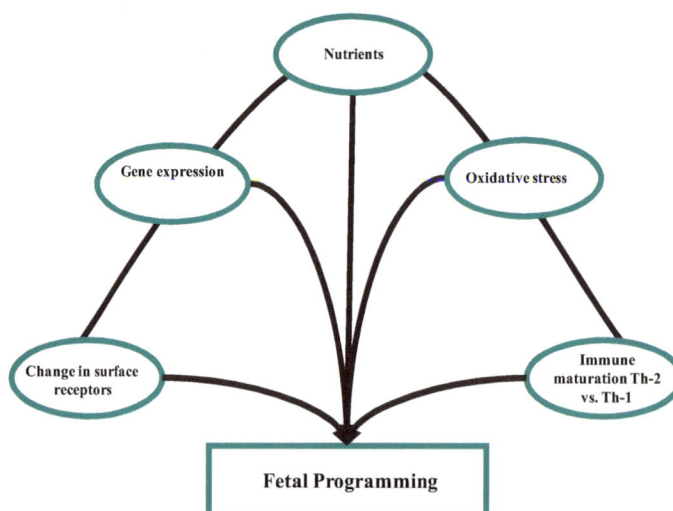

Figure 1: A Proposed Model for Fetal–Neonatal Programming.

*Address Correspondence to Hany Aly: Department of Newborn Services, The George Washington University and the Children's National Medical Center, Washington, DC, USA; Tel: (202)715-5350; Email: haly@mfa.gwu.edu

Bashir M. Matata and Maqsood M. Elahi (Eds.)

EARLY NEONATAL NUTRITION

One of the major elements that program the individual organ systems is nutrition during fetal life and the early neonatal period. Suboptimal quality and quantity of maternal nutrition can be hazardous to the fetus. The impact of a suboptimal amount of maternal nutrition on fetal programming has been demonstrated in individuals prenatally exposed to the "Dutch famine" during World War II. These individuals were born smaller and higher incidence of metabolic syndrome as adult compared to the general population [2]. Having a small for gestational age pregnancy (SGA) not only affects the future of the fetus, but the uterus is also adversely programmed. Mothers with history of SGA pregnancy have a fourfold increased risk for delivering SGA infants in subsequent pregnancies. Even if the subsequent fetus is not SGA, the neonatal mortality rate among this group of infants is much higher compared to the general population and is similar if compared to the neonatal mortality among the SGA infants. Such findings confirm that the uterus after SGA pregnancy is not the same anymore [3].

An even more interesting observation is a transgenerational effect of fetal programming that was recently demonstrated in a large cohort study. Women who were born SGA were more likely to deliver smaller infants compared with the general population [4]. The quality of maternal nutrition is not of less importance than the quantity. A recent animal study demonstrated that maternal protein restriction in rats led to the delivery of small offspring that were more likely to develop insulin resistance later in life. Moreover, a postnatal high-energy diet, in an effort to achieve a catch-up growth, only exacerbates this effect [5]. Early postnatal nutrition is also a major player in programming. Among a cohort of infants with BW of 500 to 1000 g, it was shown that infants who gained 21 g/kg/d had lower risk for cerebral palsy and neuro-developmental impairment at 18 to 20 months of corrected age compared to infants who gained 12 g/kg/d during the initial hospital stay [6]. Malnutrition has been long associated with a decreased number of brain cells and, as a result, deficits in behavior, learning, and memory [6]. However, the mechanism for adverse brain outcomes may be more complex than just a decreased number of brain cells. Malnutrition can also compromise the overall health, reducing immune response to infections and prolonging time to recovery. Poor nutrition is also associated with decreased motor development and rate of growth. On the other hand, there is strong evidence in literature that overfeeding during the initial neonatal period is associated with hypertension, obesity, and insulin resistance [7,8,9,10]. In a large cohort study that included 27,000 full-term infants, the rate of weight gain during the first 4 months of life was associated with an increased risk of obesity at 7 years of age. This association is independent of BW and weight attained at 1 year of age [10]. The over-nutrition-programmed hypertension was characteristically observed only in diastolic and mean blood pressure but not in systolic blood pressure [11]. Relative under-nutrition and slower rate of growth early in life is protective against type 2 diabetes in preterm infants. In a randomized controlled trial, using plain unfortified breast milk in preterm infants was later associated with less incidence of insulin resistance measured at 13 to 16 years of age when compared with using enriched preterm formula [12]. Not only do the rate of growth and amount of calories received during the early neonatal period matter, but the content of feeding does as well. A recent study has demonstrated that higher protein intake during the first 5 days of life has been associated with improved growth at 36 weeks of postmenstrual age and more favorable neurodevelopmental outcome at 18 months of corrected age [13]. Preterm infants who are fed breast milk have less risk for hypertension when compared with those who are fed term formula that contains calories similar to breast milk [12]. Feeding an SGA infant can be a challenge. In a randomized controlled trial on a group of term SGA infants, over-nutrition in the early postnatal life was associated with an increased risk for hypertension measured at 6 to 8 years of age [11]. The renal insufficiency known to occur in SGA animal models was successfully ameliorated when protein intake was restricted in the early postnatal life. These SGA animals survived longer with such restricted protein intake [14]. Insulin resistance in SGA rats was exacerbated when offered a high-energy diet post-natally [5]. It seems that SGA infants adapt in-utero to a different diet with low calories and low protein content and are not able to handle the relatively higher protein and calories when offered post-natally. These findings challenge the current concept of overfeeding SGA infants to achieve a catch-up growth. Nutrition of premature infants is a continuously evolving subject in neonatal management. Historically, premature infants have been classified based on BW, as extremely LBW, very LBW, and LBW, for infants weighting < 1000 g, < 1500 g, and <2500 g, respectively. Most of the clinical decisions for the daily management of these infants are based on this weight classification. However, heterogeneity of the population of premature infants, even among the same weight category, is now clearly demonstrated. The most important subgroups to consider are appropriate-for-gestational-age (AGA) and SGA preterm infants [15]. For example, an infant born with a BW of 1500 g but SGA has already undergone unfavorable prenatal programming and most likely has developed a different metabolism. This infant is more likely to respond differently to the nutrition and medical management than an infant born with the same weight of 1500 g but AGA. This concept necessitates a different approach for nutrition and management of these subgroups of infants. Multiple questions emerge on the surface that requires more exploration. What is the optimal quantity of caloric intake? What is the optimal quality or content of this nutrition? How does this optimum differ between AGA and SGA infants? A careful risk-benefit analysis needs to be conducted to determine the optimal type and amount of nutrition offered to infants during the early neonatal period. This will be used to balance the adequate growth and neurodevelopment of infants with the adverse effects of insulin resistance and high blood pressure. It has been proposed that prenatal nutrition, as indexed by BW, has a U-shaped relation with the long-term risk for insulin resistance. Based on this proposal, severe SGA and large-for-gestational (LGA) infants have the highest risk for developing diabetes [16]. We speculate that a similar *U*-shape relationship exists between early postnatal nutritional intake and the future risk of insulin resistance and hypertension (Fig. **2**). Such a U-shaped relation is likely different between AGA and SGA infants. The definition of optimal caloric intake should be redefined based on incidence of long-term complications in addition to current short-term outcomes.

INITIAL GUT FLORA AND THE USE OF PROBIOTICS

The concept that initial gut colonization shortly after birth modulates the immune system opens a wide horizon for investigations. Studies have shown that older children and adults with inflammatory bowel diseases have different bacteria in their colon when compared with the general population [17, 18]. This observation shows the relation between bacteria in the gut and immune system. Over the last five decades, the Western world has achieved substantial control over many infections such as tuberculosis, rheumatic heart disease, and typhoid fever. However, at the same time, a steep surge of autoimmune diseases, such as diabetes and asthma, has evolved [19]. The type of initial microflora depends on genetic factors, mode of delivery, maternal microflora, type of feeding, use of antibiotics, and environmental surroundings. The bacteria in the gut of breast-fed infants have high proportions (90%) of *Bifidobacteria* species, and the guts of formula-fed infants are mostly colonized with coliforms and *Bacteroides* [20]. It is well recognized that infants breast-fed during the first week of life have less risk for development of allergies in childhood compared with formula-fed infants.' Unlike in healthy individuals, the predominance of *Bifidobacteria* species is less likely to occur in the gut of children with atopy. Such difference in gut colonization has been demonstrated in the first week of life in neonates who developed atopy later in their childhood [21]. Children who spent their early infancy in rural areas have much less risk for allergies compared with those who were raised in a "clean" city environment [22]. Alteration of the initial gut bacterial inoculum can produce changes in the immune system. For example, the use of multiple courses of antibiotics during the first 2 years of life is associated with an increased risk for allergies later in life. There is a dose response relationship that shows that the more courses of antibiotics, the more severe the risk and the symptoms of allergies [23, 24, 25]. Delivery *via* caesarian section delays the initial gut colonization, which ordinarily happens when infants pass through the colonized birth canal. Infants born *via* cesarean section have more than a threefold increased risk for development of food allergies when compared with those born vaginally in a population of mothers with a history of allergies [26]. The significance of modulation of gut colonization by probiotics has been a subject of interest in research for decades. Probiotics are defined as nonpathogenic organisms in the food supply that are capable of conferring a health benefit to the host by modifying gut microflora ecology. The use of probiotics has been implemented in multiple pathologies such as, diarrhea, necrotizing enterocolitis (NEC), atopic dermatitis, and allergic rhinitis [20]. A recent systematic review has supported the use of probiotics for prevention of NEC in premature infants. However, it has not become a standard of care yet [27]. Probiotics prevent NEC in premature infants by increasing the favorable microflora at the expense of pathogenic microflora. They also modify the host immune response to these unfavorable bacteria [20].

The effects of probiotics on innate and adaptive immune systems have been repeatedly demonstrated. The major effects on innate immune system include: increased mucin production, competitive inhibition of pathogenic microflora, decreased gut permeability to pathogens, and enhanced activity of natural killer cells, macrophages, and phagocytes [28]. Effects of probiotics on adaptive immune system are characterized by increased number of immunoglobulin (Ig)A-, IgG-, and IgM secreting cells and increased concentrations of total and specific secretory IgA in serum and intestinal lumen. This prevents the adhesion of pathogens to mucosa. The use of probiotics significantly improves the production of serum-specific IgA antibody against polio and *Salmonella typhi* in response to vaccinations [29, 30]. In addition, probiotics can modulate gut inflammatory response by promoting Th-l-type lymphocyte activity and competitive inhibition of Th-2 lymphocyte activity [29]. It is important to realize that in preterm infants, the initial gut colonization is significantly delayed compared with full-term infants. The colonization process is not BW dependent, but rather depends on gestational age. It seems that the colonization of the gut in infants born before 33 weeks of gestation is significantly impaired [31]. Therefore, the use of probiotics not only will modify the colonization but also will provide the beneficial gut microflora for an infant whose gut is too premature. The effectiveness and duration of colonization provided by enteral administration of probiotics are different depending on species and available formulations. The studies have shown that probiotics, administered to infants post-natally provide only short-term gut colonization [32]. However, administration of probiotics to pregnant women during the last trimester has been shown to provide longer colonization of favorable flora in their infants' gut. This flora decreased the risk of atopic dermatitis when these infants were followed at 4 years of age [33, 34]. This option seems to be especially plausible when the infant is born prematurely and is too unstable to initiate enteral nutrition or medications. Meanwhile, a more judicious use of prophylactic and empiric antibiotics will further support the favorable gut colonization and augment its short- and long-term benefits. In a recent study, 256 women were randomized to receive either a probiotic-enriched diet or a regular diet at the first trimester of pregnancy. The study demonstrated a positive effect of probiotics on the metabolic status of their infants at 6 month of age. The proportion of infants with a high split pro-insulin, as an index for insulin resistance, was significantly lower in infants born to the mothers who received a probiotic-enriched diet [35].The increased risk of allergies in infants born *via* cesarean section to mothers with allergies should be considered before justifying the choice for elective cesarean deliveries. Research needs to focus on how to rapidly institute normal gut flora for infants born *via* cesarean section. Of note the relationship between cesarean deliveries and allergies has not been settled yet. A recent study showed a lack of association between the mode of delivery and the development of food allergy, despite an apparent trend for increased cesarean deliveries that was concomitant with an uprising in the incidence of food allergy [36]. Another study compared two cohorts of delivering mothers in the periods of 1993 and 2004, wherein cesarean deliveries significantly increased between the two cohorts and the prevalence of asthma also increased. There was a trend for increased wheezing at four years of age in girls born by cesarean section, however, that was not statistically significant [37].

INTELLIGENCE AND COGNITION IN RESPECT TO GROWTH HORMONE (GH) AND INSULIN-LIKE GROWTH FACTOR-1 (IGF-1) MEDIATED EFFECTS ON THE HUMAN BRAIN.

Intelligence is a property of mind which comprises a set of abilities for abstract thinking, understanding, communicating, learning, reasoning, planning and problem solving. It can be expressed in terms of an intelligence quotient (IQ). Intelligence and cognition is one of the major components of neuro-developmental outcome (NDO). Improvement of NDO of preterm infants and infants born small for gestation is one of the ultimate goals in neonatal management. Excluding prematurity as an independent risk factor for inferior intelligence and cognition, IQ in children born SGA is significantly lower than the IQ in children born AGA [36]. The lower the weight in SGA born infants the lower their IQ. However, the difference doesn't exceed one standard deviation (15 IQ points) [38].

Animal as well as human studies demonstrated the presence of GH and IGF-1 receptors in all cells of the brain. However, in the human brain these receptors are mainly concentrated in the choroid plexus, pituitary, hippocampus, putamen and hypothalamus [39]. The induction of neuronal and glial proliferation and differentiation by GH itself or *via* IGF-1 [39, 40, 41, 42] raises a question whether the exogenous administration of GH to premature and SGA infants will improve their cognition and intelligence? It is known that after birth the most important factor associated with better outcome in respect to intelligence and cognition is the home and school environment, socioeconomic status and parental intelligence [43, 44]. Two studies evaluating the effect of GH treatment on head circumference and IQ scores have been conducted in Europe [38] with contradictory results making the evidence that GH treatment in SGA children has an effect on IQ inconclusive. However, these data is insufficient and the beneficial effect of GH treatment needs to be further explored. Furthermore, treatments that could be related to GH such as the use of insulin to achieve euglycemia in preterm infants should be investigated for its effect on brain development. Especially, as a deleterious effect of glucocorticoids, which are anti-insulin, has become less doubtful in the last decade [45].

OTHER CLINICAL APPLICATIONS

The prenatal and postnatal management of SGA infants in lieu of the programming theory becomes more challenging. It is considered standard practice to allow a fetus with intrauterine growth restriction to grow inside the mother's womb, unless the obstetrician has a distinct indication to deliver the infant prematurely. The presence of reverse blood flow in the umbilical vein or the development of severe maternal complications could be valid reasons for premature delivery. Although postponing prematurity is definitely a noble goal, allowing further delay in the growth of the fetus may program different responses with an increased risk for several diseases. Therefore, fetal programming should be considered when calculating risks and benefits associated with delaying delivery of an SGA infant. Another scenario for possible clinical application of neonatal programming could be the management of patent ductus arteriosus in premature SGA infants. Knowing that kidneys of SGA infants are histologically abnormal, should the approach to medical treatment in these infants be different? Is it safe to administer multiple courses of non-steroidal anti-inflammatory drugs, or should a more cautious regimen be exercised? These are a few clinically applicable examples of fetal-neonatal programming. This concept can be applicable to almost every aspect of management of the newborn infant including exposure to oxygen, procedures, and different environmental stimuli.

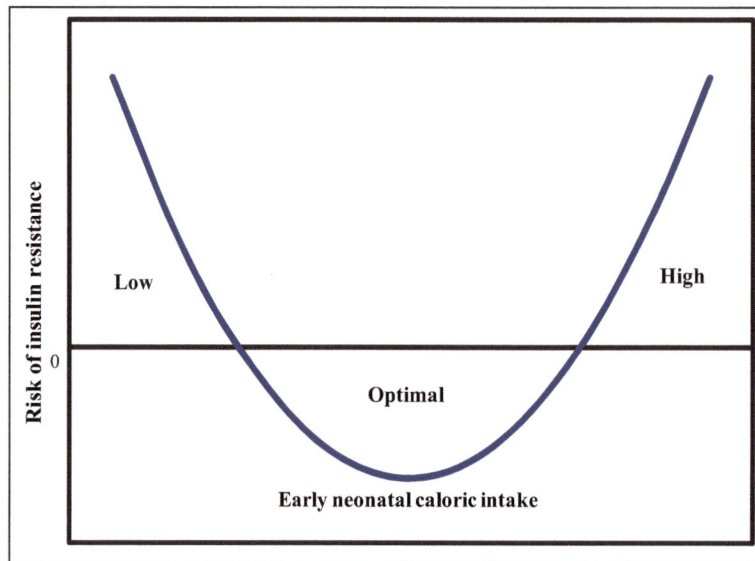

Figure 2: Proposed Relationship Between Caloric Intake in Early Neonatal Life and Development of Insulin Resistance (U-Shaped Model) Later on.

CONCLUSION

There is growing evidence to support the concept of fetal-neonatal programming. Recognition of a unique window of opportunity now exists to prevent or ameliorate the emergence of childhood and adult diseases. Programming during early neonatal life brings higher responsibilities and expectations for neonatologists, not only to stabilize the acutely ill neonates but also to shape their future health as adults. It is plausible that standards of care may change in lieu of fetal-neonatal programming to include interventions that will work to prevent adult diseases. The introduction of any new intervention or therapy should be evaluated carefully not only for its short-term efficacy but also for its possible long-term impact on general health.

ACKNOWLDEGEMENT

Parts of this chapter have been reproduced from reference (1) with permission. There is no financial interest to disclose in relation to this chapter.

REFERENCES

[1]   Nesterenko TH, Aly AZ. Fetal and neonatal programming: evidence and clinical implications. Am J Perinatol 2009; 26(3):191-8.
[2]   De Rooij SR, Painter Re, Holleman F, Bossuyt PM, Roseboom TJ. The metabolic syndrome in adults prenatally exposed to the Dutch famine. Am Clio Nutr 2007; 86: 1219-24.

[3]   Salihu HM, Mbah AK, Alio AP, Kirby RS. ACA-primed uteri compared with SGA-primed uteri and the success of subsequent in utero fetal programming. Obstet Gynecol 2008; 111; 935-43.

[4]   Selling KE, Carstensen], Finstrom 0, Sydsjo G. Intergenerational effects of preterm birth and reduced intrauterine growth: a population-based study of Swedish motheroffspring pairs. BJOC 2006; 113; 430-40.

[5]   Hales CN, Ozanne SE. The dangerous road of catch-up growth. J Physiol 2003; 547; 5-10.

[6]   Ehrenkranz RA, Dusick AM, Vohr HR, Wright LL, Wrage LA, Poole WK. Growth in the neonatal intensive care unit influences neurodevelopmental and growth outcomes of extremely low birth weight infants. Pediatrics 2006; 117:1253-61.

[7]   Hovi P, Andersson S, Ericsson JG, et al. Glucose regulation in young adults with very low birth weight. N Engl Med 2007; 356; 2053-2063.

[8]   DesRobert C, Lane R, Li N, Neu J. Neonatal nutrition and consequences of adult health. Neoreview 2005; 6:211-9.

[9]   Wells]C, Chomtho S, Fewtrell MS. Programming of body composition by early growth and nutrition. Proc Nutr Soc 2007; 66; 423-34.

[10]   Stettler N, Zemel BS, Kumanyika S, Stalling VA. Infant weight gain and childhood overweight status in a multicenter, cohort study. Pediatrics 2002; 109:194-9.

[11]   Singhal A, Cole T, Fewtrell M, et al. Promotion of faster weight gain in infants born small for gestational age: is there and adverse effect on later blood pressure. Circulation 2007; 115; 213-20.

[12]   Singhal A, Fewtrell M, Cole T, Lucas A. Low nutrient intake and early growth for later insulin resistance in adolescents born preterm. Lancet 2003; 361:1089-97.

[13]   Poindexter BB, Langer JC, Dusick AM, Ehrenkranz RA. Early provision of parenteral amino acids in extremely low birth weight infants: relation to growth and neurodevelopmental outcome. J Pediatr 2006; 148:300-5.

[14]   Jennings B, Ozanne SE, Darling MW, Hales CN. Early growth determines longevity in male rats and may be related to telomere shortening in the kidney. FEBS Lett 1999; 448:4-8.

[15]   Thureen PJ. The neonatologist's dilemma: catch-up growth or beneficial undernutrition in very low birth weight infants- what are optimal growth rates? J Pediatr Gastroenterol Nutr 2007; 45:s152-s154.

[16]   Hanson M, Gluckman P, Bier D, et al. Report on the 2nd World Congress on fetal origins of adult disease. Pediatr Res 2004; 55,894-7.

[17]   Giaffer MH, Holdsworth CD, Duerden BI. The assessment of feacal flora in patients with inflammatory bowel disease by a simplified bacteriological technique. J Med Microbial 1991; 35: 238-43.

[18]   Fabia R, Ar'Rajab A, Johanson ML, et al. Impairment of bacterial flora in human ulcerative colitis and experimental colitis in rats. Digestion 1993; 54:248-55

[19]   Bach JF. The effect of infections on susceptibility to autoimmune and allergic diseases. N Engl J Med 2002; 347:911-20.

[20]   Saavedra JM. Use of probiotics in pediatrics: rationale, mechanisms of action, and practical aspects. Nutr Clin Pract 2007; 22:351-3.

[21]   Bjorksten B, Sepp E, Julge K, Voor T, Mikelsaar M. Allergy development and the intestinal microflora during the first year of life. J Allergy Clin Immunol 2001; 108:516-20.

[22]   Raqib R, Alam DS, Sarker P, et al. Low birth weight is associated with altered immune function in rural Bangladeshi children: a birth cohort study. Am Clin Nutr 2007; 85:845-852.

[23]   Farooqi IS, Hopkin JM. Early childhood infection and atopic disorder. Thorax 1998; 53:927-32.

[24]   Wickens K, Pearce N, Crane J, Beasley R. Antibiotic use in early childhood and the development of asthma. Clin Exp Allergy 1999; 29:766-771.

[25]   Von Mutius E, Illi S, Hirsch T, Leupold W, Keil D, Weiland SK. Frequency of infections and risk of asthma, atopy and aitway hyperresponsiveness in children. Eur Respir J 1999; H4-11.

[26]   Eggesbo M, Botten G, Stigum H, Nafstad P, Magnus P. Is delivery by cesarean section a risk factor for food allergy? J Allergy Clin Immunol 2003; 112; 420-6.

[27]   Barclay AR, Stenson B, Simpson JH, Weaver LT, Wilson DC. Probiotics for necrotizing enterocolitis: a systematic review. Pediatr Gastroenterol Nutr 2007; 45:569-76.

[28]   Chiang BL, Sheih YH, Wang LH, Lian CK, Gill HS. Enhancing immunity by dietary consumption of a probiotic lactic acid bacterium (Bifidobacterium lactis HN019): optimization and definition of cellular immune responses. Eur J Clin Nutr 2000; 54:849-55.

[29]   Fukushima Y, Kawata Y, Hara H, Terada A, Mitsuoka T. Effect of probiotic formula on intestinal immunoglobulin A production in healthy children. lnt J Food Microbiol 1998;42:39-44.

[30]   Link-Amster H, Rochat F, Saudan KY, Mignot 0, Aeschlimann JM. Modulation of a specific humoral immune response and changes in intestinal flora mediated through fermented milk intake. FEMS Immunol Med Microbiol 1994; 10:55-63.

[31]   Butel M, Suau A, Campeotto F, *et al.* Conditions of bifidobacterial colonization in preterm infants: a prospective analysis. J Pediatr Gastroenterol Nutr 2007; 44: 577582.

[32]   Fukushima Y, Li S-T, Hara H, Terada A, Mitsuoka T. Effect of follow-up formula containing bifidobacteria (NANBF) on fecal flora and fecal metabolites in healthy children. Biosci Microflora 1997; 16:65-72.

[33]   Kalliomaki M, Salminen S, Arvilommi H, Kero P, Koskinen P, lsolauri E. Probiotics in primary prevention of atopic disease: a randomised placebo-controlled trial. Lancet 2001; 35:H1076-9.

[34]   Kalliomaki M, Salminen S, Poussa T, Arvilommi H, Isolauri E. Probiotics and prevention of atopic disease: 4-year follow-up of a randomized placebo-controlled trial. Lancet 2003; 36: U1869-71.

[35]   Aaltopen J, Ojala T, laitinen K, Poussa T, Ozanne S, Isolauri E. Impact of maternal diet during pregnancy and breastfeeding on infant metabolic programming: a prospective randomized controlled study. Eur J Clin Nutr 2011; 65:10-9.

[36]   Kvenshagen B, Halvorsen R, Jacobsen M. Is there an increased frequency of food allergy in children delivered by caesarean section compared to those delivered vaginally? Acta Paediatr 2009; 98(2):324-27.

[37]   Menezes AM, Hallal PC, Matijasevich AM, *et al.* Caesarean sections and risk of wheezing in childhood and adolescence: data from two birth cohort studies in Brazil. Clin Exp Allergy 2011; 41(2):218-23.

[38]   De Bie HMA, Oostrom KJ, Delemarre-van de Waal HA. Brain development, intelligence and cognitive outcome in children born small for gestational age. Horm Res Paediatr 2010; 73:6-14.

[39]   Harvey S, Hull K. Neural growth hormone: an update. J Mol Neurosci 2003;20:1-14

[40]   Lobie PE, Zhu T, Graichan R Goh EL. Growth hormone, Insulin-like growth factor 1 and the CNS: localization, function and mechanisms of action. Growth Horm IGF Res 200; 10(Suppl B):S51-S56.

[41]   Ajo R, Cacicedo L, Navarro C, Sanchez-Franco F. Growth hormone action on proliferation and differentiation of cerebral cortical cells from fetal rat. Endocrinology 2003; 144:1086-97.

[42]   Russo VC, Gluckman PD, Feldman EL, Werther GA. The insulin-like growth factor system and its pleiotrophic function in brain. Endocr Rev 2005; 26:916-43.

[43]   Theodore RF, Thompson JM, Waldie KE, *et al.* Determinants of cognitive ability at 7 years: a longitudinal case-control study of children born small-for-gestational age at term. Eur J Pediatr 2009; 168:1217-24.

[44]   Sommerfelt K, Andersson HW, Sonnander K, *et al.* Cognitive development of term small for gestational age children at five years of age. Arch Dis Child 2000; 83:25-30.

[45]   Wilson-Costello D, Walsh MC, Langer JC, *et al.* Impact of postnatal corticosteroids use on neurodevelopment at 18 to 22 months' adjusted age: effects of dose, timing, and risk of bronchopulmonary dysplasia in extremely low birth weight infants. Pediatrics 2009; 123(3):e430-7.

CHAPTER 7

Oxidative Stress and its Role in Prepubertal Children

Angelika Mohn[*], Valentina Chiavaroli and Francesco Chiarelli

Department of Pediatrics, University of Chieti, 66013 Chieti, Italy

Abstract: Oxidative stress, occurring as a consequence of imbalance between the production of oxygen free radicals and inactivation of these species by antioxidant defense system, seems to play a pivotal role in the pathophysiology of several diseases. In fact, there are numerous cellular biochemical targets for oxidative stress, all susceptible to long-lasting dangerous effects, especially if they take place early during infancy. Therefore, it is fundamental to obtain data starting in prepuberty to fully explore the intriguing relationship between precocious impairment of the oxidant-antioxidant status and organic alterations, and to preserve prepubertal children to the tracking of disease from infancy to adulthood. Nowadays the identification of children with a highly altered oxidant-antioxidant status is possible through accurate analysis. Much work still needs to be done to offer appropriate treatments aiming to guarantee a good quality of life for the young patients.

Keywords: Non-alcoholic fatty liver disease, type 1 diabetes, advanced glycation endproducts, malonildialdehyde, type 2 diabetes, hepatic steatosis, small for gestational age.

INTRODUCTION

Oxidative stress occurs as a consequence of imbalance between the production of oxygen free radicals and inactivation of these species by antioxidant defense system [1], leading to oxidative damage of lipids, proteins, and DNA. Free radical damage has been recognized as a mechanism playing a pivotal role in the pathophysiology of inflammation, endothelial dysfunction and cardiovascular disease [2-4]. In fact, a strong correlation has been described between oxidative stress and organic alterations, such as diabetes, obesity, growth hormone deficiency, juvenile idiopathic arthritis, asthma and other pathological conditions even during childhood [5-9]. In particular, prepubertal children represent a special study population because the shorter duration combined with better control of diseases eliminates confounding factors commonly present in older subjects, such as adolescents. In fact, it has clearly been demonstrated that puberty, phase of life characterized by relevant physiological hormonal changes, represents a well-known risk factor for developing disorders complications, such as obesity related complications [10]; furthermore, puberty is characterized by several environmental factors (smoking, diet and lifestyle), constituting important elements able to influence precocious impairment of the oxidant-antioxidant status. On the contrary, the prepubertal population offers the exclusive opportunity to abolish the confounding influence of these factors and to untangle whether oxidative stress explicates or not an independent effect. Therefore, it might be of crucial interest to obtain data starting in prepuberty to fully explore the intriguing relationship and to not underestimate the possible role of an impaired oxidant/antioxidant status on the development of many pathological conditions. Nowadays the identification of children with a highly altered oxidant/antioxidant status is possible through accurate analysis. A timely diagnosis is of paramount importance to offer prevention and effective treatments reducing the risk of future disease.

The aim of this chapter is to examine the most important and recent findings regarding the role of oxidative stress in the development of several pathological conditions in children during prepuberty.

OXIDATIVE STRESS AND TYPE 1 DIABETES

Type 1 diabetes (T1D) represents a chronic metabolic disorder characterized by hyperglycemia due to autoimmune destruction of insulin-producing β-cells in the pancreas. Genetic, metabolic, and environmental factors operate together leading to the onset of the disease. The increasing incidence of T1D during infancy and the onset of related complications highlight the importance of therapeutic strategies to prevent and fruitfully manage this pathological condition.

*Address correspondence to Angelika Mohn: Department of Pediatrics, University of Chieti, Via dei Vestini 5, 66013 Chieti; Tel +39 0871 358827; Fax +39 0871 584731; E-mail amohn@unich.it

In patients with T1D chronic hyperglycemia and lipid metabolism alterations produce numerous biochemical effects and early tissue damage in target organs and tissues undergoing insulin-independent glucose uptake, such as eye, kidney, heart, and peripheral nerve [11]. The Diabetic Control and Complications Trial Research Group [12] has recognized that rigorous insulin therapy successfully delays the beginning and the evolution of diabetic complications; however, the most excellent control of glycemic homeostasis does not diminish their occurrence.

Premature micro- and macrovascular disease is one of the most important complications in patients with T1D, representing the main cause of morbidity and mortality in diabetic subjects. The main risk factors for the development of microangiopathy are poor glycemic control and long diabetes duration [12]. Clinically evident diabetes-related microvascular complications are extremely rare in childhood and adolescence. However, early functional and structural abnormalities may be present a few years after the onset of the disease. Chronic hyperglycemia is central in the pathophysiology of microangiopathy and in the evolution of diabetes complications, such as diabetic nephropathy. It sets in motion a series of biochemical disturbances in critical tissue, including the kidney, leading to functional modifications followed by irreversible structural changes [13-15]. Abnormalities of endothelial functions represent the precursor of diabetic angiopathy [16]. In this respect, oxidative stress plays a fundamental role in the pathophysiology of endothelial alterations [17] as diabetic subjects experience a decrease of antioxidant systems [18] with a high production of oxygen reactive species [11]. In fact, chronic hyperglycemia promotes oxidative stress through glucose autoxidation [19], promotion of lipid peroxidation of low density lipoprotein (LDL) by a superoxide-dependent pathway [20,21], nonenzymatic glycation of proteins leading to an increased production of glucose-derived advanced glycation endproducts (AGEs) [22], and activation of NAD(P)H oxidases [23], nitric oxide (NO) synthase [24], and xanthine oxidase [25]. Therefore, oxidative stress following diabetes could be crucial in its progression and complications, including nephropathy [26].

Glucose oxidation is supposed to be the foremost font of oxygen reactive species. Firstly glucose is oxidized from its enediol form into an enediol radical anion, then is transformed into reactive ketoaldehydes and superoxide anion radicals [27]. The superoxide anion radicals undergo further biochemical reactions leading to the production of extremely reactive hydroxyl [19,28] and peroxynitrite radicals [29,30].

Furthermore, among the several pathways able to promote oxidative stress in subjects with diabetes, an interesting and important role is played by the interaction between glucose and proteins, which determines the production of AGEs. In fact, the AGEs/Receptor for AGEs (AGEs/RAGE) system has been proved to be involved in the pathogenesis of diabetic complications [22] as elicits oxidative stress generation and subsequently alters gene expression in various types of cells [31,32]. RAGE is a multiligand cell-surface receptor expressed in human cells as three major splicing variants [33]. The full-length RAGE and the N-truncated type retained in the plasma membrane. In contrast the third variant, C-truncated and known as endogenous secretory RAGE (esRAGE), lacks cytosolic and trans-membrane domains and is extracellularly secreted [33,34]. The enzymatic cleavage of the full-length cell-surface produces an additional form of extracellularly secreted RAGE, known as soluble RAGE (sRAGE). Both esRAGE as well as sRAGE can be detected in blood serum and are able to bind the circulating ligands, neutralizing their actions. In conditions characterized by high concentrations of the circulating ligands the decoy receptors are reduced drastically revealing the system function [34]. In addition, a continued proteins exposure to reactive species can cause dangerous structural changes, including the production of carbonyl proteins [35] which have cytotoxic effects on cellular metabolism. In general, oxidative and non-oxidative pathways can generate reactive carbonyl complexes from amino acids, lipids and carbohydrates leading to AGEs [36]. This process is named carbonyl stress and is thought to be implicated in the development of diabetes complications [31].

In addition, the polyol pathway accelerates aldose reductase leading to the reduction of NADPH and glutathione peroxidase (GPX), the foremost intracellular antioxidant [37,38].

Although the effects of oxidative stress have extensively been investigated in diabetic adults, the number of similar studies in children with T1D is very restricted and the pathogenic mechanisms of endothelial dysfunction and oxidative stress are not yet clear. Jos *et al.* [39] have previously suggested in young patients with T1D an association among reduced GPX activity and retinopathy. Subsequently, it has been reported in a group of well-controlled T1D subjects, with a median age of 15 years and a median diabetes duration of 5 years, the absence of a reduction into the total antioxidant status, also when patients were categorized according to complications [40]. Furthermore, a decrease in the antioxidant activity and total peroxyl radical-trapping antioxidant parameter was reported in children with T1D in relation to poor glycemic control, suggesting that a defective serum antioxidant status contributes to the increased oxidative stress [41]. In line with these data, Jakus *et al.* [42] reported that increased MDA correlated with AGEs in T1D children with poor glycemic control. Hoeldtke *et al.* [43] investigated whether lipid peroxidation, assessed by malonildialdehyde (MDA) excretion, which indicates the lipid peroxide content of LDL, is associated with oxidative damage to DNA, assessed by 8-hydroxydeoxyguanosine excretion, in patients with early T1D (mean age 20.3 years). The authors demonstrated the presence of oxidative stress in diabetic patients without confirming, however, the oxidative damage in DNA. In line with these data, a cross-sectional study [44] performed in diabetic children and adolescent showed that oxidative stress, assessed by parameters of lipoperoxidation, protein oxidation, and changes in the status of antioxidant defence systems, is present upon early onset of T1D and is increased by early adulthood. Therefore, the authors suggested that decreased antioxidant defences may augment the susceptibility of diabetic children to oxidative damage, leading to the necessity of antioxidant supply to prevent complications during the course of the disease.

Markers of oxidative stress have recently been assessed in a group of prepubertal children with T1D with a median diabetes duration less than 5 years compared to controls [45]. Oxidative stress parameters included advanced oxidation protein products, total peroxyl radical-trapping antioxidant parameter, and isoprostanes. The two groups were similar for weight, height, and metabolic tests, including creatininemia and cholesterol levels; no significant differences were detected between diabetic and control children in terms of oxidative stress markers. The authors concluded that the lack of significant differences between children with T1D and controls suggests that treatment is able to neutralize the increased generation of oxygen free radicals. Furthermore, a recent study was performed to analyze oxidative stress and anti-oxidative defences in children and adolescents with T1D, demonstrating that increased oxidative mechanisms and lipid peroxidation occur at a very early stage of diabetic disease, even if plasma antioxidative defence was not impaired [46]. Furthermore, several authors [47,48] have detected anomalous values of endothelial dysfunction markers in children with T1D without angiopathy. Later, Elhadd *et al.* [49] found in a group of prepubertal children significantly elevated levels of red cell superoxide dismutase (SOD), suggesting an activation of the enzyme as a consequence of early oxidative stress.

Also indexes of antioxidant capacity, such as levels of vitamin E and coenzyme Q10 (CoQ10), a powerful antioxidant with a pivotal role in bioenergetics of mitochondria, have been found to be increased in the presence of poor metabolic control and complications in young patients with T1D [50]. In line with these results, recently Menke *et al.* [5] conducted an open prospective study in children with T1D to evaluate concentrations of CoQ10; the authors detected an increase in plasma concentration and intracellular redox capacity of the antioxidant CoQ10, particularly in children with poor control, as a result of an adaptive body response to oxidative stress in diabetes to neutralize increased reactive oxygen species. Finally, it has recently been demonstrated that in children with T1D, chronic hyperglycemia may act through a mechanism that involves increased NO production and/or action and contributes intrarenal hemodynamic abnormalities, which are detectable by doppler ultrasonography even in early diabetic nephropathy [51].

Further studies are needed to complete clarify the oxidative stress-related T1D effects in order to develop new targets for optimal preventive and therapeutic strategies in young populations.

OXIDATIVE STRESS AND BODY WEIGHT: OBESITY VERSUS LEANNESS

Childhood obesity, defined as body mass index (BMI) higher than 2 standard deviation (SD) for the mean age and gender, is the most prominent chronic problem among youngsters in the United States and European Union [52-54]. The prevalence of childhood obesity has dramatically increased over the last two decades, reaching epidemic proportions [55]. This is of major concern because obesity tracks into adulthood, with only one third of obese boys and one fifth of obese girls able to normalize their BMI during puberty. Furthermore, childhood obesity represents a major health problem worldwide, because excessive body weight is a risk factor for future development of chronic diseases. In fact, the persistence of adult obesity is strongly related to approximately double the risk of cardiovascular disease in adulthood [52-54] with an increased morbidity and mortality, justifying a stricter clinical approach together with intensive intervention programs [56,57]. The earliest signs of coronary heart disease, such as coronary artery fatty streaks, are present even during childhood and rapidly increase through adolescence, particularly in those with elevated BMI [58,59]. The biochemical mechanisms of atherosclerosis have been extensively studied, and it has been demonstrated that oxidative stress plays a central role in its etiology [60-62]. The link between oxidative stress and atherosclerosis derives from the oxidative modifications of LDL, which represents a key step in the generation of foam cells and fatty streaks [63]. Oxidative stress seems to be tightly linked to significantly decreased insulin sensitivity. In fact, it has been suggested that insulin resistance (IR) *per se* or *via* an increased plasma concentration of free fatty acids seems to increase reactive oxygen species production through nicotinamide adenine dinucleotide phosphate oxidase activation [23]. In addition, the major source of oxygen free radical production is adipose tissue, which seems to play a key role for the development of IR and metabolic syndrome [64,65]. In fact, Keaney *et al.* [66] found in the community-based cohort, the Framingham Heart Study, a strong association between markers of oxidative stress and both BMI and waist-to-hip ratio (WHR), implicating adiposity as the main factor and suggesting that a greater fat mass determines a greater degree of oxidative stress. Several studies have clearly demonstrated the tight association between adiposity-related increased IR, oxidative stress, and inflammation in adults as well as in children [67,68]. Impaired insulin sensitivity represents an important promoting factor of atherosclerosis [69] through chronic inflammation and impaired oxidative stress, two mechanisms directly involved in the development of endothelial dysfunction and increased carotid intima media thickness (IMT), an early atherosclerotic change in the arterial wall universally accepted as a cardiovascular risk factor [68,70,71]. Isoprostanes can induce vasoconstriction in many vascular beds, promote platelet aggregation, and support proliferation of vascular smooth muscle cells, and they have been considered important pro-atherogenic factors on the arterial wall [6,72]. Recently the relationship between IMT, IR and oxidant status has been investigated in obese prepubertal children compared to healthy prepubertal subjects [68]; the authors demonstrated that obese children had higher levels of homeostasis model assessment of IR, isoprostanes and high sensitive C-reactive protein as well as an increased IMT than controls. Therefore, early changes in glucose metabolism and an alteration of oxidant-antioxidant status may be present in obese prepubertal children, leading to increase IMT and early cardiovascular disease.

A recent study was performed to determine whether systemic oxidative stress is already increased in severely obese prepubertal children and whether it is modifiable with a dietary restriction-weight loss program [6]. This study represents the first evidence of a significant altered oxidant-antioxidant status in prepubertal children affected by severe obesity, fluctuating in strict relation to a dietary restriction weight loss program. This case-control data clearly showed that lag phase was significantly shorter in obese than in normal-weight children; likewise, a significant difference was found in MDA, which was on average 2-fold greater in obese children. This increased oxidant status was associated with decreased plasma vitamin E levels when compared with control children. These data clearly demonstrate that already prepubertal severely obese children present an altered oxidant status leading to an increased consumption of antioxidant vitamins. In fact, a strong correlation between plasma vitamin E and markers of oxidant status were found, suggesting a significant imbalanced state between oxidative and anti-oxidative systems in obese children. It is alarming that it has been detected such a degree of oxidative imbalance in prepubertal children because the subsequent period of puberty might enhance the given alterations as a result of the relevant hormonal changes associated with puberty, particularly increased IR. Like previous studies in adults [73,74], through a 6-month dietary restriction-weight loss program, the authors found that the reduction of BMI, WHR, and fat mass was associated with a reduction in oxidative stress, leading to values of lag phase and MDA comparable to those of normal-weight children. The relationship between obesity and oxidative stress was additionally supported by a subsequent increase of the latter in relation to weight regain when children returned to a hypercaloric unbalanced diet. This demonstrates that a normalization of the oxidant status in obese children can be obtained, which is extremely important because it suggests that the earliest events of atherogenesis could be reversed without the use of any drugs or antioxidants. However, these data also suggest that a long-term program is of crucial importance when the weight reduction will be maintained over time. These findings raise the question whether the main cause of this fluctuation in oxidative stress is dietary variation *per se* or weight changes. Persistent overnutrition might expose children to excessive production of reactive oxidative species besides increase of fat mass, and thus diet might improve oxidative status through the reduction of the amount of food intake and a change in the food composition [73,75].

Previous studies reported decreased levels of vitamin E in obese children, and it has been suggested that this might be the result of sequestration in adipose tissue and variations in its absorption, availability, and metabolism among individuals [76,77]. Strauss *et al.* [76] documented that levels of lipophilic antioxidants vitamins, such as α-tocopherol and lycopene, were significantly reduced in a group of children with obesity. Also Mohn *et al.* [6] detected significantly lower plasma vitamin E levels in obese patients when compared to normal-weight children, although no significant improvement was found after the 6-month-hypocaloric diet. This result might suggest that the reduction of oxidants is independent of antioxidants, or more probably the antioxidant plasma pool might need a longer period to be reconstituted after the long-term consumption by the high oxidant levels.

However, also constitutional leanness, defined as BMI lower than the 2 SD for the mean age and gender, appears to induce impaired IR, oxidative stress, and chronic inflammation. In fact, Giannini *et al.* [78] have recently demonstrated, for the first time, that both prepubertal lean and obese children showed significantly impaired oxidative status compared with controls, without differences between the obese and lean groups. In fact, oxidative markers in lean children were similar to those detected in obese children, demonstrating similar effects of extremely low or high adipose tissue storage. These results suggest that impaired insulin sensitivity and altered oxidant-antioxidant status, related to adipose tissue depletion, represent key elements for the development of early abnormalities in the arterial wall in lean prepubertal children. These data appear to be supported by previous studies that reported a J-curve phenomenon between prevalence of disease, including cardiovascular complications, and BMI, suggesting a direct role of adiposity on several diseases [79,80]. Therefore, impaired adiposity stores determine an unbalanced endothelial regulation resulting in an increased risk of cardiovascular complications; thus, prepubertal lean and obese children present increased oxidative stress and impaired inflammation and insulin sensitivity, which in turn seem to result in a similar impaired endothelial dysfunction and early sign of atherosclerosis.

In conclusion, prepubertal severely obese children present a highly altered oxidant/antioxidant status, which seems to be completely reversible with dietary restriction and weight loss; both simple interventions should be encouraged and maintained over time to reduce the increased risk of future cardiovascular disease. On the other hand, also prepubertal lean children present increased oxidative stress and impaired inflammation and insulin sensitivity.

A complete elucidation of the adipose tissue-related endocrine outcomes represents an important action on the developing of new goals for therapeutic approach to prevent and restore the adiposity-related impaired status, early in childhood.

OXIDATIVE STRESS AND NAFLD

Non-alcoholic fatty liver disease (NAFLD) is one of the most important emerging liver diseases in obese children and adolescents in developed countries [81], and represents an important risk factor for the development of type 2 diabetes (T2D) and a component of the metabolic syndrome [82]. NAFLD is expected to become one of the most common causes of hepatic disease in children and young adults [83], paralleling the increasing prevalence of childhood obesity. Up to now, contrasting data for the pediatric population have been reported. However, studies from autopsies in children (aged 2-19 years) reported prevalence of fatty liver of 9.6%, with a highest rate of the disease in obese children (38%) [84]. The gold standard for the diagnosis of steatosis and various degrees of hepatic fibrosis is liver biopsy, and none of the non-invasive methods, such as computer tomography, magnetic resonance imaging, or ultrasonography, has been recognized to be able to replace liver biopsy completely, even though they have acceptable sensitivity and specificity [85].

Although a multifactorial pathogenesis for the development of NAFLD has been suggested, both IR and oxidative stress play an important role in the development of liver disease [86]. In fact, in a large cohort-based studies of adult [87,88] and adolescent populations [83,89], it has been demonstrated that IR is an essential requirement for the development of steatosis. Both obesity and IR are responsible for abnormalities in lipid storage and lipolysis in insulin sensitive tissues, leading to an increased fatty acids flux from adipose tissue to the liver [90], especially triglycerides (TG) in the hepatocytes [91]. However, few data on a similar tight correlation between steatosis and IR are available for the prepubertal age group. In fact, in consideration of the shorter duration of obesity associated with a lower degree of adiposity, IR might not be a predominant feature of obesity in this age group. D'Adamo *et al.* [92] demonstrated not only that obese prepubertal children are more IR than controls but also a significant difference in IR indexes between obese children with liver steatosis and those without steatosis. These data support the role of IR-associated hyperinsulinemia in the development of hepatic steatosis. A possible explanation for the relationship between hepatic steatosis and IR is that the reduced insulin sensitivity in adipose tissue determines the suppression of lipolysis by insulin and an increased flux of free fatty acids to the liver [93]. This effect, together with the increased hepatic lipogenesis related to hyperinsulinemia, is responsible for the accumulation of TG in the hepatocytes and for the development of steatosis [91]. Therefore, NAFLD should be recognized as an emerging problem also in prepubertal children affected by severe obesity; the high prevalence of steatosis found is especially worrying as it might be further exacerbated by the influence of puberty.

Furthermore, in a recent study it has been demonstrated that metabolic syndrome is common even among prepubertal obese children, particularly when liver steatosis is included among the diagnostic criteria [94]; therefore, screening for the metabolic syndrome should be performed in this age group and hepatic steatosis should be considered as an additional diagnostic criterion.

Regarding to the role of oxidative stress in the pathogenesis of NAFLD, it is well known that the increased fat deposition within the liver is followed by an excessive fatty acid oxidation. This process generates reactive oxygen species, damaging hepatocytes and causing fibrogenesis due to cytokines. Furthermore, the pro-inflammatory factors seem to be responsible for the progression from NAFLD to the following necro-inflammatory condition named non-alcoholic steatohepatitis (NASH) [95]. In fact, among the potential mediators contributing to NASH, an increased microsomal and peroxisomal oxidation has been included, leading to a high production of reactive oxygen species. Mandato *et al.* [96] have investigated the role of oxidative mediators in pediatric obesity-related NAFLD through the evaluation of antioxidant reserve by quantifying erythrocytic GPX activity, important in protecting cells from lipid peroxidation; the authors found a major GPX activity in children with steatosis than in children without, suggesting that toxic injuries stimulate enzymes during the early phase of steatosis. Furthermore, a recent study has demonstrated that oxidative stress not only has a high prevalence in children diagnosed with biopsy-proven NAFLD but is also related to an augmented severity of steatohepatitis [97]. In addition, there is evidence that esRAGE and sRAGE are reliable biomarkers of liver injury [98]. In this respect, it has recently been documented in a group of obese prepubertal children that both esRAGE and sRAGE levels were significantly lower in children affected by liver steatosis and were independently related to its presence [99]. Therefore, these findings suggest that AGE-RAGE pathway plays an independent role in the development of liver injury, even in this age group.

Life style changes, consisting in weight loss and increased physical activity, represent the primary current approaches for treatment of NAFLD in obese children and adults, although they are recognised to be difficult to be realized. For this reason, many therapies have been proposed for hepatopathic obese subjects. Antioxidants represent a valid treatment to reduce oxidative stress and the evolution from NAFLD to cirrhosis [100]. Among antioxidants, vitamin E has a protective role for cellular membranes against lipid peroxidation, with beneficial effects on transaminase values, and liver inflammation [101]. A recent study performed by Sanyal *et al.* [102] demonstrated that vitamin E therapy was superior to placebo for the treatment of NASH in adults. In this respect, Lavine *et al.* [103] performed an open-label pilot study recruiting obese children with diagnosis of non-alcoholic steatohepatitis to detect the effects of oral vitamin E from 400 to 1200 units/daily for 2-4 months; the author demonstrated that this supplementation was able to normalize alanine aminotransferase values in all obese children. A beneficial effect was also reported by Vajro *et al.* [104] who detected a reduction of transaminase levels in obese children with liver disease adherent to oral vitamin E therapy.

In conclusion, the presented data underlie the importance of screening for metabolic complications of obesity including NAFLD, even in young children, as a misdiagnosis represents a serious risk factor for the development of further persistent and exacerbated metabolic abnormalities. Furthermore, there is an urgent need to elucidate the role of oxidative stress into the development of liver disease in order to identify optimal therapeutic strategies across young population at greater risk.

OXIDATIVE STRESS AND BIRTH WEIGHT

Size at birth has been recognized to be predictive of an increased risk for developing chronic cardio-metabolic diseases later in life [105,106], which represent the long-term effects of an adverse fetal environment leading to permanent metabolic changes [107]. In this respect, there is a large body of evidence showing that children born small for gestational age (SGA), defined as neonates whose birth weight (BW) or birth crown-heel length was at least 2 SD below the mean for gestational age, are known to be at increased risk of adult degenerative disease, such as cardiovascular dysfunction and the metabolic syndrome, a combination of T2D, hypertension, dyslipidemia, and obesity [108]. Most of these dysfunctions are related to rapid postnatal catch-up growth [109]. This phenomenon, described in nearly 90% of subjects born SGA, determines changes in body proportions due to enhanced central fat deposition [110] and leading thereby to a relevant increase of the BMI. This determines changes in insulin sensitivity and is associated with a higher predisposition to develop IR.

In addition, Boney *et al.* [111] demonstrated that children who were large for gestational age (LGA) at birth, defined as neonates whose BW was greater than the 90th percentile for gestational age, and were exposed to an intrauterine environment of either diabetes or maternal obesity, were at increased risk of metabolic syndrome during childhood. Therefore, during intrauterine life, both infants born SGA and LGA experience metabolic derangements leading to adaptive responses and pathophysiological alterations, [112,113] which might predispose them to dangerous consequences.

Impaired insulin sensitivity has been described in normal-weight, prepubertal SGA [114] and LGA children, [115] suggesting that this metabolic alteration might play a key role in linking BW to long-term consequences. Most importantly, in individuals born SGA the development of impaired insulin sensitivity has been found to be significantly independent by confounding factors, such as BMI, age, and family history of diabetes [116]. Interestingly, children born LGA are at risk of developing IR as well [115]. Previous studies have reported a U-shaped relation between fasting insulin levels and size at birth [117,118]. However, in LGA subjects it is still not clear whether IR is due only to genetic factors or also to fetal hyperinsulinemia as a consequence of overt or hidden maternal hyperglycemia [114]. These changes in insulin sensitivity are positively correlated with obesity [119,120]. Evidence from several childhood studies has shown that a high BMI value is a strong predictor for the development of IR during the prepubertal period [121,122]. In fact, it has recently been documented that obese SGA and LGA children have lower insulin sensitivity than obese appropriate for gestational age (AGA) children, defined as neonates whose BW or birth crown-heel length between the 10th to 90th percentile for gestational age; interestingly, the LGA group had higher fasting insulin levels and a worse IR status than SGA children, although no significant differences were observed between these groups [123]. These data underline the strong role of a greater amount of fat mass as an independent factor in exacerbating the pathophysiological background of SGA and LGA children. However, despite the phenomenon of catch-up growth, SGA children tend to remain slimmer than LGA infants throughout early childhood [124]. In fact, infants born LGA frequently experienced an increasing fat accumulation in infancy, reflecting an inherited susceptibility to obesity. As highlighted in previous studies, a critical role seems to be played by an early adiposity rebound, a phenomenon that has been reported in around 30% of LGA children and is strictly associated with larger size in childhood [125,126]. Recently, it has been demonstrated in a cohort of obese children born LGA an increased risk for metabolic syndrome during infancy when compared with AGA children [111].

On the other hand, oxidative stress seems to play a fundamental role in the pathophysiology of size at birth-related effects. Previous studies have assessed the status of oxidative stress in SGA children revealing a high generation of reactive oxygen species strictly related to increased oxidative damage [127,128]. An impaired oxidant-antioxidant status has been found in normal-weight SGA children even during the prepubertal age, suggesting a background oxidative derangement strongly exacerbated by IR induced by catch-up growth [129,130]. In addition, it is well known that oxidant/ antioxidant status is influenced by the obese state. In fact, recent data have demonstrated a strong association between oxidative stress and BMI, implicating adipose tissue as the main factor. In line with these data, a recent study evaluated possible alterations in the oxidant/antioxidant status in prepubertal SGA and LGA children compared with AGA children [123]. This study is the first to show evidence of an independent effect of BW and obesity on increased oxidative stress and IR in prepubertal children born SGA and LGA. In fact, an impaired oxidant/antioxidant status has been documented in normal-weight SGA and LGA subjects. In addition, these data have clearly shown that oxidative stress and IR were even higher in obese SGA and LGA children than obese AGA children. Therefore, a greater fat mass in SGA and LGA subjects leads to a greater degree of impaired oxidant/antioxidant status and insulin sensitivity compared with obese AGA children. Similarly, Park [131] reported that overweight children born with higher birth weight might have altered metabolism of CoQ10 and catalase activity compared to those children with low BW, which may contribute to the resulting risk of the complications related to obesity. The authors also demonstrated that overweight children born full term SGA showed increased ghrelin levels and IR, while overweight children born LGA experienced decreased CoQ10 concentration and catalase activity. In addition, BW was negatively associated with ghrelin, IR, and CoQ10 in overweight children. Although the reasons underlying alterations of the oxidant/antioxidant status remain speculative, there are several hypotheses that might explain the worse oxidant/antioxidant status in these two risk groups. The available data strongly support the hypothesis that normal-weight subjects born SGA and LGA seem to be prone to elevated oxidative stress, most likely because of both an adverse intrauterine environment and the linked reduced insulin sensitivity. The background oxidative derangement related to BW can be further exacerbated by the development of excessive fat mass.

These data underline the importance of careful follow-up of SGA and LGA children to detect the development of metabolic abnormalities during childhood.

OXIDATIVE STRESS AND GROWTH HORMONE DEFICIENCY

Linear growth is a central process during infancy and several biological factors are necessary to guarantee a normal growth. The growth hormone (GH)/insulin-like growth factor-1 (IGF-1) axis is of paramount importance in the complex process of linear growth in children. Their levels fluctuate during the life span: postnatal GH and IGF-1 levels are low but rise before puberty followed by a gradual reduction [132,133].

Growth hormone deficiency (GHD) represents an important endocrine condition affecting about one in 10.000 adults [134]. The prevalence in the pediatric population is almost threefold, being about one in 3000 to one in 4000 [135]. GHD can be due to genetic defects or acquired during infancy as a result of hypothalamic-pituitary tumors, cranial irradiation, infections, or trauma.

The cardiovascular system is an important target organ for both GH and IGF-1. In fact, GHD and low levels of IGF-1 in adults are associated with several atherosclerotic factors including altered body composition [136], IR [137] and dyslipidemia [138], increasing the risk for cardiovascular and cerebrovascular diseases. As oxidative stress plays a central role in the aetiology of atherosclerosis, it has extensively been demonstrated that the increased cardiovascular morbidity and mortality in adults with GH/IGF-1 axis alterations is tightly correlated to enhanced oxidative stress [139,140]. Subjects with GHD experienced lipid profile mutations, including TG enrichment of LDL and production of dense LDL particles characterized by being vulnerable to oxidative modification [141,142] and, consequently, by being extremely atherogenic as support foam cells development into the endothelium [143].

In adults and animal models, the GH/IGF-1 axis seems to play a pivotal role into the regulation of vascular redox homeostasis. In fact, adverse effects have been described on vascular endothelial and smooth muscle cells in laboratory animals and adults with GH/IGF-1 deficiency. A recent study assessed vascular effects of life span-extending peripubertal GH replacement (rGH) therapy in Lewis dwarf rats, model of human GHD having a normal pituitary function except for a selective genetic GH deficiency [144]. The authors demonstrated that peripubertal GH/IGF-1 deficiency has pro-oxidative cellular environment, accelerating vascular impairments later in life; however, a prevention of these adverse vascular effects has been reported by peripubertal rGH therapy with normalization of IGF-1 levels. In the pediatric populations, up to now only one study is available on the relationship between GHD and oxidative stress, performed by Mohn *et al.* [7] who evaluated the presence of oxidant/antioxidant alterations in children with GHD and the effects of 12 months of rGH therapy on the oxidant/antioxidant status. These case-control data have shown that lag phase, index inversely related to oxidative stress, is significantly lower in GH-deficient than in normal children. Likewise, a significant difference was found in MDA, which was twofold greater in GH-deficient children. This increased status of oxidative stress was associated with decreased plasma vitamin E levels when compared with control children. These data suggest that the increased oxidative stress might lead to increased consumption of antioxidant vitamins, demonstrating a significant imbalance between oxidant and antioxidants sterns in GHD children. Through a 12-month rGH trial, further evidence for a cause-and-effect relationship between the GH-deficient state and oxidative stress was obtained. A complete reversion of the altered oxidant /antioxidant status has been detected, together with values of lag phase, MDA and vitamin E reaching levels comparable to those of control children. These results are in agreement with previous data reported by Evans *et al.* [145,146] who demonstrated, in eight GHD adults, a significant increase in lipid-derived free radicals and an improvement in indices of oxidative stress and endothelial function after rGH therapy.

Nonetheless, controversy persists as to whether oxidative stress is a major feature of the pro-atherogenic state of GHD patients as no changes in these parameters have been found before and after GH treatment in one study [147].

However, in the latter report, oxidative stress was studied with electron paramagnetic spectroscopy and, as acknowledged by the authors, methodological differences between studies can lead to different results. The main cause of possible increased oxidative stress in GHD subjects has not been completely elucidated and remains speculative. Nevertheless, it has been proposed that the well-known alteration of the GH-IGF-1 axis in these subjects might cause an increased oxidative load by inducing a dysmetabolic state [136-138] or low IGF-1 levels [148]. However, Mohn *et al.* [7] reported no significant difference in terms of BMI and lipid profile between the two studied groups; therefore, these data might indicate that in these young study population a dysmetabolic state plays a secondary role. On the contrary, the authors found a significant correlation between indices of oxidative stress and IGF-1 levels suggesting, in line with previous studies, that impaired levels of IGF-1 might play the major role in the induction of oxidative stress. In fact, it has widely been demonstrated that low IGF-1 levels are directly responsible for increased production and decreased elimination-of free-radicals. This key role has been proven by two independent *in vivo* studies [149,150] where IGF-1 was found to induce a direct production of NO by endothelial cells and by smooth vascular muscle cells. Moreover, Serri *et al.* [148,151] showed that the lipoprotein lipase mass could be significantly reduced *in vitro* by IGF-1 treatment. The same effect was not observed after exposure to rGH, suggesting that the key role of the proatherosclerotic state of macrophages belongs to the IGF-1 system. This is in agreement with the results of Mohn *et al.* [7], where rGH induced a significant improvement in IGF-1 levels that was associated with a similar trend in markers of oxidant/antioxidant status. In conclusion, this study demonstrates that, as in adults, children who lack GH also have unfavourable alterations in oxidant/antioxidant status, which is easily restored by rGH therapy. Therefore, timely treatment positively influences the levels of GH surrogates, allowing not only growth recovery but also restoration of a normal balance in oxidant/antioxidant load.

Further, larger and longer studies are needed to confirm these data and to establish more fully the effect of GHD on oxidative stress in prepubertal children.

OXIDATIVE STRESS AND JUVENILE IDIOPATHIC ARTHRITIS

Juvenile idiopathic arthritis (JIA) represents the most common rheumatic disorder during infancy and comprises all chronic arthritis of unknown origin beginning before the age of 16 years [152]. Different classification criteria have been suggested to define clinical subsets that could correspond to different diseases [153]. The International League of Associations for Rheumatology (ILAR) provided the most recent classification, which divides patients with JIA in homogeneous subgroups. Three main categories were recognised on the basis of features detectable during the first 6 months of illness: systemic onset JIA (s-JIA), pauciarticular JIA (< 5 joints involved) and polyarticular JIA (> 5 joints involved) [154]. In all these different categories, chronic inflammation of the synovial joints as well as monocytes/macrophages enrollment in the synovial fluid represent the main characteristics, leading to joint damage and disability [155]. Many inflammatory markers have been detected increased in patients with JIA, including tumor necrosis factor (TNF)-alpha, interleukin (IL)-6, IL-12 [156,157], and it has been documented a concomitant rise in the synovial fluid in matrix metalloproteinase (MMP)-2, MMP-3 and MMP-9 [158,159]. An immune cell-mediated pathogenesis has been suggested, with a significant role played by the interaction between genetic and environmental factors. Recently, it has been recognized that oxidative stress is of paramount importance not only in the pathogenic mechanism of JIA, but also in its progression. In fact, in adult patients with inflammatory joint disease it has been observed excessive levels of oxygen free radicals and NO [160]. Furthermore, it has been suggested that inflamed joints, with the alternation of activity and relax, experience cycles of hypoxia-reperfusion leading to a highly reactive species [161-163].

In children with JIA, just few data on oxidative stress are available. One of the first evidence of an impaired oxidant-antioxidant status was reported by Honkanen *et al.* [164] who found low total cholesterol and vitamin E levels in children with JIA when compared to controls, suggesting that defective vitamin E and reduced antioxidant protection contribute to low cholesterol levels. Subsequently, Sklodowska *et al.* [165] confirmed the supposition of an impaired oxidant-antioxidant status in the development of JIA even during childhood, after documenting a significant increase of thiobarbituric acid reactive substances and a significant low antioxidant levels in terms of SOD activity and vitamin E concentrations in JIA children. Araujo *et al.* [166] detected significantly higher MDA and hydroperoxide levels in children with polyarticular and s-JIA when compared to controls; in addition, plasma vitamin E and beta-carotene levels of the JIA children were lower in all JIA types. A further study evaluated both enzymatic and non-enzymatic antioxidant status in children with JIA, documenting significantly reduced albumin, ceruloplasmin, vitamin C, vitamin E as well as erythrocyte SOD and GPX activities concentrations [167]. In 2000 Renke *et al.* [168] assessed free radical reactions in children with different types of JIA, evaluating carbonyl groups' content in plasma proteins; compared to healthy subjects, JIA children showed significantly higher carbonyls levels, especially in patients with high-disease activity than in children with medium- or low-disease activity. In addition, children with oligoarthritis showed lower carbonyls levels than children with systemic and polyarthritis JCA. The authors concluded that carbonyls levels represent a helpful marker of inflammatory process activity in children with diagnosis of JIA.

It has also been suggested an elevated *in situ* NO production in JIA children, supporting the implication of nitrogen and oxygen species in the joint damage in subjects with JIA [169]. In 2006, Zurawa-Janicka *et al.* [170] investigated which fraction of proteins was mostly damaged by oxidative stress, by estimating the carbonyl derivatives of plasma proteins in JIA children. The authors demonstrated that γ-globulins were preferentially oxidized, without involvement of the majority of the other proteins; furthermore, oxidative proteins alterations were linked to the type of JIA. These data could support carbonyls as good markers of inflammatory progression in young patients with different JIA categories. Recently, Brik *et al.* [155] investigated the composition of salivary glands and the antioxidant profile in young patients with JIA. Twenty-two children and adolescents (10 oligoarticular, 7 polyarticular, and 5 systemic-category) and 15 controls were recruited. The authors documented a major increase in antioxidant enzyme activity (peroxidase activity, SOD) both in serum and in saliva of JIA patient; furthermore, children with oligoarticular JIA showed significant damage of salivary glands compared to controls and also to other JIA subjects. In 2010, the same study group [8] confirmed that children with JIA showed a higher salivary antioxidant activity and lower MMP values. In addition, anti-TNF treatment was related to an additional reduction in MMP in JIA children's saliva, whereas an active state of JIA was linked to a further augment in the salivary antioxidant activity. Therefore, it is verisimilar that anti-TNF therapy may modulate the degradation progression through arthritis by inhibition of the activity of MMP.

It has also been investigated whether determination of antioxidant enzyme levels can be used as following marker for immunosuppressive therapy in young patients with JIA. Gotia *et al.* [171] documented low antioxidant enzymes at diagnosis, with a parallel high MDA, SOD and inflammatory tests. In the majority of patients, after 6 weeks of anti-inflammatory therapy, antioxidant enzymes were still low, also in cases that need immunomodulatory activity, in comparison to inflammatory tests that became normal. Furthermore, it has been reported in a year follow-up study that level of plasma protein oxidation products remains higher in children with JIA than controls; however, the lack of further accumulation of plasma protein carbonyls should represent the result of an efficient proteolysis in infancy during anti-inflammatory treatment [172].

In conclusion, further studies are needed to elucidate the oxidative stress-related injury effect as well as to develop high-quality markers helpful in monitoring the clinical treatment of young children suffering from JIA.

OXIDATIVE STRESS AND ASTHMA

Over the past several decades the rates of childhood asthma, a complex chronic inflammatory disorder of the airways, has steadily increased. In fact, the Centers for Disease Control National Surveillance for Asthma [173] revealed that its prevalence in children has risen from 3.5% to 7.5% over a period ranging from 2001 to 2003. Accordingly, the World Health Organization [174] includes asthma among the major chronic disorders representing worldwide public health priorities. The genesis of chronic inflammation of the airway system [175] observed in asthma is characterized by persistent infiltration of eosinophils, T-lymphocytes and mast cells combined with different cytokines. Currently, there is an increasing body of literature on the discovery of those genes coding for proteins involved in inflammation of asthma [176]. Glutathione S-transferase (GST) is a candidate gene due to its role in protection against oxidative stress, as recently demonstrated by Babusikova *et al.* [177] who found that the GST-T1 null genotype was more frequent among asthma patients. Very recently, also Ercan *et al.* [178] reported in a large group of children that asthma was associated with a very strong systemic oxidative stress, that increased in parallel with the severity of the disease; furthermore, the authors reported that, from the GST supergene family, GSTP1 val/val genotype at GSTP1 Ile105Val locus was a significant determinant of the degree of oxidant injury in this population. In this respect, there is a growing evidence that asthma is related to oxidative stress. Many studies have been performed to clarify the association between asthma and oxidative stress, as a high production of reactive oxygen species has been detected in numerous cells in the lungs of asthmatic patients [179]. Consequently, this high pulmonary amount of reactive oxygen species, linked to hyperresponsiveness degree, leads to an impaired oxidant/antioxidant status with exacerbation of inflammation. In this respect, leukotriene B4 and 8-isoprostane concentrations have been found increased in asthmatic children compared to healthy subjects, with differences detected for degrees of asthma severity [180]. The oxidative stress has been investigated not only in the systemic circulation but also locally in the airways system [9]. In fact, children with severe asthma have increased biomarkers of oxidant stress also in the epithelial lining fluid, which are associated with increased formation of glutathione disulfide and a shift in the glutathione redox potential toward the more oxidized state [181]. Also Dut *et al.* [9] detected significantly higher levels of MDA and lower levels of reduced glutathione in asthmatic children compared with controls, without difference between mild and moderate asthmatics. Recently, as severe asthmatic children have poor symptom control and elevated markers of airway oxidative and nitrosative stress, a study has been performed evaluating the relationship between asthma pathology and the depletion of S-nitrosothiols (SNOs) [182]. SNOs represents a class of endogenous airway smooth muscle relaxants, resulting from increased activity of an enzyme that both reduces SNOs to ammonia and oxidizes formaldehyde to formic acid, a volatile carboxylic acid more easily detectable in exhaled breath condensate (EBC) than SNOs. The authors found that EBC formate concentration was significantly higher in the breath of children with asthma than in those without asthma. In addition, among asthmatics, formate was elevated in the breath of those with severe asthma compared to those with mild-to-moderate asthma. It has been suggested that this difference is related to asthma pathology and may be a product of increased catabolism of endogenous S-nitrosothiols. Exhaled NO (eNO) has been shown to tightly reflect this airway inflammation [183] and its fractional concentration in exhaled air (FeNO) has been recently accepted by the PRACTALL Consensus Report for the Diagnosis, Management and Treatment of Childhood Asthma as a logical complementary item in the follow-up of bronchial inflammation [184]. Recent results have indicated that children with elevated FeNO are at increased risk for new-onset asthma, especially if they have no parental history of asthma [185]. In addition, in schoolchildren with asthma the major serum antioxidant albumin levels have been found reduced and associated with increased FeNO, while poorly controlled asthma has been associated with decreased vitamin E levels [186].

Oxidative stress can be not just caused by airway inflammation but is able as well to worsen it [179]. An impaired oxidant/antioxidant status can alter the T helper 1/T helper 2 immune response leading to NF-κβ activation, a key oxidative stress inducible inflammatory marker and potent inducer of pro-inflammatory genes [176]. In fact, an important aspect is the genetic susceptibility to an impaired oxidant/antioxidant status [187], and antioxidant enzymes polymorphisms represent possible and considerable risk factors for airway inflammation. In addition, the exposure of respiratory tract to air pollution and tobacco smoke causes oxidative stress and can trigger asthma, especially in children [176]. In fact, two important risk factors for unfavorable respiratory outcomes are represented by prenatal and postnatal tobacco smoke exposure. In particular, maternal smoking during pregnancy has adverse effects on lung function of infants and children. It has been recently demonstrated that GSTs genes may be especially important during fetal development because they may modify, through proficient detoxification, the effects of *in utero* maternal smoke exposure on AR and lung function in infants during the first year of life [188]. However, it has also been reported that, although the detrimental effect of intrauterine tobacco smoke exposure on childhood lung function are confirmed, there is no strong evidence of modification by maternal genotype for important antioxidant genes, such as GST. Therefore, it has been suggested that adverse effects of fetal exposure to tobacco smoke on the respiratory health of children may be mediated by pathways other than oxidative stress [189].

Some authors have explored the oxidative stress implications regarding therapy. In fact, respiratory diseases are more common in those adults with scarce dietary intake of vegetables, fruit and antioxidants [190,191]. Many studies have investigated the effects of diet on respiratory health during infancy [192-194]. It has been reported that low fish intake represented the most consistent predictor of poor respiratory health, while fruit and vegetable intake showed stronger associations with cough than with wheeze [192]. Gilliland *et al.* [193] found that low intakes of orange and other fruit juices, which were the largest source of vitamin C, were associated with deficits in forced vital capacity and forced expiratory volume in 1 second in boys, evidencing lower lung function levels in children with inadequate dietary antioxidant vitamin intake. Furthermore, as previously shown by several epidemiological studies [192,195], a recent study has demonstrated in children aged 8-13 years that the intake of whole grain products and fish was inversely associated with asthma, suggesting that these products may have a protective effect against asthma in children [194]. However, the supplementation of current pharmacological strategies with dietary interventions, finalized to reduce oxidative stress and prevent or minimize asthma, is not supported by many randomized, placebo-controlled studies [196].

In conclusion, a better understanding of the intricate relationship between asthma and oxidative stress is required to augment the therapeutic approaches.

CONCLUSION

Oxidative stress is strongly implicated in the pathogenesis of many diseases, with deleterious systemic consequences already in young subjects. There are numerous cellular biochemical targets for oxidative stress, all susceptible to long-lasting dangerous effects especially if they take place early during infancy. In fact, childhood per se represents a phase of life of paramount importance, during which many fundamental processes happen. In particular, prepubertal children offer the advantage to have no confounding factors, such as pubertal development and the duration of disease. Furthermore, children who experience adverse systemic events are potentially exposed to a high risk for developing permanent and severe complications, while a timely good metabolic control has long-term beneficial effects. This process has been named "metabolic memory" and refers to diabetic complications, as the concept that early glycemic environment is memorized in target organs and has persistent influence on the progression of T1D and T2D complications [197,198]. Metabolic memory has emerging as a complex process and recent evidence has suggested that oxidative stress plays a central role [199]. In fact, oxygen reactive species are of paramount importance in developing hyperglycemia-related diabetic complications, clarifying why the risk for complications still persists after reaching a good glycemic control. In both human and animal models it has been demonstrated that oxidative stress damages mitochondria, leading to impaired cellular functions for long time. The potential adverse consequences of oxidative stress may concern not only the diabetes status but potentially all disorders characterized by an impaired oxidant-antioxidant status. For this reason, it is fundamental to reduce intracellular exposition of oxidative stress to switch off early the metabolic memory and preserve prepubertal children to the tracking of systemic alterations from infancy to adolescence and, then, to adulthood. Therefore, an early diagnosis of children with a highly altered oxidant/antioxidant status related to organic disease is crucial. Much work still needs to be done to offer appropriate treatments aiming to guarantee a good quality of life for the young patients.

REFERENCES

[1]   Rice-Evans C, Burdon R. Free radical-lipid interactions and their pathological consequences. Prog Lipid Res 1993; 32(1): 71-110.

[2]   Ceconi C, Boraso A, Cargnoni A, Ferrari R. Oxidative stress in cardiovascular disease: myth or fact? Arch Biochem Biophys 2003; 420(2): 217-21.

[3]   Delbosc S, Paizanis E, Magous R, *et al.* Involvement of oxidative stress and NADPH oxidase activation in the development of cardiovascular complications in a model of insulin resistance, the fructose-fed rat. Atherosclerosis 2005; 179(1): 43-9.

[4]   Hansen LL, Ikeda Y, Olsen GS, Busch AK, Mosthaf L. Insulin signaling is inhibited by micromolar concentrations of H(2)O(2). Evidence for a role of H(2)O(2) in tumor necrosis factor alphamediated insulin resistance. J Biol Chem 1999; 274(35): 25078-84.

[5]   Menke T, Niklowitz P, Wiesel T, Andler W. Antioxidant level and redox status of coenzyme Q10 in the plasma and blood cells of children with diabetes mellitus type 1. Pediatr Diabetes 2008; 9(6): 540-5.

[6]   Mohn A, Catino M, Capanna R, Giannini C, Marcovecchio M, Chiarelli F. Increased oxidative stress in prepubertal severely obese children: effect of a dietary restriction-weight loss program. J Clin Endocrinol Metab 2005; 90(5): 2653-8.

[7]   Mohn A, Marzio D, Giannini C, Capanna R, Marcovecchio M, Chiarelli F. Alterations in the oxidant-antioxidant status in prepubertal children with growth hormone deficiency: effect of growth hormone replacement therapy. Clin Endocrinol (Oxf) 2005; 63(5): 537-42.

[8]   Brik R, Rosen I, Savulescu D, Borovoi I, Gavish M, Nagler R. Salivary antioxidants and metalloproteinases in juvenile idiopathic arthritis. Mol Med 2010; 16(3-4): 122-8.

[9]   Dut R, Dizdar EA, Birben E, *et al.* Oxidative stress and its determinants in the airways of children with asthma. Allergy 2008; 63(12): 1605-9.

[10]   Guzzaloni G, Grugni G, Mazzilli G, Moro D, Morabito F. Comparison between beta-cell function and insulin resistance indexes in prepubertal and pubertal obese children. Metabolism 2002; 51(8): 1011-6.

[11]   Wolff SP. Diabetes mellitus and free radicals. Free radicals, transition metals and oxidative stress in the aetiology of diabetes mellitus and complications. Br Med Bull 1993; 49(3): 642-52.

[12]   The Diabetes Control and Complications Trial Research Group. The effect of intensive treatment of diabetes on the development of long-term complications in insulin-dependent diabetes mellitus. N Engl J Med 1993; 329: 977-86.

[13] Chiarelli F, Cipollone F, Romano F, *et al.* Increased circulating nitric oxide in young patients with type 1 diabetes and persistent microalbuminuria: relation to glomerular hyperfiltration. Diabetes 2000; 49: 1258-63.

[14] Danne T, Kordonouri O, Hovener G, Weber B. Diabetic angiopathy in children. Diabet Med 1997; 14: 1012-25.

[15] Larkins RG, Dunlop ME. The link between hyperglycemia and diabetic nephropathy. Diabetologia 1992; 35: 499-504.

[16] Cohen RA. Dysfunction of the vascular endothelium in diabetes mellitus. Circulation 1993; 87: 67-76.

[17] Tesfamariam B. Free radicals in diabetic endothelial dysfunction. Free Radical BioMed 1991; 10: 339-52.

[18] Sinclair AJ, Taylor PB, Lunec J, Girling AJ, Barnett AH. Low plasma ascorbate level in patients with type 2 diabetes mellitus consuming adequate dietary vitamin C. Diabet Med 1994; 11: 893-8.

[19] Wolff SP, Dean RT. Glucose autooxidation and protein modification. The potential role of autoxidative glycosylation in diabetes. Biochem J 1987; 245: 243-50.

[20] Obrosova IG, Van Hysen C, Fathallah L, Cao X, Greene DA, Stevens MJ. An aldose reductase inhibitor reverses early diabetes-induced changes in peripheral nerve function, metabolism and antioxidative defense. FASEB J 2002; 16: 123-5.

[21] Kawamura M, Heinecke JW, Chait A. Pathophysiological concentrations of glucose promote oxidative modification of low density lipoprotein by a superoxidedependent pathway. J Clin Invest 1994; 94(2): 771-8.

[22] Brownlee M, Cerami A, Vlassara H. Advanced glycosylation end products in tissue and the biochemical basis of diabetic complications. N Engl J Med 1988; 318: 1315-21.

[23] Inoguchi T, Li P, Umeda F, *et al.* High glucose level and free fatty acid stimulate reactive oxygen species production through protein kinase C-dependent activation of NAD(P)H oxidase in cultured vascular cells. Diabetes 2000; 49: 1939-45.

[24] Cosentino F, Hishikawa K, Katusic ZS, Luscher TF. High glucose increases nitric oxide synthase expression and superoxide anion generation in human aortic endothelial cells. Circulation 1997; 96: 25-8.

[25] Desco MC, Asensi M, Marquez R, *et al.* Xanthine oxidase is involved in free radical production in type 1 diabetes: protection by allopurinol. Diabetes 2002; 51: 1118-24.

[26] Giugliano D, Ceriello A, Paolisso G. Oxidative stress and diabetic vascular complications. Diabetes Care 1996; 19: 257-67.

[27] Maritim AC, Sanders RA, Watkins JB 3rd. Diabetes, oxidative stress, and antioxidants: a review. J Biochem Mol Toxicol 2003; 17(1): 24-38.

[28] Jiang ZY, Woollard AC, Wolff SP. Hydrogen peroxide production during experimental protein glycation. FEBS Lett 1990; 268(1): 69-71.

[29] Halliwell B, Gutteridge JM. Role of free radicals and catalytic metal ions in human disease: An overview. Meth Enzymol 1990; 186: 1-85.

[30] Hogg N, Kalyanaraman B, Joseph J, Struck A, Parthasarathy S. Inhibition of low-density lipoprotein oxidation by nitric oxide. Potential role in atherogenesis. FEBS Lett 1993; 334(2): 170-4.

[31] Baynes JW, Thorpe SR. Role of oxidative stress in diabetic complications: a new perspective on an old paradigm. Diabetes 1999; 48: 1-9.

[32] Baynes JW. Role of oxidative stress in development of complications in diabetes. Diabetes 1991; 40: 405-12.

[33] Vazzana N, Santilli F, Cuccurullo C, Davì G. Soluble forms of RAGE in internal medicine. Intern Emerg Med 2009; 4: 389-401.

[34] Koyama H, Yamamoto H, Nishizawa Y. RAGE and Soluble RAGE: Potential Therapeutic Targets for Cardiovascular Diseases. Mol Med 2007; 13: 625-35.

[35] Stadtman ER. Protein oxidation and aging. Science 1992; 257: 1220-4.

[36] Martín-Gallán P, Carrascosa A, Gussinyé M, Domínguez C. Biomarkers of diabetes-associated oxidative stress and antioxidant status in young diabetic patients with or without subclinical complications. Free Radic Biol Med 2003; 34(12): 1563-74.

[37] Williamson JR, Chang K, Frangos M, *et al.* Hyperglycemic pseudohypoxia and diabetic complications. Diabetes 1993; 42: 801-13.

[38] De Mattia G, Laurenti O, Bravi C, Ghiselli A, Iuliano L, Balsano F. Effect of aldose reductase inhibition on glutathione redox status in erythrocytes of diabetic patients. Metabolism 1994; 43(8): 965-8.

[39] Jos J, Rybak M, Patin PH, Robert JJ, Boitard C, Thevenin R. Etude des enzymes anti-oxydantes dans le diabète insulino-dépendant de l'enfant et de l'adolescent. Diabete Metab 1990; 16: 498-503.

[40] Willems D, Dorchy H, Dufrasne D. Serum antioxidant status and oxidized LDL in well-controlled young type 1 diabetic patients with and without subclinical complications. Atherosclerosis 1998; 137: S61-4.

[41] Asayama K, Uchida N, Nakane T, *et al.* Antioxidants in the serum of children with insulin-dependent diabetes mellitus. Free Radic Biol Med 1993; 15: 597-602.

[42] Jakus V, Bauerova K, Michalkova D, Carsky J. Values of markers of early and advanced glycation and lipoxidation in serum proteins of children with diabetes mellitus. Bratisl Lek Listy 2000; 101: 484-9.

[43] Hoeldtke RD, Bryner KD, Corum LL, Hobbs GR, Van Dyke K. Lipid peroxidation in early type 1 diabetes mellitus is unassociated with oxidative damage to DNA. Metabolism 2009; 58(5): 731-4.

[44] Domínguez C, Ruiz E, Gussinye M, Carrascosa A. Oxidative stress at onset and in early stages of type 1 diabetes in children and adolescents. Diabetes Care 1998; 21(10): 1736-42.

[45] Gleisner A, Martinez L, Pino R, *et al.* Oxidative stress markers in plasma and urine of prepubertal patients with type 1 diabetes mellitus. J Pediatr Endocrinol Metab 2006; 19(8): 995-1000.

[46] Wittenstein B, Klein M, Finckh B, Ullrich K, Kohlschütter A. Plasma antioxidants in pediatric patients with glycogen storage disease, diabetes mellitus, and hypercholesterolemia. Free Radic Biol Med 2002; 33(1): 103-10.

[47] Khan F, Elhadd TA, Lichfield S, Greene SA, Belch JJF. Cutaneous vascular responses to endothelium dependent and independent vasodilators in children with IDDM. Diabet Med 1996; 13(Suppl. 7): S51.

[48] Belch JJF, Greene SA, Littleford R, Jennings PE, Khan F. Impaired skin blood flow response to heat in children with insulin-dependent diabetes. Int Angio 1996; 15: 189-191.

[49] Elhadd TA, Khan F, Kirk G, *et al.* Influence of puberty on endothelial dysfunction and oxidative stress in young patients with type 1 diabetes. Diabetes Care 1998; 21(11): 1990-6.

[50] Salardi S, Zucchini S, Elleri D, *et al.* High glucose levels induce an increase in membrane antioxidants, in terms of vitamin E and coenzyme Q10, in children and adolescents with type 1 diabetes. Diabetes Care 2004; 27(2): 630-1.

[51] Savino A, Pelliccia P, Schiavone C, *et al.* Serum and urinary nitrites and nitrates and doppler sonography in children with diabetes. Diabetes Care 2006; 29(12): 2676-81.

[52] Rocchini AP. Childhood obesity and a diabetes epidemic. N Engl J Med 2002; 346: 854-5.

[53] Must A, Jacques PF, Dallal GE, Bajema CJ, Dietz WH. Long-term morbidity and mortality of overweight adolescents. A follow-up of the Harvard Group Study of 1922 to 1935. N Engl J Med 1992; 327: 1350-5.

[54] Freedman DS, Kettel Khan L, Dietz WS, Srinivasan SR, Berenson GS. Relationship of childhood obesity to coronary heart disease risk factors in adulthood: the Bogalusa Heart Study. Pediatrics 2001; 108: 712-8.

[55] Chinn S, Rona RJ. Prevalence and trends in overweight and obesity in three cross sectional studies of British Children, 1974-94. BMJ 2001; 322(7277): 24-6.

[56] Laitinen J, Power C, Jarvelin MR. Family social class, maternal body mass index, childhood body mass index, and age at menarche as predictors of adult obesity. Am J Clin Nutr 2001; 74(3): 287-94.

[57] Whitaker RC, Wright JA, Pepe MS, Seidel KD, Dietz WH. Predicting obesity in young adulthood from childhood and parental obesity. N Engl J Med 1997; 337(13): 869-73.

[58] McGill HC, McMahan CA, Malcolm GT, Oalmann MC, Strong JP. Relation of glycohemoglobin and adiposity to atherosclerosis in youth. Pathobiological Determinants of Atherosclerosis in Youth (PDAY) Research Group. Arterioscler Thromb Vasc Biol 1995; 15: 431-40.

[59] Berenson GS, Srinivasan SR, Bao W, Newman WP, Tracy RE, WattigneyWA. Association between multiple cardiovascular risk factors and atherosclerosis in children and young adults. N Engl J Med 1998; 338: 1650-6.

[60] Berliner JA, Heinecke JW. The role of oxidized lipoprotein in atherogenesis. Free Radic Biol Med 1996; 20: 707-27.

[61] Chisolm GM, Steinberg D. The oxidative modification hypothesis of atherogenesis: an overview. Free Radic Biol Med 2000; 28: 1815-26.

[62] Steinberg D, Witzum JL. Is the oxidative modification hypothesis relevant to human atherosclerosis? Circulation 2002; 105: 2107-11.

[63] Yokoyama M. Oxidant stress and atherosclerosis. Curr Opin Pharmacol 2004; 4: 110-5.

[64] Furukawa S, Fujita T, Shimabukuro M, *et al.* Increased oxidative stress in obesity and its impact on metabolic syndrome. J Clin Invest 2004; 114: 1752-61.

[65] Weinbrenner T, Schroder H, Escurriol V, *et al.* Circulating oxidized LDL is associated with increased waist circumference independent of body mass index in men and women. Am J Clin Nutr 2006; 83: 30-5.

[66] Keaney Jr JF, Larson MG, Vasan RS, *et al*; Framingham Study. Obesity and systemic oxidative stress: clinical correlates of oxidative stress the Framingham Study. Arterioscler Thromb Vasc Biol 2003; 23: 434-9.

[67] Raitakari OT, Juonala M, Kahonen M, *et al.* Cardiovascular risk factors in childhood and carotid artery intima-media thickness in adulthood: the Cardiovascular Risk in Young Finns Study. Journal of the American Medical Association 2003; 290: 2277-83.

[68] Giannini C, de Giorgis T, Scarinci A, *et al.* Obese related effects of inflammatory markers and insulin resistance on increased carotid intima media thickness in pre-pubertal children. Atherosclerosis 2008; 197: 448-56.

[69] Yudkin JS. Abnormalities of coagulation and fibrinolysis in insulin resistance. Evidence for a common antecedent? Diabetes Care 1999; 22: C25-30.

[70]   Ford ES. C-reactive protein concentration and cardiovascular disease risk factors in children: findings from the National Health and Nutrition Examination Survey 1999–2000. Circulation 2003; 108: 1053-8.

[71]   Jarvisalo MJ, Harmoinen A, Hakanen M, *et al.* Elevated serum C-reactive protein levels and early arterial changes in healthy children. Arteriosclerosis, Thrombosis, and Vascular Biology 2002; 22: 1323-8.

[72]   Nigro J, Osman N, Dart AM, Little PJ. Insulin resistance and atherosclerosis. Endocrine Reviews 2006; 27: 242-59.

[73]   Dandona P, Mohanty P, Ghanim H, *et al.* The suppressive effect of dietary restriction and weight loss in the obese on the generation of reactive oxygen species by leukocytes, lipid peroxidation, and protein carbonylation. J Clin Endocrinol Metab 2001; 86: 355-62.

[74]   Davi G, Guagnano MT, Ciabattoni G, *et al.* Platelet activation in obese women. JAMA 2002; 288: 2008-14.

[75]   Mohanty P, Hamouda W, Garg R, Aljada A, Ghanim H, Dandona P. Glucose challenge stimulates reactive oxygen species (ROS) generation by leucocytes. J Clin Endocrinol Metab 2000; 85: 2970-3.

[76]   Strauss RS. Comparison of serum concentration of α-tocopherol and β-carotene in a cross-sectional sample of obese and non obese children (NHANES III). J Pediatr 1999; 134: 160-5.

[77]   Kuno T, Hozumi M, Morinobu T, Murata T, Mingci, Tamai H. Antioxidant vitamin levels in plasma and low density lipoprotein of obese girls. Free Radic Res 1998; 28: 81-6.

[78]   Giannini C, de Giorgis T, Scarinci A, *et al.* Increased carotid intima-media thickness in pre-pubertal children with constitutional leanness and severe obesity: the speculative role of insulin sensitivity, oxidant status, and chronic inflammation. Eur J Endocrinol 2009; 161(1): 73-80.

[79]   Adams KF, Schatzkin A, Harris TB, *et al.* Overweight, obesity, and mortality in a large prospective cohort of persons 50 to 71 years old. New England Journal of Medicine 2006; 355: 763-78.

[80]   Pischon T, Boeing H, Hoffmann K, *et al.* General and abdominal adiposity and risk of death in Europe. N Engl J Med 2008; 359: 2105-20.

[81]   Angulo P. Non alcoholic fatty liver disease. N Engl J Med 2002; 346: 1221-31.

[82]   Marchesini G, Brizi M, Bianchi G, *et al.* Nonalcoholic fatty liver disease a feature of the metabolic syndrome. Diabetes 2001; 50: 1844-50.

[83]   Nobili V, Marcellini M, Devito R, *et al.* NAFLD in children: a prospective clinical-pathological study and effect of lifestyle advice. Hepatology 2006; 44: 458-65.

[84]   Schwimmer JB, Deutsch R, Kahen T, Lavine JE, Stanley C, Behling C. Prevalence of fatty liver in children and adolescents. Pediatrics 2006; 118: 1388-93.

[85]   Agawal N, Sharma BC. Insulin resistance and clinical aspects of non-alcoholic steatohepatitis (NASH). Hepatol Res 2005; 33: 92-6.

[86]   Fabbrini E, Sullivan S, Klein S. Obesity and nonalcoholic fatty liver disease: biochemical, metabolic, and clinical implications. Hepatology 2010; 51: 679-89.

[87]   Angelico F, Del Ben M, Conti R, *et al.* Non-alcoholic fatty liver syndrome: a hepatic consequence of common metabolic diseases. J Gastroenterol Hepatol 2003; 18: 588-94.

[88]   Angelico F, Del Ben M, Conti R, *et al.* Insulin resistance, the metabolic syndrome and non-alcoholic fatty liver disease. J Clin Endocrinol Metab 2005; 90: 1578-82.

[89]   Burgert TS, Taksali SE, Dziura J, *et al.* Alanine aminitransferase levels and fatty liver in childhood obesity: associations with insulin resistance, adiponectin, and visceral fat. J Clin Endocrinol Metab 2006; 91: 2487-94.

[90]   Day CP, James OF. Steatohepatitis: a tale of two "hits"? Gastronterology 1998; 114: 842-5.

[91]   Browning JD, Horton JD. Molecular mediators of hepatic steatosis and liver injury. J Clin Invest 2004; 114: 147-52.

[92]   D'Adamo E, Impicciatore M, Capanna R, *et al.* Liver steatosis in obese prepubertal children: a possible role of insulin resistance. Obesity (Silver Spring) 2008; 16(3): 677-83.

[93]   Garg A, Misra A. Hepatic steatosis, insulin resistance, and adipose tissue disorders. J Clin Endocrinol Metab 2002; 87: 3019-22.

[94]   D'Adamo E, Marcovecchio ML, Giannini C, *et al.* The possible role of liver steatosis in defining metabolic syndrome in prepubertal children. Metabolism 2010; 59(5): 671-6.

[95]   Oh MK, Winn J, Poordad F. Review article: diagnosis and treatment of non-alcoholic fatty liver disease. Aliment Pharmacol Ther 2008; 28(5): 503-22.

[96]   Mandato C, Lucariello S, Licenziati MR, *et al.* Metabolic, hormonal, oxidative, and inflammatory factors in pediatric obesity-related liver disease. J Pediatr 2005; 147(1): 62-6.

[97]   Nobili V, Parola M, Alisi A, *et al.* Oxidative stress parameters in paediatric non-alcoholic fatty liver disease. Int J Mol Med 2010; 26(4): 471-6.

[98]   Yilmaz Y. The AGEs-RAGE axis and nonalcoholic steatohepatitis: the evidence mounts. J Gastroenterol 2010; 45: 782-3.

[99]   D'Adamo E, Giannini C, Chiavaroli V, *et al.* What is the significance of soluble and endogenous secretory receptor for advanced glycation end products in liver steatosis in obese pre-pubertal children? Antioxid Redox Signal 2010 [Epub ahead of print].

[100] Barshop NJ, Sirlin CB, Schwimmer JB, Lavine JE. Review article: epidemiology, pathogenesis and potential treatments of paediatric non-alcoholic fatty liver disease. Aliment Pharmacol Ther 2008; 28(1): 13-24.

[101] Bugianesi E, Gentilcore E, Manini R, *et al.* A randomized controlled trial of metformin versus vitamin E or prescriptive diet in nonalcoholic fatty liver disease. Am J Gastroenterol 2005; 100(5): 1082-90.

[102] Sanyal AJ, Chalasani N, Kowdley KV, *et al*, NASH CRN. Pioglitazone, vitamin E, or placebo for nonalcoholic steatohepatitis. N Engl J Med 2010; 362(18): 1675-85.

[103] Lavine JE. Vitamin E treatment of nonalcoholic steatohepatitis in children: a pilot study. J Pediatr 2000; 136(6): 734-8.

[104] Vajro P, Mandato C, Franzese A, *et al.* Vitamin E treatment in pediatric obesity-related liver disease: a randomized study. J Pediatr Gastroenterol Nutr 2004; 38(1): 48-55.

[105] Levy-Marchal C, Jaquet D. Long-term metabolic consequences of being born small for gestational age. Pediatr Diabetes 2004; 5(3): 147-53.

[106] Pietiläinen KH, Kaprio J, Räsänen M, Winter T, Rissanen A, Rose RJ. Tracking of body size from birth to late adolescence: contributions of birth length, birth weight, duration of gestation, parents' body size, and twinship. Am J Epidemiol 2001; 154(1): 21-9.

[107] Reynolds RM, Phillips DI. Long-term consequences of intrauterine growth retardation. Horm Res 1998; 49(suppl 2): 28-31.

[108] Chatelain P. Children born with intra-uterine growth retardation (IUGR) or small for gestational age (SGA): long term growth and metabolic consequences. Endocr Regul 2000; 34: 33-6.

[109] Mericq V, Ong KK, Bazaes R, *et al.* Longitudinal changes in insulin sensitivity and secretion from birth to age three years in small- and appropriate-for-gestational-age children. Diabetologia 2005; 48: 2609-14.

[110] Ong KK, Ahmed ML, Emmett PM, Preece MA, Dunger DB. Association between postnatal catch-up growth and obesity in childhood: prospective cohort study. BMJ 2000; 320: 967-71.

[111] Boney CM, Verma A, Tucker R, Vohr BR. Metabolic syndrome in childhood: association with birth weight, maternal obesity, and gestational diabetes mellitus. Pediatrics 2005; 115(3). Available at: www.pediatrics.org/cgi/content/full/115/3/e290.

[112] McCance DR, Pettitt DJ, Hanson RL, Jacobsson LT, Knowler WC, Bennett PH. Birth weight and non-insulin dependent diabetes: thrifty genotype, thrifty phenotype, or surviving small baby genotype? BMJ 1994; 308(6934): 942-5.

[113] Langer O. Fetal macrosomia: etiologic factors. Clin Obstet Gynecol 2000; 43(2): 283-97.

[114] Sancakli O, Darendeliler F, Bas F, *et al.* Insulin, adiponectin, IGFBP-1 levels and body composition in small for gestational age born non-obese children during prepubertal ages. Clin Endocrinol (Oxf) 2008; 69(1): 88-92.

[115]. Evagelidou EN, Kiortsis DN, Bairaktari ET, *et al.* Lipid profile, glucose homeostasis, blood pressure, and obesity-anthropometric markers in macrosomic offspring of nondiabetic mothers. Diabetes Care 2006; 29(6): 1197-201.

[116] Jaquet D, Gaboriau A, Czernichow P, Levy-Marchal C. Insulin resistance early in adulthood in subjects born with intrauterine growth retardation. J Clin Endocrinol Metab 2000; 85(4): 1401-6.

[117] Murtaugh MA, Jacobs DR Jr, Moran A, Steinberger J, Sinaiko AR. Relation of birth weight to fasting insulin, insulin resistance, and body size in adolescence. Diabetes Care 2003; 26(1): 187-92.

[118] Dabelea D, Pettitt DJ, Hanson RL, Imperatore G, Bennett PH, Knowler WC. Birth weight, type 2 diabetes, and insulin resistance in Pima Indian children and young adults. Diabetes Care 1999; 22(6): 944-50.

[119] Saenger P, Czernichow P, Hughes I, Reiter EO. Small for gestational age: short stature and beyond. Endocr Rev 2007; 28(2): 219-51.

[120] Wang X, Liang L, Junfen FU, Lizhong DU. Metabolic syndrome in obese children born large for gestational age. Indian J Pediatr 2007; 74(6): 561-5.

[121] Yensel CS, Preud'homme D, Curry DM. Childhood obesity and insulin-resistant syndrome. J Pediatr Nurs 2004; 19(4): 238-46.

[122] Hirschler V, Aranda C, Calcagno Mde L, Maccalini G, Jadzinsky M. Can waist circumference identify children with the metabolic syndrome? Arch Pediatr Adolesc Med 2005; 159(8): 740-4.

[123] Chiavaroli V, Giannini C, D'Adamo E, de Giorgis T, Chiarelli F, Mohn A. Insulin resistance and oxidative stress in children born small and large for gestational age. Pediatrics 2009; 124(2): 695-702.

[124] Hediger ML, Overpeck MD, McGlynn A, Kuczmarski RJ, Maurer KR, Davis WW. Growth and fatness at three to six years of age of children born small-or large-for-gestational age. Pediatrics 1999; 104(3). Available at: www.pediatrics.org/cgi/content/full/104/3/e33

[125] Rolland-Cachera MF, Deheeger M, Akrout M, Bellisle F. Influence of macronutrients on adiposity development: a follow up study of nutrition and growth from 10 months to 8 years of age. Int J Obes Relat Metab Disord 1995; 19(8): 573-8.

[126] Whitaker RC, Pepe MS, Wright JA, Seidel KD, Dietz WH. Early adiposity rebound and the risk of adult obesity. Pediatrics 1998; 101(3). Available at: www.pediatrics.org/cgi/content/full/101/3/e5.

[127] Gupta P, Narang M, Banerjee BD, Basu S. Oxidative stress in term small for gestational age neonates born to undernourished mothers: a case control study. BMC Pediatr 2004; 4: 14.

[128] Luo ZC, Fraser WD, Julien P, *et al.* Tracing the origins of "fetal origins" of adult diseases: programming by oxidative stress? Med Hypotheses 2006; 66(1): 38-44.

[129] Lee YS, Chou YH. Antioxidant profiles in full term and preterm neonates. Chang Gung Med J 2005; 28(12): 846-51.

[130] Mohn A, Chiavaroli V, Cerruto M, *et al.* Increased oxidative stress in prepubertal children born small for gestational age. J Clin Endocrinol Metab 2007; 92(4): 1372-8.

[131] Park E. Birth weight was negatively correlated with plasma ghrelin, insulin resistance, and coenzyme Q10 levels in overweight children. Nutr Res Pract 2010; 4(4): 311-6.

[132] Argente J, Barrios V, Pozo J, *et al.* Normative data for insulin-like growth factors (IGFs), IGF-binding proteins, and growth hormone-binding protein in a healthy Spanish pediatric population: age- and sex-related changes. J Clin Endocrinol Metab 1993; 77(6): 1522-8.

[133] Sonntag WE, Lynch CD, Cooney PT, Hutchins PM. Decreases in cerebral microvasculature with age are associated with the decline in growth hormone and insulin-like growth factor 1. Endocrinology 1997; 138(8): 3515-20.

[134] Regal M, Paramo C, Sierra JM. Garcia-Mayor RV. Prevalence and incidence of hypopituitarism in adult Caucasian population in northwestern Spain. Clin Endocrinol 2001; 55: 735-40.

[135] Lindsay R, Feldkamp M, Harris D, Robertson J, Rallison M. Utah growth study: growth standards and prevalence of growth hormone deficiency. J Pediatrics 1994; 125: 29-35.

[136] Salomon F, Cuneo RC, Hesp R, Sonksen PH. The effects of treatment with recombinant human growth hormone on body composition and metabolism in adults with growth hormone deficiency. N Engl J Med 1989; 321: 1797-803.

[137] Johansson J0, Fowelin J, Landin K, Lager I, Bengtsson BA. Growth hormone-deficient adults are insulin-resistant. Metabolism 1995; 44: 1126-9.

[138] Russell-Jones DL, Watts GF, Weissberger A, *et al.* The effect of GH replacement on serum lipids, lipoproteins, apolipoproteins and cholesterol precursors in adult GHD patients. Clin Endocrinol 1994; 41: 345-50.

[139] Thomas AM, Berglund L. Growth hormone and cardiovascular disease: an area in rapid growth. J Clin Endocrinol Metab 2001; 86: 1871-3.

[140] Bulow B, Hagmar L, Mikoczy Z, Nordstrom CH, Erfurth EM. Increased cerebrovascular mortality in patients with hypopituitarism. Clin Endocrinol 1997; 46: 75-81.

[141] O'Neal D, Few FL, Sikaris K, Ward G, Alford F, Best JD. Low density lipoprotein particle size in hypopituitary adults receiving conventional hormone replacement therapy. J Clin Endocrinol Metab 1996; 81: 2448-54.

[142] Tribble DL, Holl LG, Wood PD, Krauss RM. Variations in oxidative susceptibility among six low density lipoprotein subfractions of varying size and density. Atherosclerosis 1992; 93: 189-199.

[143] Ungvari Z, Gautam T, Koncz P, *et al.* Vasoprotective effects of life span-extending peripubertal GH replacement in Lewis dwarf rats. J Gerontol A Biol Sci Med Sci 2010; 65(11): 1145-56.

[144] Steinberg D, Parthasarathy S, Carew TE, Khoo JC, Witzum JL. Beyond cholesterol: modifications of LDL that increase its atherogenicity. N Engl J Med 1989; 320: 915-24.

[145] Evans LM, Davies JS, Goodfellow J, Rees JA, Scanlon MF. Endothelial dysfunction in hypopituitary adults with growth hormone deficiency. Clini Endocrinol 1999; 50: 457-64.

[146] Evans LM, Davies JS, Anderson RA, *et al.* The effect of GH replacement on endothelial function and oxidative stress in adult growth hormone deficiency. Eur J Endocrinol 2000; 142: 254-62.

[147] Smith JC, Lang D, McEneny J, *et al.* Effects of GH on lipid peroxidation and neutrophil superoxide anion-generating capacity in hypopituitary adults with GH deficiency. Clin Endocrinol 2002, 56: 449-55.

[148] Serri 0, Li L, Maingrette F, Jaffry N, Renier G. Enhanced lipoprotein lipase secretion and foam cell formation by macrophages of patients with growth hormone deficiency: possible contribution to increased risk of atherogenesis? J Clin Endocrinol Metab 2004; 89: 979-85.

[149] Tsukahara H, Gordienko DV, Tonshoff B, Gelato MC, Goligorsky MS. Direct demonstration of insulin like growth factor-I-induced nitric oxide production by endothelial cells. Kidney Intern 1994; 45: 598-604.

[150] Boger RH, Skamira C, Bode-Boger SM, Brabant G, von zur Muhlen A, Frolich JC. Nitric oxide may mediate the hemodynamic effects of recombinant growth hormone in patients with acquired growth hormone deficiency. A double-blind, placebo-controlled study. J Clin Investig 1996; 98: 2706-13.

[151] Serri 0, St-Jaques P, Sartippour M, Renier G. Alterations of monocyte function in patients with growth hormone (GH) deficiency: effect of substitutive GH therapy. J Clin Endocrinol Metab 1999; 84: 58-63.

[152] Martini A, Lovell DJ. Juvenile idiopathic arthritis: state of the art and future perspectives. Ann Rheum Dis 2010; 69(7): 1260-3.

[153] Ravelli A, Martini A. Juvenile idiopathic arthritis. Lancet 2007; 369: 767-8.

[154] Petty RE, Southwood TR, Manners P, *et al.* International League of Associations for Rheumatology classification of juvenile idiopathic arthritis: second revision, Edmonton, 2001. J Rheumatol 2004; 31: 390-2

[155] Brik R, Livnat G, Pollack S, Catz R, Nagler R. Salivary gland involvement and oxidative stress in juvenile idiopathic arthritis: novel observation in oligoarticular-type patients. J Rheumatol 2006; 33(12): 2532-7.

[156] Moore TL. Immunopathogenesis of juvenile rheumatoid arthritis. Curr Opin Rheumatol 1999; 11: 377-83.

[157] De Benedetti F, Robbioni P, Massa M, Viola S, Albani S, Martini A. Serum interleukin-6 levels and joint involvement in polyarticular and pauciarticular juvenile chronic arthritis. Clin Exp Rheumatol 1992; 10: 493-8.

[158] Peake NJ, Khawaja K, Myers A, *et al.* Levels of matrix metalloproteinase (MMP)-1 in paired sera and synovial fluids of juvenile idiopathic arthritis patients: relationship to inflammatory activity, MMP-3 and tissue inhibitor of metalloproteinases-1 in a longitudinal study. Rheumatology 2005; 44: 1383-9.

[159] Gattorno M, Vignola S, Falcini F, *et al.* Serum and synovial fluid concentrations of matrix metalloproteinases 3 and its tissue inhibitor 1 in Juvenile Idiopathic Arthritis. J Rheumatol 2002; 29: 826-31.

[160] Vasanthi P, Nalini G, Rajasekhar G. Status of oxidative stress in rheumatoid arthritis. Int J Rheum Dis 2009; 12(1): 29-33.

[161] Halliwell B. Oxygen radicals, nitric oxide and human inflammatory joint disease. Annals of the Rheumatic Diseases 1995; 54: 505-10.

[162] Merry P, Grootveld M, Lunec J, Blake D R. Oxidative damage to lipids within the inflamed human joint provides evidence of radical-mediated hypoxicreperfusion injury. Am J Clin Nutr 1991; 56: 362-9S.

[163] Simonini G, Matucci Cerinic M, Cimaz R, *et al.* Evidence for immune activation against oxidized lipoproteins in inactive phases of juvenile chronic arthritis. J Rheumatol 2001; 28(1): 198-203.

[164] Honkanen VE, Pelkonen P, Konttinen YT, Mussalo-Rauhamaa H, Lehto J, Westermarck T. Serum cholesterol and vitamins A and E in juvenile chronic arthritis. Clin Exp Rheumatol 1990; 8(2): 187-91.

[165] Sklodowska M, Gromadzińska J, Biernacka M, *et al.* Vitamin E, thiobarbituric acid reactive substance concentrations and superoxide dismutase activity in the blood of children with juvenile rheumatoid arthritis. Clin Exp Rheumatol 1996; 14(4): 433-9.

[166] Araujo V, Arnal C, Boronat M, Ruiz E, Domínguez C. Oxidant-antioxidant imbalance in blood of children with juvenile rheumatoid arthritis. Biofactors 1998; 8(1-2): 155-9.

[167] Ashour M, Salem S, Hassaneen H, *et al.* Antioxidant status in children with juvenile rheumatoid arthritis (JRA) living in Cairo, Egypt. Int J Food Sci Nutr 2000; 51(2): 85-90.

[168] Renke J, Popadiuk S, Korzon M, Bugajczyk B, Wozniak M. Protein carbonyl groups' content as a useful clinical marker of antioxidant barrier impairment in plasma of children with juvenile chronic arthritis. Free Radic Biol Med 2000; 29(2): 101-4.

[169] Lotito AP, Muscará MN, Kiss MH, *et al.* Nitric oxide-derived species in synovial fluid from patients with juvenile idiopathic arthritis. J Rheumatol 2004; 31(5): 992-7.

[170] Zurawa-Janicka D, Renke J, Popadiuk S, *et al.* Preferential immunoglobulin oxidation in children with juvenile idiopathic arthritis. Scand J Rheumatol 2006; 35(3): 193-200

[171] Goţia S, Popovici I, Hermeziu B. Antioxidant enzymes levels in children with juvenile rheumatoid arthritis. Rev Med Chir Soc Med Nat Iasi 2001; 105(3): 499-503.

[172] Renke J, Szlagatys A, Hansdorfer-Korzon R, *et al.* Persistence of protein oxidation products and plasma antioxidants in juvenile idiopathic arthritis. A one-year follow-up study. Clin Exp Rheumatol 2007; 25(1): 112-4.

[173] Moorman JE, Rudd RA, Johnson CA, *et al.* Centers for Disease Control and Prevention (CDC). MMWR Surveill Summ 2007; 56; 1-54.

[174] World Health Organization. Preventing chronic diseases: a vital investment. Geneva, Switzerland,WHO, 2005.

[175] Visser M, Bouter LM, McQuillan GM, Wener MH, Harris TB. Elevated C-reactive protein levels in overweight and obese adults. JAMA 1999; 282: 2131-5.

[176] Dozor AJ. The role of oxidative stress in the pathogenesis and treatment of asthma. Ann N Y Acad Sci 2010; 1203: 133-7.

[177] Babusikova E, Jesenak M, Kirschnerova R, Banovcin P, Dobrota D. Association of oxidative stress and GST-T1 gene with childhood bronchial asthma. J Physiol Pharmacol 2009; 60 Suppl 5: 27-30.

[178] Ercan H, Birben E, Dizdar EA, *et al.* Oxidative stress and genetic and epidemiologic determinants of oxidant injury in childhood asthma. J Allergy Clin Immunol 2006; 118(5): 1097-104.

[179] Riedl MA, Nel AE. Importance of oxidative stress in the pathogenesis and treatment of asthma. Curr Opin Allergy Clin Immunol 2008; 49-56.

[180] Caballero Balanzá S, Martorell Aragonés A, Cerdá Mir JC, *et al.* Leukotriene B4 and 8-isoprostane in exhaled breath condensate of children with episodic and persistent asthma. J Investig Allergol Clin Immunol 2010; 20(3): 237-43.

[181] Fitzpatrick AM, Teague WG, Holguin F, Yeh M, Brown LA. Severe Asthma Research Program. Airway glutathione homeostasis is altered in children with severe asthma: evidence for oxidant stress. J Allergy Clin Immunol 2009; 123(1): 146-152.e8.

[182] Greenwald R, Fitzpatrick AM, Gaston B, Marozkina NV, Erzurum S, Teague WG. Breath formate is a marker of airway S-nitrosothiol depletion in severe asthma. PLoS One 2010; 5(7): e11919.

[183] Payne DN, Adcock IM, Wilson NM, Oates T, Scallan M, Bush A. Relationship between exhaled nitric oxide and mucosal eosinophilic inflammation in children with difficult asthma, after treatment with oral prednisolone. Am J Respir Crit Care Med 2001; 164: 1376-81.

[184] Bacharier LB, Boner A, Carlsen K-H, *et al.* European Pediatric Asthma Group. Diagnosis and treatment of asthma in childhood: a PRACTALL Consensus Report. Allergy 2008; 63: 5-34.

[185] Bastain TM, Islam T, Berhane KT, *et al.* Exhaled nitric oxide, susceptibility and new-onset asthma in the children's health study. Eur Respir J 2011; 37(3): 523-31.

[186] Bakkeheim E, Mowinckel P, Carlsen KH, Burney P, Lødrup Carlsen KC. Altered oxidative state in schoolchildren with asthma and allergic rhinitis. Pediatr Allergy Immunol. 2011; 22(2): 178-85.

[187] London SJ. Gene-Air pollution interactions in asthma. Proc Am Thor Soc 2007; 4: 217-20.

[188] Murdzoska J, Devadason SG, Khoo SK, *et al. In utero* smoke exposure and role of maternal and infant glutathione s-transferase genes on airway responsiveness and lung function in infancy. Am J Respir Crit Care Med 2010; 181(1): 64-71.

[189] Henderson AJ, Newson RB, Rose-Zerilli M, Ring SM, Holloway JW, Shaheen SO. Maternal Nrf2 and gluthathione-S-transferase polymorphisms do not modify associations of prenatal tobacco smoke exposure with asthma and lung function in school-aged children. Thorax 2010; 65(10): 897-902.

[190] Shaheen SO, Sterne JA, Thompson RL, *et al.* Dietary antioxidants and asthma in adults: population-based case-control study. Am J Respir Crit Care Med 2001; 164: 1823-8.

[191] Patel BD, Welch AA, Bingham SA, *et al.* Dietary anti-oxidants and symptomatic asthma in adults. Thorax 2006; 61: 388-93.

[192] Antova T, Pattenden S, Nikiforov B, *et al.* Nutrition and respiratory health in children in six Central and Eastern European countries. Thorax 2003; 58: 231-6.

[193] Gilliland FD, Berhane KT, Li YF, *et al.* Children's lung function and antioxidant vitamin, fruit, juice, and vegetable intake. Am J Epidemiol 2003,158; 576-84.

[194] Tabak C, Wijga AH, de Meer G, *et al.* Diet and asthma in Dutch school children (ISAAC-2). Thorax 2005; 61: 1048-53.

[195] Nafstad P, Nystad W, Magnus P, *et al.* Asthma and allergic rhinitis at 4 years of age in relation to fish consumption in infancy. J Asthma 2003; 40: 343-8.

[196] Riccioni G, Barbara M, Bucciarelli T, di Ilio C, D'Orazio N. Antioxidant vitamin supplementation in asthma. Ann Clin Lab Sci 2007; 37(1): 96-101.

[197] Ceriello A, Ihnat MA, Thorpe JE. Clinical review 2: The "metabolic memory": is more than just tight glucose control necessary to prevent diabetic complications? J Clin Endocrinol Metab 2009; 94(2): 410-5.

[198] Nathan DM, Cleary PA, Backlund JY, *et al.* Diabetes Control and Complications Trial/Epidemiology of Diabetes Interventions and Complications (DCCT/EDIC) Study Research Group. Intensive diabetes treatment and cardiovascular disease in patients with type 1 diabetes. N Engl J Med 2005; 353; 2643-53.

[199] Ihnat MA, Thorpe JE, Kamat CD, *et al.* Reactive oxygen species mediate a cellular 'memory' of high glucose stress signalling. Diabetologia 2007; 50: 1523-31.

CHAPTER 8

Maternal and Fetal Metabolic Dysfunction in Pregnancy Diseases Associated with Vascular Oxidative and Nitrative Stress

Marcelo González[1,2], Ernesto Muñoz[1], Carlos Puebla[1], Enrique Guzmán-Gutiérrez[1], Fredi Cifuentes[1,3], Jyh K Nien[4], Fernando Abarzúa[1,5], Andrea Leiva[1], Paola Casanello[1] and Luis Sobrevia[1,*]

[1]*Cellular and Molecular Physiology Laboratory (CMPL) and Perinatology Research Laboratory (PRL), Division of Obstetrics and Gynecology, School of Medicine, Faculty of Medicine, Pontificia Universidad Católica de Chile, P.O. Box 114-D, Santiago, Chile;* [2]*Vascular Physiology Laboratory, Department of Physiology, Faculty of Biological Sciences, Universidad de Concepción, Concepción, Chile;* [3]*Experimental Physiology Laboratory, Department of Biomedicine, Faculty of Health Sciences, Universidad de Antofagasta, Antofagasta, Chile;* [4]*Department of Obstetrics and Gynecology, Clínica Dávila, Santiago, Chile and* [5]*Division of Obstetrics and Gynecology, School of Medicine, Faculty of Medicine, Pontificia Universidad Católica de Chile, Santiago, Chile*

Abstract: Molecular mechanisms are increasingly being reported allowing a better understanding of the mother health and fetal metabolic abnormalities in pregnancies that are affected by diseases. Most aspects of cellular function are regulated by a tuned equilibrium between the ability of cells to synthesize oxidants and antioxidants, and preventing the formation or blocking the actions of antioxidants. Oxidative and nitrative stresses are causative agents in human pregnancy-related disorders, including preeclampsia, intrauterine growth restriction, pre-gestational and gestational diabetes and premature delivery. An equilibrium between abundance and/or activity of reactive oxygen (ROS) and nitrogen (RNS) derived species, and antioxidant and nitrative enzyme systems are crucial in gestation. Hydrogen peroxide and superoxide radicals as well as NADPH oxidase and nitric oxide synthases (NOS) play significant contributions to maintain this physiological equilibrium in the human fetoplacental endothelium. Alterations in this relationship lead to abnormal cell function, where the endothelium is one of the targeted cells affected by these pathological conditions. Thus, altered ROS and RNS production, *i.e.*, over the physiological permitted levels, leads to altered endothelial function, a phenomenon associated with endothelial dysfunction in pregnancy diseases. This chapter briefly reviews general aspects of oxidative and nitrative stress in the vasculature in diseases of pregnancy, and a role to NADPH oxidase, NOS and adenosine is summarized.

Keywords: Placental dysfunction, pregnancy-related disorders, oxidative and nitrative stresses, fetal metabolic abnormalities, preeclampsia, intrauterine growth restriction, pre-gestational diabetes, gestational diabetes, endothelial dysfunction in pregnancy.

INTRODUCTION

A large number (~15%) of the women who get pregnant will develop complications leading to maternal or fetal vital risk. More than 500 thousand women die each year in the world due to complications during their pregnancies or at delivery. The perinatal diseases with major impact are intrauterine growth restriction (IUGR), pre-eclampsia (PE), preterm delivery (PTD), diabetes mellitus and gestational diabetes (GD). The incidence of these pathologies varies between 2-15%, with evident consequences for clinical care (*i.e.*, assistance) and social support (*i.e.*, familiar aspects and quality of life) of patients. The etiology of these pathologies is multiple, but unfortunately a significant number of these diseases are idiopathic, with not a clear cause.

Placental dysfunction is a common condition for several of these pregnancy diseases, where altered placental function is associated particularly with vascular and endothelial dysfunction, and/or a local condition limiting oxygenation to the developing fetus [1-6]. Even when the existence of alterations in the placenta in these pathologies is known, there is no concluding information regarding the intrinsic mechanisms of the etiology. This is potentially

---

*Address correspondence to Luis Sobrevia: Cellular and Molecular Physiology Laboratory (CMPL), Division of Obstetrics and Gynecology, School of Medicine, Pontificia Universidad Católica de Chile, P.O. Box 114-D, Santiago, Chile; Tel: +562-3548118; Fax: +562-6321924; E-mail: sobrevia@med.puc.cl

evidenced in the unequal therapeutical approach that is at present used to treat patients with these pregnancy-related pathologies associated with placental dysfunction.

The normal development of the placenta is crucial to sustain the adequate fetal development and growth. The human feto-placental circulation under physiological conditions exhibits a high blood flow and low vascular resistance. Since it lacks of autonomic innervation [7,8], circulating and locally released vasoactive molecules, such as nitric oxide (NO), are crucial to maintain the control of feto-placental hemodynamics [5,6]. The alteration in this process, where the placental function is not preserved, referred as 'placental dysfunction', leads to different clinical manifestations of diseases of pregnancy diagnosed alone or associated with other diseases in a same patient, leading to multiple clinical possibilities, maternal and/or fetal symptoms, as well as different short and long term prognosis.

Oxidative stress has been suggested as a causative agent in human pregnancy-related disorders, such as embryonic resorption, recurrent pregnancy loss, PE, IUGR and fetal death [5, 9]. It has been suggested that reactive oxygen species (ROS) and antioxidant enzyme systems are important for reproduction and gestation. For example, hydrogen peroxide (H_2O_2) and superoxide radicals, such as the superoxide anion ($O_2^{\bullet-}$), play important roles in the control of uterine contraction [10,11], and in implantation and development of the fetus. In these phenomena a fine regulation of ROS levels by oxidases and antioxidant enzymes activity in cells from placental tissues is seen. Several markers of oxidative stress like higher levels of pro-inflammatory cytokines, 8-isoprostane, H_2O_2 and $O_2^{\bullet-}$ in the plasma and the placenta have been detected in PE [9]. Although measurements of markers of oxidative stress in maternal blood and urine show that pregnancy *per se* is a state of oxidative stress, this is heightened in pregnancies complicated by PE, IUGR or diabetes [3, 5]. Placenta production of $O_2^{\bullet-}$ is increased in PE and there is evidence for an increase in $O_2^{\bullet-}$ production in the placenta that is dependent on homologues of the cytochrome subunit of the phagocyte NADPH oxidase (NOX) [12]. Nox1 and Nox5 isoforms of the NOX family were initially cloned in human trophoblast, and the expression of these isoforms increased in the syncytiotrophoblast, vascular endothelium and estromal cells of the placenta in PE [5,13], suggesting that these isoforms could be required for the state of 'oxidative stress' in this pathology [3, 5]. In addition to ROS, it has been shown that in maternal circulating leucocytes from 16th week of gestation there is an elevation of nitrative stress. The prolonged nitrative stress in GD patients may be involved in the development of carbohydrate intolerance later in life or in the development of late cardiovascular complications [14]. In patients with GD or PE there is a decrease in the antioxidant defense paralleled by increased levels of protein oxidation markers associated with oxidative stress [15]. In addition, in placental endothelial cells from PE there is a decrease in the expression of the inducible NO synthase (iNOS) isoform related with high levels of extracellular adenosine and oxidative stress. This phenomenon could be involved in the reduced placental blood flow in PE where a pivotal role seems to be played by vascular macro and microvascular endothelium [3, 4, 6].

Vascular Function and Reactive Oxygen (ROS) and Nitrative (RNS) Species

Endothelial cells are involved in regulation of vascular tone through the release of vasoactive substances, such as prostacyclins (PGI_2) [16], endothelin-1 [17] and NO [16,18]. The broad functions of NO include regulation of vascular tone, cell proliferation, vascular remodeling, inflammation and thrombotic balance [19,20]. In other hands, ROS are important vascular signaling molecules or mediators of oxidative stress [21]. ROS modulate signaling of growth factors and transcription factors controlling gene expression associated with proliferation, differentiation and apoptosis. Under normal physiological conditions, ROS degradation by antioxidant enzymes is enough to maintain a controlled activation of signaling cascades (Fig. **1**).

ROS include a number of highly chemically reactive molecules including $O_2^{\bullet-}$, hydroxyl radical ($^{\bullet}OH$), peroxide radicals ($ROO^{\bullet}$), carbon monoxide (CO), and certain non-radicals molecules that are either oxidizing agents and are easily converted into radicals, such as hypochlorous acid (HOCl), ozone (O_3), singlet oxygen ($^1O_2$) and hydrogen peroxide (H_2O_2) [22]. The $O_2^{\bullet-}$ can be synthesized by NOX, xanthine oxidoreductase (XOR), complexes I and III of the electron transport chain, uncoupled NOS [19], heme-oxygenase (HO), the P_{450} enzymes family and enzymes of the arachidonic acid metabolism [23]. NOS synthesize $O_2^{\bullet-}$ only when adopt the "uncoupled" form due to several conditions including reduced availability of cofactors such as tetrahydrobiopterine (BH_4) (Fig. **1**).

In addition, reactive nitrative species (RNS) relates mainly to $NO^{\bullet}$, which is synthesized by NOS in normal conditions, but depending on its environment, it can be transformed into other species such nitrosonium cation

(NO$^+$), nitroxyl anion (NO$^-$) and peroxynitrite (ONOO$^-$) [24]. The latter could also be considered as ROS since is the product of a reaction between NO and O$_2$$^{\bullet-}$. Similarly, there are several antioxidant systems that control the potential damage that could produce an environment of oxidative stress. Non-enzymatic antioxidant mechanisms are important in the defense or protection against the deleterious effects of oxidative agents. Examples of these molecules include ascorbic acid (vitamin C), α-tocopherol (vitamin E) and glutathione (GSH). GSH is the major cellular redox buffer and its intracellular concentration is in mM range [25]. In addition, cells express enzyme systems to control oxidative stress, such as superoxide dismutase (SOD), which converts O$_2$$^{\bullet-}$ into H$_2$O$_2$ and O$_2$. SOD uses metals as cofactors (Zn and Cu in the cytoplasm, and Mn in the mitochondria). Glutathione peroxidase (GPx) catalyzes the reduction of H$_2$O$_2$ oxidizing GSH to oxidized glutathione (GSSG), which oxidizes cysteine residues of proteins [26], a modification referred as *S*-glutathiolation. Catalase (CAT) metabolizes H$_2$O$_2$ to form O$_2$ and H$_2$O. Thus, cells handle abnormal increases in ROS under stress conditions; however, in pathological circumstances the antioxidant capacity is exceeded by oxidative stress leading to cell damage.

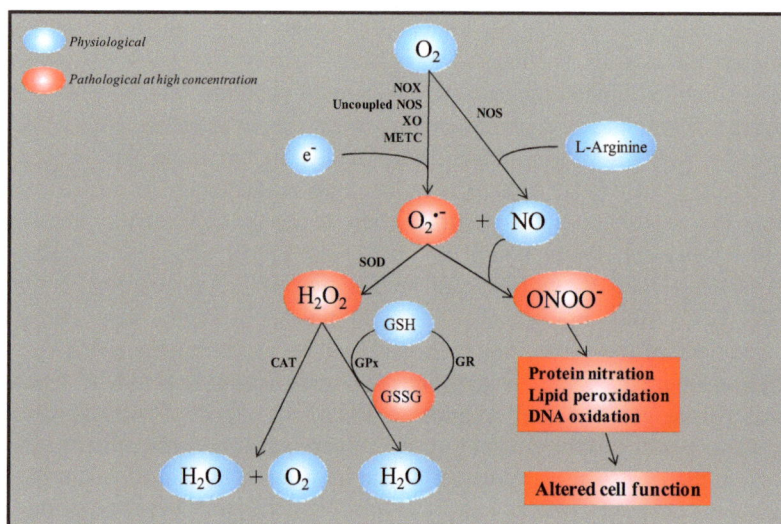

Figure 1: Enzyme systems involved in the generation and control of oxidative and nitrative stress. Overproduction of superoxide anion (O$_2$$^-$) by NADPH oxidases (NOX), uncoupled nitric oxide synthase (NOS), xanthine oxidase (XO) and mitochondrial electron transport chain (METC) and further reaction with nitric oxide (NO) results in the formation of peroxynitrite (ONOO-), which changes several molecules in the cell leading to altered cell function. On the other hand, O$_2$$^{\bullet-}$ accumulation is avoided by the action of superoxide dismutase (SOD) that converts it into hydrogen peroxide (H$_2$O$_2$), which is finally degraded into water by catalase (CAT) and glutathione cycle system preventing cell damage. Light blue shows a physiological condition, while red refers to pathological conditions due to abnormally elevated levels. GSH, glutathione; GSSG, glutathione disulfide; GPx, glutathione peroxidase; GR, glutathione reductase.

SYNTHESIS OF ROS IN THE VASCULAR ENDOTHELIUM

Among all sources of endothelial ROS, NOX are the only enzymes whose primary function is the generation of ROS and play an important role in redox signaling [27]. The activity of NOX may cause uncoupling of eNOS as a secondary effect to the oxidative degradation of tetrahydrobiopterin (BH$_4$), leading to the synthesis of O$_2$$^{\bullet-}$ in detrimental of NO synthesis [28,29], a phenomena implicated in hyperglycemia-associated oxidative stress [30] (Fig. **2**).

Once synthesized, O$_2$$^{\bullet-}$ it is used as a substrate by SOD to generate H$_2$O$_2$ which has greater stability and capacity to cross biological membranes and act as a modulator of signal transduction pathways [31]. In addition, the O$_2$$^{\bullet-}$ reacts rapidly with NO to generate ONOO$^-$ [32], a powerful oxidizing agent that induces DNA fragmentation and lipid oxidation [33]. Currently, it is postulated that the mechanism by which oxygen 'hijack' the NO plays a central role in the development of endothelial dysfunction in diseases such as diabetes mellitus [34-36], PE [3,37] and hypertension [38]. In diabetes, it has been reported that activation of NOX is dependent of the protein kinase C (PKC) activation [39], advance glycation-end products (AGEs) and angiotensin II [30]. The mechanism by which NOX-derived ROS causes biological effects include stimulation of angiogenesis [40], activation of phospholipase A$_2$ [41], and increased PKC [42] and nuclear factor κB (NFκB) [43] activity.

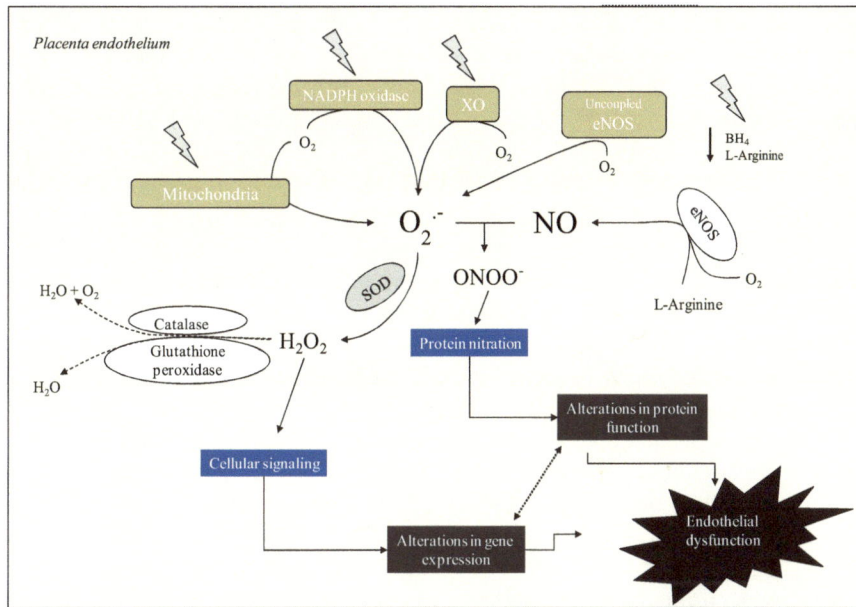

Figure 2: Sources of oxidative stress in the human fetoplacental endothelium. In endothelium exposed to a stressful situation (grey arrows) there is an up regulation of NADPH oxidase and xanthine oxidase (XO), increased mitochondrial activity and/or altered (uncoupling) function of the endothelial nitric oxide synthase (eNOS) due to reduced supplementation of tetrahydrobiopterin (BH$_4$) or L-arginine. This phenomenon leads to increased synthesis of superoxide anion (O$_2^{\bullet-}$) in detrimental of nitric oxide (NO) synthesis. With a physiological L-arginine and cofactors availability to eNOS, this enzyme releases NO, which in the presence of elevated levels of O$_2^{\bullet-}$ is converted into peroxynitrite (ONOO$^-$). The latter is a highly reactive molecule involved in protein nitration leading to altered function in several proteins in vascular endothelium of the human fetoplacental circulation. Alternatively an increase in the activity of superoxide dismutases (SOD) leading to synthesis of a more stable reactive specie, hydrogen peroxide (H$_2$O$_2$), plays a role in regulation of intracellular signaling pathways involved in changes of genes expression modifying expression of proteins involved in redox and NO metabolism. This phenomenon is accelerated if there is a decrease in the activity of catalase and glutathione peroxidase. If these phenomena are chronic, endothelial dysfunction and vascular damage in placental and fetal vessels is the final result.

Several studies indicate that persisting oxidative stress renders endothelial NOS (eNOS) dysfunctional, such that it ceases to produce NO and produces O$_2^{\bullet-}$ instead [19,22]. Pro-oxidant action of NO is attributed to reactive nitrogen intermediates rather than NO itself [9]. In addition to the interaction with NO, ROS have important direct effects through the modulation of diverse redox-sensitive pathways in endothelium [29]. In human umbilical vein endothelial cells (HUVEC), ROS pathway mediated by the activity of NOX is involved in the cellular effect of high extracellular concentration of D-glucose, related with changes in the expression and activity of proteins involved in the L-arginine transport and NO synthesis [44]. The cellular damage induced by ROS in the endothelium generates a reduced bioavailability of NO, leading to endothelial dysfunction [45-48]. If these alterations are maintained for long periods of time (*i.e.*, chronically), endothelial dysfunction resulting of this condition is associated with structural alterations in blood vessels resulting in altered vascular tone, remodeling the vascular wall, platelet aggregation and inflammation. All these phenomena would trigger clinical complications such as myocardial infarction, heart attack, ischemia and cardiac congestive failure [20, 49].

In the vasculature, the major sources of O$_2^{\bullet-}$ come from the activity of membrane and intracellular oxidases (NOX, XOR), mitochondrial activity and the uncoupled eNOS. NOX complexes, the major molecular sources of O$_2^{\bullet-}$, consist of four essential subunits, membrane subunits gp91phox and p22phox and cytosolic subunits p47phox and p67phox; in addition, a cytosolic subunit p40phox has also been described [50]. Among the gp91phox isoforms, there is consensus that Nox2 and Nox4 are expressed in endothelium and that Nox1, Nox2 and Nox4 are expressed in vascular smooth muscle cells (VSMC) [29, 50]. Recently, expression and activity of Nox5 has been reported in endothelium and placental cells [5, 13], but its physiological role in these tissues remains to be established. In arteries from placental chorionic plate, H$_2$O$_2$ causes an increase in vascular tone, an effect blocked by activation of CAT [51]. Also, vitamin C decreases the contractile response of placental vessels to the thromboxane A$_2$ mimetic U46619 [51], a molecule that increases ROS levels, and SOD and CAT activity in vascular smooth muscle cells

[52]. Similar effects has been described in umbilical vein and in the microcirculation of the human placenta, suggesting a potential relation between oxidative stress and changes in the vascular tone leading to vasoconstriction in a mechanism mediated by increases in ROS synthesis from oxidative enzymes and related with higher activity of cellular antioxidant mechanism [5].

SYNTHESIS OF RNS AND PROTEIN NITRATION IN THE VASCULAR ENDOTHELIUM

NO Synthesis

NO is a gas synthesized in endothelial cells from the semi-essential cationic amino acid L-arginine [44, 53], which is transported from the extracellular space into the endothelial cell by a family of cationic amino acid transporters (*i.e.*, CATs) [44, 54-56]. In fact, there is evidence that NOS activity may depend on the ability of endothelial cells to take up its specific substrate L-arginine *via* a variety of membrane transporters systems [44,57-60]. Endothelial cells transport L-arginine through the transport systems y^+, y^+L, $b^{0,+}$ and $B^{0,+}$ [2,44,54,55,57]. NO is synthesized from L-arginine in a metabolic reaction leading to equimolar formation of L-citrulline and NO [53, 55, 61]. This reaction requires the activity of NOS, a group of enzymes conformed by, at least, three isoforms, *i.e.*, neuronal NOS (nNOS or type 1), inducible NOS (iNOS or type 2) and endothelial NOS (eNOS or type 3) [1,44,62]. The NO diffuses from endothelium to vascular smooth muscle cells leading to cyclic GMP (cGMP)-dependent vasodilatation [55, 63]. In vessels without innervations, as the distal segment of the umbilical cord [7, 8], vascular tone is regulated by the synthesis and release of vasoconstrictors and vasodilators from endothelial cells [64,65]. Thus, quiescent endothelial cells express a vasodilator, anticoagulant and anti-adhesive phenotype, whereas endothelial cells exposed to physiological stress have pro-coagulant, pro-adhesive and vasocontractile properties [66]. The reduced ability of the endothelium to stimulate vasodilatation mediated by NO is one of the events that triggers the endothelial dysfunction, which is strongly correlated with cardiovascular risk factors [67] and with early states of chronic diseases such as hypertension, hypercholesterolemia, diabetes mellitus, hyperhomocysteinemia, chronic renal failure, chronic cardiac failure [45-47].

Protein Nitration

Nitronio ion derives from $ONOO^-$ and produces nitration of tyrosine residues in proteins, a reaction used as a marker for $ONOO^-$ formation *in vivo*. A higher abundance of nitrotyrosine in proteins has been described in several diseases, including GD [68] as well as in atherosclerotic lesions of human coronary arteries, post-ischemic heart, and in the placenta of pregnancies with PE [69]. Equally, it has been proposed that cell death by apoptosis in response to high extracellular D-glucose is associated with increased formation of nitrotyrosine in HUVEC [70], and formation of $ONOO^-$ reduces mitochondrial activity in several cell types [53]. Interestingly, adenosine uptake is an essential step protecting mitochondrial function against the deleterious effects of increased $ONOO^-$ in rat astrocytes [71]. Thus, potential alterations induced by $ONOO^-$ on adenosine transport capacity in endothelial cells could be determinant limiting the attributed antioxidant role of adenosine [72-74].

It has been shown that although adenosine did not limit the formation of ROS, this nucleoside decreased the deleterious cellular consequences produced by ROS in rat hippocampus slices [75]. This effect of adenosine occurs *via* different adenosine receptors. In rats a protective effect of the A_1 adenosine receptor agonist phenylisopropyl adenosine (PIA) in brain oxidative stress has been shown [76], and in isolated rat hearts perfused with H_2O_2 a selective protective effect of A_1 adenosine receptor activation with N^6-cyclopentyladenosine (CPA) against the cardiac toxicity of H_2O_2, where the presence of A_{2A} receptor agonist CGS-21680 has no effect, was reported [77]. This antioxidant effect of adenosine is not only in the presence of H_2O_2, since adenosine and A_1 adenosine receptor stimulation with CPA attenuated ischemic intestinal injury *via* decreasing oxidative stress, lowering neutrophil infiltration, and increasing reduced glutathione content [78]. Moreover, in PC12 cells the A_{2A} adenosine receptors activation prevented oxidative stress trough a PKA-dependent pathway, thus possibly playing a role in preventing apoptosis [79]. In the human cell line HK-2 treated with H_2O_2, adenosine protected against H_2O_2-induced injury through the activation of A_1 and A_{2A} adenosine receptors, apparently through different signaling pathways, i.e., A_1 adenosine receptors-associated protection involves pertussis toxin-sensitive G proteins and PKC, whereas A_{2A} adenosine receptors involves PKA [80]. A different signaling pathway is described in adult rat cardiomyocytes, where adenosine protects mitochondria from oxidant damage in response to H_2O_2 through a pathway involving A_{2A} adenosine receptors, Src tyrosine kinase, phosphatidyl inositol 3-kinase (PI3k)/protein kinase B (Akt), eNOS and NO [81]. There is also evidence that adenosine is functionally involved in the regulation of cardiac ROS production under physiological conditions. The knockout mice or pharmacological blockade of the A_{2A} in vivo was associated with cardiac ROS production by NOX through mitogen activated protein kinases (MAPK) activation [82]. The latter group described that inhibition of A_{2A} adenosine receptors with SCH58261, knockdown of A_{2A} adenosine receptors using siRNA in the endothelial cell line SVEC4-10 or using a knockout mice effectively inhibits basal and acute angiotensin II-induced ROS production by Nox2 [83].

Since it has been proposed that extracellular levels of adenosine are mainly maintained in the physiological range by the ability of endothelial cells to take up this nucleoside, nucleoside membrane transporters play a pivotal role in modulating biological effects of this purine nucleoside [1,4,6]. Nucleoside transporters grouped into two families mediate extracellular adenosine removal: equilibrative nucleoside transporters (ENTs) and concentrative nucleoside transporters (CNTs) [1,4,6,84,85]. At present four members of the ENTs family of solute carriers (SLC29A genes) have been cloned from human tissues (i.e., ENT1, ENT2, ENT3 and ENT4). Under physiological conditions, in primary cultures of HUVEC adenosine transport is mainly (~80%) mediated by the human ENT1 (hENT1) [86, 87], and in a minor fraction (~20%) by hENT2 [87,88]. hENT1 is a protein of 456 amino acids, encoded by SLC29A1, with apparent K_m values in the range of 50-200 μM for purine and pyrimidine nucleosides transport. hENT2 is a protein of 456 amino acids, encoded by SLC29A2. In addition to purine and pyrimidine nucleosides, hENT2 also transports nucleobases and exhibits apparent K_m values varying from 40 to 150 μM for adenosine. hENT1-mediated transport is inhibited by <1 μM nitrobenzylmercapto purine riboside (NBMPR) while higher NBMPR concentrations inhibit hENT2-mediated transport [84,87,88].

Separating hENT1- and hENT2-mediated transport from overall adenosine transport has been essential to characterize the kinetic transport parameters of these proteins when co-expressed in mammalian cells. hENT1 and hENT2 proteins exhibit tyrosine residues that are phosphorylated to maintain its transport function [89]. However, it is unknown whether these sites are nitrated and what would be the potential effects of nitration reactions in the transport activity of these proteins [2,6]. The amino acid sequence of hENT1 and hENT2 contain tyrosine residues in the positions Y^{11}, Y^{172}, Y^{232} and Y^{234} for hENT1, and Y^{11}, Y^{159}, Y^{221}, Y^{222} and Y^{350} for hENT2. There are not existing studies addressing the potential nitration of these sites in hENT1 or hENT2 [4,6], thus we would expect that these sites will be nitrated in diseases where NO synthesis is increased, such as GD [1,2,4,6,44]. In addition, whether nitration of tyrosine is a post-translational modification associated with changes in transport function in HUVEC and in human placental microvascular endothelial cells (HPMEC) from pregnancy diseases, including GD and PE, or in cells from normal pregnancies exposed to hypoxia or hyperglycemia is at present a phenomenon without a clear answer. Since adenosine transport mediated *via* hENT1 (and potentially *via* hENT2) is under strong regulation by the activity of PKC and NO in primary cultures of HUVEC [87,88,90-94] it is expected a potential nitration of these cell signaling proteins or other proteins (perhaps the proper membrane transport proteins) in response to activation of these signaling molecules [2,4,6].

OXIDATIVE AND NITRATIVE STRESS IN PREGNANCY DISORDERS INTRAUTERINE GROWTH RESTRICTION (IUGR)

This syndrome is generally defined as the inability of the fetus to reach its potential intrauterine growth, and clinically defined as the estimated fetal weight under the 10th percentile [2]. IUGR has been associated with prenatal disturbances, including fetal asphyxia, prematurity and neurological disabilities. Gathering the available information regarding IUGR-induced long-term morbidity, known as 'fetal programming', we can at this point remark an association of IUGR and chronic diseases such as obesity, dyslipidemia, hypertension, type 2 diabetes and coronary disease. Studies in IUGR and placental dysfunction show that in primary cultures of HUVEC derived from this syndrome there is a reduced uptake of L-arginine [58,88] related to down-regulation of the expression of hCAT-1 (isoform 1 of human CATs) mRNA and protein levels as well as membrane depolarization which represents one of the proposed mechanisms explaining this phenomenon in IUGR. Only recently it has been shown that HUVEC derived from IUGR pregnancies over-express arginase II, an enzyme that also metabolizes L-arginine, leading to a functional competition for this substrate with eNOS, thus reducing NOS activity and NO levels [95]. These results highlight the fact that altered L-arginine transport and NO synthesis in the placenta endothelium may be crucial in the pathophysiological processes involved in the etiology of this disease in human pregnancy.

An elevated oxidative stress level and reduced antioxidant activity has been reported in placentas from pregnancies with IUGR compared with normal pregnancies [2] (Fig. **3**). In the placenta of women with preeclampsia and IUGR there is an increase in nitrated protein tyrosine residues, which is correlated with higher generation of $O_2^{\bullet-}$ forming

ONOO. The ONOO⁻ also causes oxidation of tyrosine residues, changes that could lead to activation, suppression or have no effect on the function of nitrated proteins [96]. To date, it has been reported that nitration of human SOD by ONOO- inhibits its activity [97], but ONOO⁻ inhibits XO activity [98], thereby controlling the synthesis of additional ONOO⁻. These posttranslational modifications might be relevant to placental dysfunction seen in IUGR. However, the relationship between nitrated proteins and impaired placental function is still poorly understood [5]. Interestingly, it has been reported that SOD expression in placentas from pregnancies with IUGR, is not significantly different from placentas from normal pregnancies [99]. Other studies show that IUGR is associated with altered activity of SOD, GPx, CAT and XO in human microvillus tissue explants, in addition to altered levels of these molecules at the fetal and maternal plasma [100]. These findings are complemented with reports suggesting that reduced SOD activity correlates with elevated concentrations of cadmium, arsenic and lead in placenta homogenates from IUGR pregnancies [101]. Interestingly, it has been possible to cause *in vitro* an increase in the formation of syncytial knots by hypoxia and hyperoxia (1 and 20% O_2, respectively) compared with normoxia (6% O_2) or H_2O_2 treatment, which is similar to those observed in placentas from IUGR. Thus, an oxidative stress stage is closely associated with placental dysfunction in IUGR by still not very well characterized mechanisms involving ROS and/or RNS [2, 5, 102].

PRE-ECLAMPSIA (PE)

This syndrome refers to several vascular alterations characterized by maternal hypertension and proteinuria [103]. PE is a cause of maternal mortality, and one of the main causes of perinatal mortality and neurological sequelae as well as prematurity [2,3,5]. PE is characterized by poor perfusion of the maternal and fetal circulations of the placenta, which thus affects fetal growth and development, and, even though it is epidemiologically important, the etiology of preeclampsia has not been clearly established [3,5,104]. PE is characterized by profound dysfunction of the vascular endothelium, a phenomenon that could be secondary to oxidative stress [105]. There is abundant evidence [5, 99, 106, 107] that placental function is altered in PE and reductions in total radical trapping antioxidant capacities such as the scavenger activity of SOD and CAT, glutathione metabolism and/or vitamin E levels, as well as an increase in lipid peroxides, are seen in preeclamptic [108] or diabetic patients [109] together with the presence of nitrotyrosine residues [5] in villous tissue. The placenta may be exposed to intermittent perfusion causing ischemia/reperfusion injury [110] mediated mainly through the generation of cytotoxic ROS [111]. Several studies show increased production of ROS as well as RNS in preeclamptic placenta [112-114], and increased maternal [115-118] and fetal [119-121] plasma level, which is a phenomenon thought to scavenge NO to decrease its bioavailability [103,122] (Fig. **3**). Interestingly, blocking ROS generation would be beneficial in PE improving the deteriorated endothelial function [123], including the fetal and maternal vascular endothelium [2, 3, 6].

Since adenosine plays a key role as a vasoactive molecule leading to local vasodilatation in most vascular beds, including placental vessels [1,4,6] and acts as antioxidant [55,57] a role has also been assigned to this nucleoside in PE [100]. It has been shown that PE is associated with increased plasma adenosine concentration with the subsequent alteration of endothelial cell function due to the biological actions of this nucleoside. Adenosine, likely acting *via* A_{2A} adenosine receptors increases intracellular cAMP level and reduces the nuclear factor κB (NF-κB) binding to *NOS2A* promoter gene leading to reduced transcriptional activity of this gene and reduced expression of iNOS in hPMEC [3]. This phenomenon could explain, at least in part, the reduced placental blood flow characteristic of PE. The impact of the potential role of adenosine on the etiology of PE-induced feto-placental endothelial dysfunction is strengthened when placental hypoxic lesions, a phenomenon well documented as a condition increasing extracellular adenosine [6], are clinically manifested in this pathology. Thus, a mechanism associated with altered adenosine handling by the feto-placental vasculature, particularly at the micro and macrovascular placenta endothelium, has been proposed [4,6]. This concept could be the base for future design and application of new therapeutic protocols considering adenosine and its several biological effects, including its potential as antioxidant (a very poorly documented property) and as pro-angiogenic factor in the placenta, in the critical care of patients with preeclampsia to secure a less stressed development and growth of the fetus.

PRE-GESTATIONAL DIABETES

Pre-gestational diabetes is a state of endothelial dysfunction where ROS and RNS contribute to the progression of diabetes [124,125]. Oxygen-free radicals including $O_2^{•-}$ are thought to result from prolonged periods of exposure to hyperglycemia [44], a condition known to cause non-enzymatic glycation of plasma proteins [126]. The $O_2^{•-}$ in the absence of appropriate levels of scavengers may lead to an imbalance between pro-oxidants and antioxidants and produce a state of oxidative stress [4-6,44]. Diabetes mellitus type 2 (DMT2) is a chronic diseases leading to a high number of deaths resulting from alterations of the endothelial dysfunction, and the World Health Organization, considering the gradual increasing in the rates of obesity, aging and urbanization of world population, estimates that in 2030 the diabetes mellitus prevalence will reach ~4.4% of the world population, increasing the number of people affected by this disease to more than 300 million [127]. In addition, about 2.9 million people die annually from diseases whose origin is attributed to the development of diabetes mellitus, being the vascular diseases the leading cause of morbidity and mortality in these patients [128,129]. Remarkable, it is well known that the development of diabetes in the pregnancy (i.e., gestational diabetes) has repercussion in the development of DMT2 [130,131] or is associated with a high susceptibility to cardiovascular diseases [4,132,133] later in life in both mother and child [2, 4, 6, 134].

The development of cardiovascular disease in diabetic patients is associated with increased oxidative stress [48] caused by higher activity of the enzymes NOX and XOR, together with the uncoupling of eNOS. These phenomena induce cell dysfunction through oxidation of lipoproteins, nucleic acids, carbohydrates and proteins [20, 48, 135]. However, prior to endothelial dysfunction and cardiovascular complications in diabetes mellitus, the greatest risk factor is chronic hyperglycemia [6, 44, 129, 136, 137]. It has been shown that insulin resistance, resulting from hyperglycemia, is present in metabolic and chronic diseases (*i.e.*, obesity, hypertension and metabolic syndrome), which increases the risk for developing cardiovascular events [35]. Clinical studies have shown that the reduction of the hyperglycemia in patients with DMT1 and DMT2 is associated with a delay in the establishment and progression of retinopathy, nephropathy, neuropathy and cardiac complications [138,139].

The main mechanism for endothelial dysfunction induced by diabetes mellitus and high extracellular D-glucose is the oxidative stress resulting from the synthesis of ROS (Fig. 3) [35,140,141].

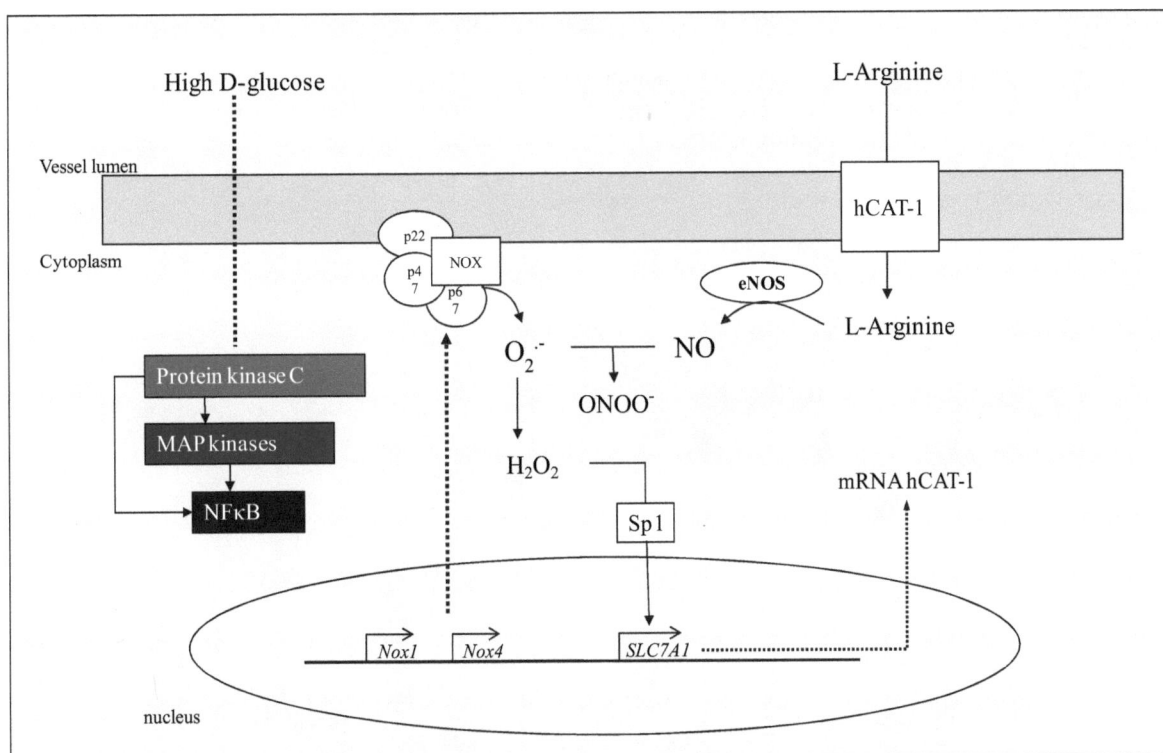

Figure 3: Transcriptional regulation of NADPH oxidase and hCAT-1 in vascular endothelium exposed to high D-glucose. In HUVEC exposed to high extracellular concentrations of D-glucose there is an increased activity of diacylglycerol-dependent isoforms of protein kinases C, mitogen activated protein (MAP) kinases and transcriptional factors such as the nuclear factor kappa B (NFkB), leading to increased NADPH oxidase (NOX) expression and activity mediated by an increase of promoter activity of *Nox1* and *Nox4* genes in human fetoplacental vascular endothelium. A higher level of hydrogen peroxide (H_2O_2) released from NOX activity leads to activation of the general transcription factor specific protein 1 (Sp1). This mechanism induces an increase in the promoter activity of *SLC7A1* gene, leading to increased human cationic amino acid transporter 1

(hCAT-1) expression and higher L-arginine transport and Nitric oxide (NO) synthesis from this amino acid *via* endothelial NO synthase (eNOS). Concomitant to these cellular events, accumulation of nitrogen reactive species (including peroxynitrite ($ONOO^-$)) could be involved in high D-glucose triggered endothelial dysfunction and vascular pathology in the human fetoplacental circulation [44].

It has been established that in vascular endothelium the major source of ROS is the activity of NOX [142], and the intracellular $O_2^{\bullet-}$ is one of the most powerful factors associated with reduction in NO bioavailability induced by D-glucose [143]. In HUVEC, 33 mM D-glucose increases intracellular accumulation of ROS after 48 hours of exposure [144], while 25 mM D-glucose for 24 hours increases the accumulation of ROS and PKC activity [145]. Additionally, the increase in the synthesis of ROS by high D-glucose has been associated with higher L-arginine transport; an effect blocked by co-incubation with insulin or ascorbic acid in HUVEC. The experimental data reported in primary cultures of endothelial and vascular smooth muscle cells from umbilical vessels and from placental vessels, show that high extracellular concentration of D-glucose and gestational diabetes are associated with increased ROS synthesis with detrimental actions of NO, being this mechanism a key factor to the development of endothelial dysfunction [2,6,44].

GESTATIONAL DIABETES

This is a syndrome characterized by glucose intolerance, leading to maternal hyperglycemia, first recognized during pregnancy, associated with abnormal fetal development and perinatal complications, such as macrosomia, neonatal hypoglycemia, and neuroconginitive and behavior disorders [72,146-149]. GD is one of the diseases of pregnancy with highest incidence, depending on the diagnostic criteria used, varying between 3-8% of the total of pregnant women in developing countries [150,151]. The main perinatal complications are late fetal mortality, fetal macrosomia associated with delivery complications, metabolic alterations in the neonatal period such as poliglobulia, hypoglycemia, hypocalcaemia. GD is characterized by abnormal regulation of the vascular tone in placental and fetal tissues. GD also alters adenosine metabolism [152] and leas to abnormal regulation of the vascular tone in placental and fetal tissues [153,154], a phenomenon associated with higher NO synthesis [1,2,86,93]. GD alterations of fetal endothelial function, including reduced adenosine transport and increased NO synthesis, are mimicked by exposure of HUVEC from normal pregnancies to elevated extracellular D-glucose (>5 mM, high D-glucose) [155], a condition associated with increased formation of $O_2^{\bullet-}$ [156]. These findings are thought important in diabetes mellitus where episodes of elevated D-glucose plasma levels can occurs leading to endothelial dysfunction (Fig. **4**).

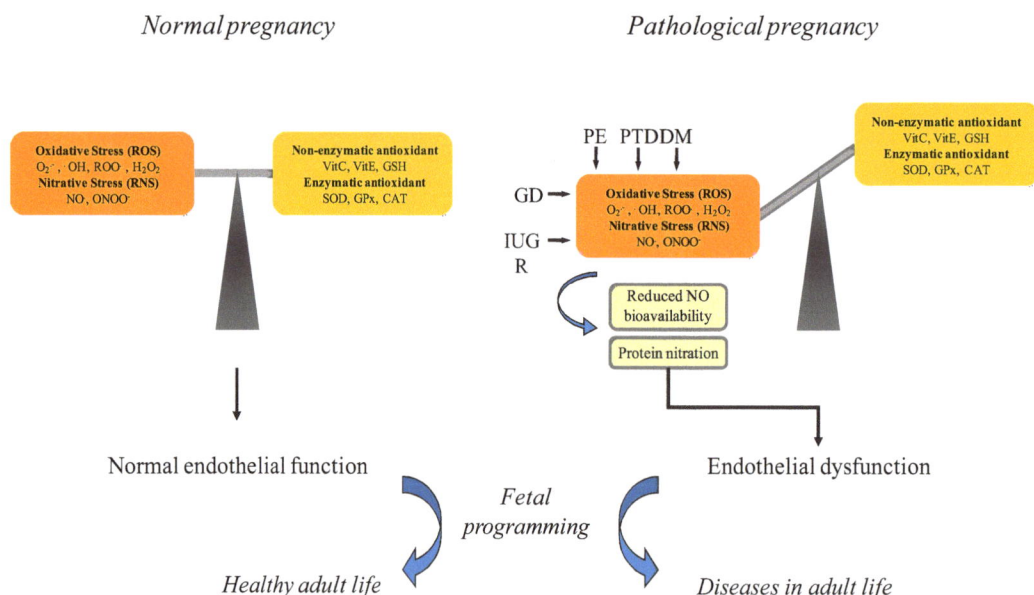

Figure 4: Acute equilibrium between oxidant and antioxidant species in endothelial function. A perfect equilibrium between oxidative (ROS) and nitrative (RNS) reactive species synthesis and bioactivity, and non-enzymatic and enzymatic antioxidant mechanisms are required to maintain a normal function of the endothelium. This phenomenon is considered as the bases of a

programming *in uterus* ('fetal programming') of a healthy state at adult life. When this equilibrium changes due to different factors associated with diseases of pregnancy, such as preeclampsia (PE), preterm delivery (PTD), pre-gestational diabetes mellitus (DM), gestational diabetes (GD) or intrauterine growth restriction (IUGR), a direct consequence is a reduced availability of nitric oxide (NO), therefore limiting its several biological effects, due either to reduced synthesis or increased formation of nitrative reactive species leading to protein nitration. The latter could ends in endothelial dysfunction, characteristic of the mentioned diseases. Following this abnormal cell function an increased risk of developing diseases is expected during the adult life of babies from women with pregnancies affected by these diseases. In this case the concept of fetal programming is validated and becomes crucial. $O_2^{\cdot-}$, superoxide anion; $^{\cdot}OH$, hydroxyl radical; $ROO\bullet$, peroxide radicals; H_2O_2, hydrogen peroxide; NO^-, nitroxyl anion; $ONOO^-$, peroxynitrite, VitC, vitamin C; VitE, vitamin E; GSH, reduced glutathione; SOD, superoxide dismutase; GPx, glutathione peroxidase; CAT, catalase.

GD is associated with oxidative stress [157-159], where an overproduction of ROS and free radicals is characteristic. In this phenomenon in GD, several enzymes are involved including NOX and XO [157], and phenomena such as lipidic peroxidation products (*i.e.*, malondialdehyde, thiobarbituric acid reactive subtances, lipid hydroperoxide), which interrupt the electron flow in the mitochondrial respiratory chain [160-162], and protein oxidation (*i.e.*, carbonylation, nitration of tyrosine and methionine sulphoxide formation) leading to proteolytic degradation [163]. In addition, RNS derived from NO leads to nitration and nitrosilation of several molecules, including DNA nitration leading to apoptosis [164], protein nitration influencing enzyme activities [165], and lipid nitration influencing several signaling pathways [166,167].

Studies in the last decade have proposed that GD alters adenosine transport *via* hENT1 and hENT2, and L-arginine transport *via* hCAT-1 in HUVEC, suggesting that these pathological conditions alter cell signaling cascades involving PI3K, PKC (most likely PKCα), NO and p42 and p44 MAPK (p42/p44^{mapk}) [1,2,4,6,86,93,94]. One of the consequences of the stimulation of this pathway is the activation of transcription factors inhibiting promoter activity of *SLC29A1* (for hENT1) leading to reduced transcript and protein abundance with the subsequent reduced adenosine uptake. This could be a mechanism by which adenosine antioxidant properties could be facilitated since increasing concentrations of this nucleoside are reported in the umbilical vein blood from GD [4,6]. Less is known regarding expression and activity of hENT2 in this cell type, thus not really a clear contribution to this transport system has been reported regarding adenosine actions as a protective factor in ROS and RNS generation and biological effects in the fetoplacental circulation in this syndrome. It has been proposed that NO is not involved in the modulation of hENT2 in HUVEC, but nothing is clear regarding the implications of the proposed signaling pathway in the promoter activity of *SLC29A2* in GD (and/or hyperglycemia). Interestingly, GD effects in the microcirculation of the human placenta remain unknown [4, 6].

PRE-TERM DELIVERY (PTD)

This is the most frequent cause of neonatal mortality and one of the main causes of neurological damage, including cerebral palsy. The risk of death is increasing not only in the prenatal period but also in the first year of postnatal life. Excluding congenital malformations, 75% of perinatal deaths and 50% of neurological damage of infants are associated directly to prematurity [168]. In this pathology the uterus exhibits limited forms to express a response to a noxa or stimulus: uterine contractions (with the corresponding myometrium modifications) and altered structural composition of the cervix (resulting in softening, effacement and dilatation). Around 30% of the PTD are secondary to preterm rupture of the membranes (PROM) mainly due to maternal and fetal infectious compromise [169]. Biochemical mechanisms have been described involving metalloproteinases (MMPs) and interleukins, and more recently it has been proposed an indirect role of the placental endothelium [170,171]. In addition, the existence of mechanisms leading to spontaneous rupture of the membranes by unknown causes has been proposed. The period between the rupture of membranes and labor, known as the latency period, could lead to increased risk of intrauterine infection. These mechanisms are completely unknown in terms of cellular physiology of the membranes, as well as cell dysfunction that could act at distance to modulate localized phenomena in the membranes. One of the proposed alternatives is that PROM occurs after generation of a weakening area (a 'weak zone') as a result of changes in the trans- and extra versus intracellular ionic equilibrium. This region, also called 'zone of altered morphology (ZAM)', has been observed in membranes at the cervix after term vaginal deliveries, before labor and after preterm birth [172]. In addition, cytokines, prostaglandins and oxidative stress are proposed to be involved mechanisms leading to PROM [173,174]. Increased synthesis of ROS is associated with apoptosis [175], and cytochrome c release from mitochondria (marker of apoptosis) [173] is apparently largely mediated by

ROS action. In addition to this, oxidant stress caused by ROS and/or antioxidant depletion (for example adenosine depletion) may damage amnion epithelium causing PROM [176]. It has been reported that antioxidant treatment reduces lipopolysaccharide (LPS)-stimulated MMP-9 enzyme activity and glutathione peroxidase, glutathione reductase, and SOD activity in amnion and chorion [177]. This phenomenon is associated with reduced antioxidant enzyme activity leading to oxidative stress and collagen degradation.

CONCLUDING REMARKS

There are diverse evidences that are briefly discussed in this chapter that strongly suggest the relevance of proper regulation of oxidative and nitrative stress in gestation to reduce the critical consequences in the development of human pregnancy pathologies. Several aspects of pregnancy diseases, including PE, IUGR, diabetes mellitus as well as PTD, point out to the general idea that oxidative/nitrative stress are highly interdependent mechanisms which will be altered leading to endothelial dysfunction (see Fig. **4**). These alterations could be crucial in the 'programming' of the appearance of diseases in adult life. It is evident the need of a characterization of cellular and molecular mechanisms involved in the etiology of these diseases of pregnancy and research focused in the signaling pathways that are activated or inhibited in endothelium, vascular smooth muscle cells and syncytiotrophoblast from the placenta is required. This has been the main topic of interest in recent scientific world congresses of related societies, *i.e.*, the International Federation of Placenta Associations (IFPA) [178], and the Developmental Origins of Health and Diseases (DOHaD) Society [179]. The need of this future knowledge addressing some aspects particularly associated with oxidative and nitrative stress of the etiology of these syndromes, will be valuable information to understand vascular mechanisms supporting current and/or future therapeutic approaches for treatment of patients (i.e, the baby and the mother) [6].

ACKNOWLEDGEMENTS

We thank the researchers at the Cellular and Molecular Physiology Laboratory (CMPL) and Perinatology Research Laboratory (PRL) of the Division of Obstetrics and Gynecology at the Faculty of Medicine from Pontificia Universidad Católica de Chile for their contribution in the production of the experimental data that has been cited throughout the text. Authors also thank Mrs Ninoska Muñoz for excellent secretarial assistance, and the personnel of the Hospital Clínico Pontificia Universidad Católica de Chile labor ward for supply of placentas.

Fondo Nacional de Desarrollo Científico y Tecnológico (FONDECYT 1110977, 1070865, 1080534, 11100192); Programa de Investigación Interdisciplinario (PIA) from Comisión Nacional de Investigación en Ciencia y Tecnología (CONICYT)(Anillos ACT-73), Chile; Dirección de Investigación Universidad de Concepción (DIUC 210.033.103-1.0), Concepción, Chile; Dirección de Investigación (DI-1339-07) y Vicerrectoría Académica (Anillos ACT-73 postdoctoral research associate at CMPL-PRL, Pontificia Universidad Católica de Chile), Universidad de Antofagasta, Chile; Fellowship Apoyo Realización de Tesis Doctoral from CONICYT AT-23070213, AT-24090190. C Puebla, E Guzmán-Gutiérrez and E Muñoz hold CONICYT-PhD (Chile) fellowships.

REFERENCES

[1]   San Martín R, Sobrevia L. Gestational diabetes and the adenosine/L-arginine/nitric oxide (ALANO) pathway in human umbilical vein endothelium. Placenta 2006;27:1-10.

[2]   Casanello P, Escudero C, Sobrevia L. Equilibrative nucleoside (ENTs) and cationic amino acid (CATs) transporters: implications in foetal endothelial dysfunction in human pregnancy diseases. Curr Vasc Pharmacol 2007; 5:69-84.

[3]   Escudero C, Sobrevia L. A hypothesis for preeclampsia: adenosine and inducible nitric oxide synthase in human placental microvascular endothelium. Placenta 2008; 29:469-83.

[4]   Westermeier F, Puebla C, Vega J, *et al.* Equilibrative nucleoside transporters in fetal endothelial dysfunction in diabetes mellitus and hyperglycaemia. Curr Vasc Pharmacol 2009; 7:435-49.

[5]   Myatt L. Reactive oxygen and nitrogen species and functional adaptation of the placenta. Placenta 2010; 31:S66-9.

[6]   Sobrevia L, Abarzúa F, Nien JK, Salomón C, *et al.* Differential placental macrovascular and microvascular endothelial dysfunction in gestational diabetes. Placenta 2011; 32:S159-64.

[7]   Fox SB, Khong TY. Lack of innervation of human umbilical cord. An immunohistological and histochemical study. Placenta 1990; 11:59-62.

[8]   Marzioni D, Tamagnone L, Capparuccia L, *et al.* Restricted innervation of uterus and placenta during pregnancy: evidence for a role of the repelling signal Semaphorin 3A. Dev Dyn 2004; 231:839-48.

[9]   Al-Gubory KH, Fowler PA, Garrel C. The roles of cellular reactive oxygen species, oxidative stress and antioxidants in pregnancy outcomes. Int J Biochem Cell Biol 2010;42:1634-50.

[10]   Cherouny PH, Ghodgaonkar RB, Niebyl JR, Dubin NH. Effect of hydrogen peroxide on prostaglandin production and contractions of the pregnant rat uterus. Am J Obstet Gynecol 1988; 159:1390-4.

[11]   Warren AY, Matharoo-Ball B, Shaw RW, Khan RN. Hydrogen peroxide and superoxide anion modulate pregnant human myometrial contractility. Reproduction 2005; 130:539-44.

[12]   Raijmakers MT, Peters WH, Steegers EA, Poston L. NAD(P)H oxidase associated superoxide production in human placenta from normotensive and pre-eclamptic women. Placenta 2004; 25A:S85-9.

[13]   Cui XL, Brockman D, Campos B, Myatt L. Expression of NADPH oxidase isoform 1 (Nox1) in human placenta: involvement in preeclampsia. Placenta 2006; 27:422-31.

[14]   Horváth EM, Magenheim R, Kugler E, *et al.* Nitrative stress and poly(ADP-ribose) polymerase activation in healthy and gestational diabetic pregnancies. Diabetologia 2009; 52:1935-43.

[15]   Karacay O, Sepici-Dincel A, Karcaaltincaba D, *et al.* A quantitative evaluation of total antioxidant status and oxidative stress markers in preeclampsia and gestational diabetic patients in 24-36 weeks of gestation. Diab Res Clin Pract 2010; 89:231-8.

[16]   Moncada S, Palmer RMJ, Higgs EA. The discovery of nitric oxide as the endogenous nitrovasodilator. Hypertension 1988;12:365-72.

[17]   Yanagisawa M, Kurihara H, Kimura S, Goto K, Masaki T. A novel peptide vasoconstrictor, endothelin, is produced by vascular endothelium and modulates smooth muscle Ca^{2+} channels. J Hypertens 1988; 6:S188-91.

[18]   Ignarro LJ, Buga GM, Wood KS, Byrns RE, Chaudhuri G. Endothelium-derived relaxing factor produced and released from artery and vein is nitric oxide. Proc Natl Acad Sci USA 1987; 84:9265-9.

[19]   Förstermann U. Oxidative stress in vascular disease: causes, defense mechanisms and potential therapies. Nat Clin Pract Cardiovasc Med 2008; 5:338-49.

[20]   Pepine CJ. The impact of nitric oxide in cardiovascular medicine: untapped potential utility. Am J Med 2009; 122:10-5.

[21]   Szasz T, Thakali K, Fink GD, Watts SW. A comparison of arteries and veins in oxidative stress: producers, destroyers, function, and disease. Exp Biol Med (Maywood) 2007; 32:27-37.

[22]   Bedard K, Krause KH. The NOX family of ROS-generating NADPH oxidases: physiology and pathophysiology. Physiol Rev 2007;87:245-313.

[23]   Michaelis UR, Falck JR, Schmidt R, Busse R, Fleming I. Cytochrome P4502C9-derived epoxyeicosatrienoic acids induce the expression of cyclooxygenase-2 in endothelial cells. Arterioscler Thromb Vasc Biol 2005; 25:321-6.

[24]   Stamler JS, Singel DJ, Loscalzo J. Biochemistry of nitric oxide and its redox-activated forms. Science 1992; 258:1898-902.

[25]   Masella R, Di Benedetto R, Varì R, Filesi C, Giovannini C. Novel mechanisms of natural antioxidant compounds in biological systems: involvement of glutathione and glutathione-related enzymes. J Nutr Biochem 2005; 16:577-86.

[26]   Hidalgo C, Aracena P, Sanchez G, Donoso P. Redox regulation of calcium release in skeletal and cardiac muscle. Biol Res 2002;35:183-93.

[27]   Lambeth JD. NOX enzymes and the biology of reactive oxygen. Nat Rev Immunol 2004;4:181-9.

[28]   Antoniades C, Shirodaria C, Warrick N, *et al.* 5-methyltetrahydrofolate rapidly improves endothelial function and decreases superoxide production in human vessels: effects on vascular tetrahydrobiopterin availability and endothelial nitric oxide synthase coupling. Circulation 2006;114:1193-201.

[29]   Dworakowski R, Alom-Ruiz SP, Shah AM. NADPH oxidase-derived reactive oxygen species in the regulation of endothelial phenotype. Pharmacol Rep 2008;60:21-8.

[30]   Gao L, Mann GE. Vascular NAD(P)H oxidase activation in diabetes: a double-edged sword in redox signalling. Cardiovasc Res 2009;82:9-20.

[31]   Li JM, Shah AM. Endothelial cell superoxide generation: regulation and relevance for cardiovascular pathophysiology. Am J Physiol 2004;287:R1014-30.

[32]   Gewaltig MT, Kojda G. Vasoprotection by nitric oxide: mechanisms and therapeutic potential. Cardiovasc Res 2002;55:250-60.

[33]   Carr AC, McCall MR, Frei B. Oxidation of LDL by myeloperoxidase and reactive nitrogen species: reaction pathways and antioxidant protection. Arterioscler Thromb Vasc Biol 2000; 20:1716-23.

[34]   Rolo AP, Palmeira CM. Diabetes and mitochondrial function: role of hyperglycemia and oxidative stress. Toxicol Appl Pharmacol 2006; 212:167-78.

[35] Hadi HA, Suwaidi JA. Endothelial dysfunction in diabetes mellitus. Vasc Health Risk Manag 2007; 3:853-76.

[36] Rask-Madsen C, King GL. More sugar, less blood vessels: another piece in the puzzle of increased cardiovascular risk in diabetes. Arterioscler Thromb Vasc Biol 2008; 28:608-10.

[37] Gu Y, Lewis DF, Zhang Y, Groome LJ, Wang Y. Increased superoxide generation and decreased stress protein Hsp90 expression in human umbilical cord vein endothelial cells (HUVECs) from pregnancies complicated by preeclampsia. Hypertens Pregnancy 2006; 25:169-82.

[38] Harrison DG, Cai H, Landmesser U, Griendling KK. Interactions of angiotensin II with NAD(P)H oxidase, oxidant stress and cardiovascular disease. J Renin Angiotensin Aldosterone Syst 2003; 4:51-61.

[39] Inoguchi T, Sonta T, Tsubouchi H, et al. Protein kinase C-dependent increase in reactive oxygen species (ROS) production in vascular tissues of diabetes: role of vascular NAD(P)H oxidase. J Am Soc Nephrol 2003;14:S227-32.

[40] Ushio-Fukai M, Nakamura Y. Reactive oxygen species and angiogenesis: NADPH oxidase as target for cancer therapy. Cancer Lett 2008; 266:37-52.

[41] Zhu D, Hu C, Sheng W, et al. NADPH oxidase-mediated reactive oxygen species alter astrocyte membrane molecular order via phospholipase A2. Biochem J 2009; 421:201-10.

[42] Nishikawa T, Araki E. Impact of mitochondrial ROS production in the pathogenesis of diabetes mellitus and its complications. Antioxid Redox Signal 2007;9:343-53.

[43] Rutledge AC, Adeli K. Fructose and the metabolic syndrome: pathophysiology and molecular mechanisms. Nutr Rev 2007; 65:S13-23.

[44] Sobrevia L, González M. A role for insulin on L-arginine transport in fetal endothelial dysfunction in hyperglycaemia. Curr Vasc Pharmacol 2009; 7:467-74.

[45] De Meyer GR, Herman AG. Vascular endothelial dysfunction. Prog Cardiovasc Dis 1997; 39:325-42.

[46] Kurowska EM. Nitric oxide therapies in vascular diseases. Curr Pharm Des 2002; 8:155-66.

[47] Yang Z, Kaye DM. Endothelial dysfunction and impaired L-arginine transport in hypertension and genetically predisposed normotensive subjects. Trends Cardiovasc Med 2006;16:118-24.

[48] Kaneto H, Katakami N, Matsuhisa M, Matsuoka TA. Role of reactive oxygen species in the progression of type 2 diabetes and atherosclerosis. Mediators Inflamm 2010; 2010:453892.

[49] Triggle CR, Ding H. A review of endothelial dysfunction in diabetes: a focus on the contribution of a dysfunctional eNOS. J Am Soc Hypertens 2010;4:102-15.

[50] Muller G, Morawietz H. NAD(P)H oxidase and endothelial dysfunction. Horm Metab Res 2009;41:152-8.

[51] Mills TA, Wareing M, Shennan AH, Poston L, Baker PN, Greenwood SL. Acute and chronic modulation of placental chorionic plate artery reactivity by reactive oxygen species. Free Radic Biol Med 2009;47:159-66.

[52] Zhang M, Dong Y, Xu J, et al. Thromboxane receptor activates the AMP-activated protein kinase in vascular smooth muscle cells via hydrogen peroxide. Circ Res 2008;102:328-37.

[53] Moncada S, Higgs EA. Nitric oxide and the vascular endothelium. Handb Exp Pharmacol 2006;176:213-54.

[54] Devés R, Boyd CA. Transporters for cationic amino acids in animal cells: discovery, structure, and function. Physiol Rev 1998;78:487-545.

[55] Mann GE, Yudilevich DL, Sobrevia L. Amino acid and glucose transporters in vascular endothelial and smooth muscle cells. Physiol Rev 2003;83:183–252.

[56] Verrey F, Closs EI, Wagner CA, Palacin M, Endou H, Kanai Y. CATs and HATs: the SLC7 family of amino acid transporters. Eur J Physiol 2004;447:532-42.

[57] Sobrevia L, Mann GE. Dysfunction of the nitric oxide signalling pathway in diabetes and hyperglycaemia. Exp Physiol 1997;82:423-52.

[58] Casanello P, Sobrevia L. Intrauterine growth retardation is associated with reduced activity and expression of the cationic amino acid transport systems y+/hCAT-1 and y+/hCAT-2B and lower activity of nitric oxide synthase in human umbilical vein endothelial cells. Circ Res 2002;91:127–34.

[59] Flores C, Rojas S, Aguayo C, et al. Rapid stimulation of L-arginine transport by D-glucose involves p42/44mapk and nitric oxide in human umbilical vein endothelium. Cir Res 2003;92:64–72.

[60] Arancibia-Garavilla Y, Toledo F, Casanello P, Sobrevia L. Nitric oxide synthesis requires activity of the cationic and neutral amino acid transport system y+L in human umbilical vein endothelium. Exp Physiol 2003;88:699–710.

[61] Guyao W, Morris SM. Arginine metabolism: nitric oxide and beyond. Biochem J 1998;336:1-17.

[62] Alderton WK, Cooper CE, Knowles RG. Nitric oxide synthases: structure, function and inhibition. Biochem J 2001;357:593–615.

[63] Carvajal JA, Germain AM, Huidobro-Toro JP, Weiner CP. Molecular mechanism of cGMP-mediated smooth muscle relaxation. J Cell Physiol 2000;184:409-20.

[64]   Olsson RA, Pearson JD. Cardiovascular purinoceptors. Physiol Rev 1990;70:761-845.

[65]   Pearson JD. Endothelial cell function and thrombosis. Baillieres Best Pract Res Clin Haematol 1999;12:329-41.

[66]   Aird WC. Endothelium in health and disease. Pharmacol Rep 2008;60:139-43.

[67]   Wierzbicki AS, Chowienczyk PJ, Cockcroft JR, *et al.* Cardiovascular risk factors and endothelial dysfunction. Clin Sci (Lond) 2004;107:609-15.

[68]   Mazzanti L, Nanetti L, Vignini A, *et al.* Gestational diabetes affects platelet behaviour through modified oxidative radical metabolism. Diabet Med 2004;21:68-72.

[69]   Webster RP, Brockman D, Myatt L. Nitration of p38 MAPK in the placenta: association of nitration with reduced catalytic activity of p38 MAPK in pre-eclampsia. Mol Hum Reprod 2006;12:677-85.

[70]   Quagliaro L, Piconi L, Assaloni R, Martinelli L, Motz E, Ceriello A. Intermittent high glucose enhances apoptosis related to oxidative stress in human umbilical vein endothelial cells: the role of protein kinase C and NAD(P)H-oxidase activation. Diabetes 2003;52:2795-804.

[71]   Choi JW, Yoo BK, Ryu MK, Choi MS, Park GH, Ko KH. Adenosine and purine nucleosides prevent the disruption of mitochondrial transmembrane potential by peroxynitrite in rat primary astrocytes. Arch Pharm Res 2005;28:810-15.

[72]   Poston L, Taylor PD. Glaxo/MRS Young Investigator Prize. Endothelium-mediated vascular function in insulin-dependent diabetes mellitus. Clin Sci (Lond) 1995;88:245-55.

[73]   Burnstock G. Purinergic signalling--an overview. Novartis Found Symp 2006;276:26-48.

[74]   Manjunath S, Sakhare PM. Adenosine and adenosine receptors: Newer therapeutic perspective. Ind J Pharmacol 2009;41:97-105.

[75]   Almeida CG, Mendonça A, Cunha RA, Ribeiro JA. Adenosine promotes neuronal recovery from reactive oxygen species induced lesion in rat hippocampal slices. Neurosci Lett 2003;339:127–30.

[76]   Kalkan S, Ozdemir D, Ergur BU, Hazardin NU, Akgun A, Topcu A, Kaplan YC, Hocaoglu N, Oransay K, Tuncok Y. Protective effect of an adenosine a1 receptor agonist against metamidophos-induced toxicity and brain oxidative stress. Toxicol Mech Methods 2009;19:148–53.

[77]   Karmazyn M, Cook MA. Adenosine A1 receptor activation attenuates cardiac injury produced by hydrogen peroxide. Circ Res 1992;71:1101-10.

[78]   Ozacmak VH, Sayan H. Pretreatment with adenosine and adenosine A1 receptor agonist protects against intestinal ischemia-reperfusion injury in rat. World J Gastroenterol 2007;13:538-47.

[79]   Huang N. Adenosine A2A receptors regulate oxidative stress formation in rat pheochromocytoma PC12 cells during serum deprivation. Neurosci Lett 2003;350: 127–31.

[80]   Lee HT, Emala CW. Adenosine attenuates oxidant injury in human proximal tubular cells *via* A_1 and A_{2a} adenosine receptors. Am J Physiol 2002; 282:F844-52.

[81]   Xu Z, Park SS, Mueller RA, Bagnell RC, Patterson C, Boysen PG. Adenosine produces nitric oxide and prevents mitochondrial oxidant damage in rat cardiomyocytes. Cardiovasc Res 2005; 65:803-12.

[82]   Ribé D, Sawbridge D, Thakur S, Hussey M, Ledent C, Kitchen I, Hourani S, Li JM. Adenosine A2A receptor signaling regulation of cardiac NADPH oxidase activity. Free Radic Biol Med 2008; 44:1433-42.

[83]   Thakur S, Du J, Hourani S, Ledent C, Li JM. Inactivation of adenosine A2A receptor attenuates basal and angiotensin II-induced ros production by NOX2 in endothelial cells. J Biol Chem. 2010; 285:40104-13.

[84]   Baldwin SA, Beal PR, Yao SY, King AE, Cass CE, Young JD. The equilibrative nucleoside transporter family, SLC29. Pflügers Arch 2004; 447:735-43.

[85]   Pastor-Anglada M, Molina-Arcas M, Casado FJ, Bellosillo B, Colomer D, Gil J. Nucleoside transporters in chronic lymphocytic leukaemia. Leukemia 2004; 18:385-93.

[86]   Vásquez G, Sanhueza F, Vásquez R, *et al.* Role of adenosine transport in gestational diabetes-induced L-arginine transport and nitric oxide synthesis in human umbilical vein endothelium. J Physiol 2004; 560:111-22.

[87]   Aguayo C, Casado J, González M, *et al.* Equilibrative nucleoside transporter 2 is expressed in human umbilical vein endothelium, but is not involved in the inhibition of adenosine transport induced by hyperglycaemia. Placenta 2005; 26:641-53.

[88]   Casanello P, Torres A, Sanhueza F, *et al.* Equilibrative nucleoside transporter 1 expression is downregulated by hypoxia in human umbilical vein endothelium. Circ Res 2005; 97:16-24.

[89]   Huang Y, Anderle P, Bussey KJ, *et al.* Membrane transporters and channels: role of the transportome in cancer chemosensitivity and chemoresistance. Cancer Res 2004; 64:4294-301.

[90]   Montecinos VP, Aguayo C, Flores C, *et al.* Regulation of adenosine transport by D-glucose in human fetal endothelial cells: involvement of nitric oxide, protein kinase C and mitogen-activated protein kinase. J Physiol 2000; 529:777-90.

[91]   Parodi J, Flores C, Aguayo C, Rudolph MI, Casanello P, Sobrevia L. Inhibition of nitrobenzylthioinosine-sensitive adenosine transport by elevated D-glucose involves activation of P_{2Y2} purinoceptors in human umbilical vein endothelial cells. Circ Res 2002; 90:570-7.

[92]   Muñoz G, San Martín R, Farías M, *et al.* Insulin restores glucose inhibition of adenosine transport by increasing the expression and activity of the equilibrative nucleoside transporter 2 in human umbilical vein endothelium. J Cell Physiol 2006; 209:826-35.

[93]   Farías M, San Martín R, Puebla C, *et al.* Nitric oxide reduces adenosine transporter ENT1 gene (SLC29A1) promoter activity in human fetal endothelium from gestational diabetes. J Cell Physiol 2006; 208:451-60.

[94]   Farías M, Puebla C, Westermeier F, *et al.* Nitric oxide reduces SLC29A1 promoter activity and adenosine transport involving transcription factor complex hCHOP-C/EBPalpha in human umbilical vein endothelial cells from gestational diabetes. Cardiovasc Res 2010; 86:45-54.

[95]   Prieto CP, Sobrevia L, Casanello P. RHOA/ROCK signalling pathway is not implicated in eNOS inactivation by hypoxia in human umbilical vein endothelial cells. Placenta 2010;31:A12.

[96]   Webster RP, Roberts VH, Myatt L. Protein nitration in placenta - functional significance. Placenta 2008; 29:985-94.

[97]   MacMillan-Crow LA, Crow JP, Thompson JA. Peroxynitrite-mediated inactivation of manganese superoxide dismutase involves nitration and oxidation of critical tyrosine residues. Biochemistry 1998; 37:1613-1622.

[98]   Lee CI, Liu X, Zweier JL. Regulation of xanthine oxidase by nitric oxide and peroxynitrite. J Biol Chem 2000; 275:9369-76.

[99]   Myatt L, Eis AL, Brockman DE, Kossenjans W, Greer IA, Lyall F. Differential localization of superoxide dismutase isoforms in placental villous tissue of normotensive, pre-eclamptic, and intrauterine growth-restricted pregnancies. J Histochem Cytochem 1997; 45:1433-8.

[100]   Biri A, Bozkurt N, Turp A, Kavutcu M, Himmetoglu O, Durak I. Role of oxidative stress in intrauterine growth restriction. Gynecol Obstet Invest 2007; 64:187-92.

[101]   Llanos MN, Ronco AM. Fetal growth restriction is related to placental levels of cadmium, lead and arsenic but not with antioxidant activities. Reprod Toxicol 2009;27:88-92.

[102]   Krause B, Sobrevia L, Casanello P. Epigenetics: new concepts of old phenomena in vascular physiology. Curr Vasc Pharmacol 2009; 7:513-20.

[103]   Terán E, Escudero C, Vivero S, Enriquez A, Calle A. Intraplatelet cyclic guanosine-3',5'-monophosphate levels during pregnancy and preeclampsia. Hypertens Pregnancy 2004; 23:303-8.

[104]   Redman CW, Sargent IL. Latest advances in understanding preeclampsia. Science 2005; 308:1592-4.

[105]   Roberts JM. Endothelial dysfunction in preeclampsia. Semin Reprod Endocrinol 1998; 16:5-15.

[106]   Desoye G, Myatt L. The Placenta. In: Coustan D (ed), Diabetes in Women. Philadelphia: Lippincott, Williams and Wilkins, 2003.

[107]   Myatt L. The Placenta in Preeclampsia. Endocrine 2002; 19:103-11.

[108]   Walsh SW. Maternal-placental interactions of oxidative stress and antioxidants in preeclampsia. Semin Reprod Endocrinol 1998; 16:93-104.

[109]   Maxwell SR, Thomason H, Sandler D, *et al.* Poor glycaemic control is associated with reduced serum free radical scavenging (antioxidant) activity in non-insulin-dependent diabetes mellitus. Ann Clin Biochem 1997; 34:638-44.

[110]   Hung TH, Skepper JN, Burton GJ. *In vitro* ischemia-reperfusion injury in term human placenta as a model for oxidative stress in pathological pregnancies. Am J Pathol 2001; 159:1031-43.

[111]   Matsubara K, Matsubara Y, Hyodo S, Katayama T, Ito M. Role of nitric oxide and reactive oxygen species in the pathogenesis of preeclampsia. J Obstet Gynaecol Res 2010; 36:239-47.

[112]   Myatt L, Rosenfield RB, Eis AL, Brockman DE, Greer I, Lyall F. Nitrotyrosine residues in placenta. Evidence of peroxynitrite formation and action. Hypertension 1996; 28:488-93.

[113]   Stanek J, Eis AL, Myatt L. Nitrotyrosine immunostaining correlates with increased extracellular matrix: evidence of postplacental hypoxia. Placenta 2001;22:S56-62.

[114]   Siddiqui IA, Jaleel A, Tamimi W, Al Kadri HM. Role of oxidative stress in the pathogenesis of preeclampsia. Arch Gynecol Obstet 2010; 282:469-74.

[115]   Davidge ST, Signorella AP, Lykins DL, Gilmour CH, Roberts JM. Evidence of endothelial activation and endothelial activators in cord blood of infants of preeclamptic women. Am J Obstet Gynecol 1996; 175:1301-6.

[116]   Terán E, Racines-Orbe M, Vivero S, Escudero C, Molina G, Calle A. Preeclampsia is associated with a decrease in plasma coenzyme Q10 levels. Free Radic Biol Med 2003; 35:1453-6.

[117]   Terán E, Escudero C, Moya W. Abnormal release of nitric oxide from nitrosoprotein in preeclampsia. Int J Gynaecol Obstet 2006; 92:260-1.

[118] Karacay O, Sepici-Dincel A, Karcaaltincaba D, *et al.* A quantitative evaluation of total antioxidant status and oxidative stress markers in preeclampsia and gestational diabetic patients in 24-36 weeks of gestation. Diab Res Clin Pract 2010; 89:231-8.

[119] Kulkarni AV, Mehendale SS, Yadav HR, Kilari AS, Taralekar VS, Joshi SR. Circulating angiogenic factors and their association with birth outcomes in preeclampsia. Hypertens Res 2010; 33:561-7.

[120] Tastekin A, Ors R, Demircan B, Saricam Z, Ingec M, Akcay F. Oxidative stress in infants born to preeclamptic mothers. Pediatr Int 2005; 47:658-62.

[121] Kim YH, Kim CH, Cho MK, *et al.* Total peroxyl radical-trapping ability and anti-oxidant vitamins of the umbilical venous plasma and the placenta in pre-eclampsia. J Obstet Gynaecol Res 2006; 32:32-41.

[122] Myatt L. Placental adaptive responses and fetal programming. J Physiol 2006; 572:25-30.

[123] Chappell LC, Seed PT, Briley AL, Kelly FJ, *et al.* Effect of antioxidants on the occurrence of pre-eclampsia in women at increased risk: a randomised trial. Lancet 1999; 354:810–6.

[124] Honing ML, Morrison PJ, Banga JD, Stroes ES, Rabelink TJ. Nitric oxide availability in diabetes mellitus. Diabetes Metab Rev 1998; 14:241-9.

[125] Rösen P, Du X, Tschöpe D. Role of oxygen derived radicals for vascular dysfunction in the diabetic heart: prevention by alpha-tocopherol? Mol Cell Biochem 1998; 188:103-11.

[126] Tames FJ, Mackness MI, Arrol S, Laing I, Durrington PN. Non-enzymatic glycation of apolipoprotein B in the sera of diabetic and non-diabetic subjects. Atherosclerosis 1992; 93:237-44.

[127] Wild S, Roglic G, Green A, Sicree R, King H. Global prevalence of diabetes: estimates for the year 2000 and projections for 2030. Diab Care 2004; 27:1047-53.

[128] De Vriese AS, Stoenoiu MS, Elger M, *et al.* Diabetes-induced microvascular dysfunction in the hydronephrotic kidney: role of nitric oxide. Kidney Int 2001; 60:202-10.

[129] Aryangat AV, Gerich JE. Type 2 diabetes: postprandial hyperglycemia and increased cardiovascular risk. Vasc Health Risk Manag 2010;6:145-55.

[130] Damm P. Future risk of diabetes in mother and child after gestational diabetes mellitus. Int J Gynaecol Obstet 2009;104:S25-6.

[131] Pirkola J, Pouta A, Bloigu A, *et al.* Prepregnancy overweight and gestational diabetes as determinants of subsequent diabetes and hypertension after 20-year follow-up. J Clin Endocrinol Metab 2009;95:772-8.

[132] Ben-Haroush A, Yogev Y, Hod M. Epidemiology of gestational diabetes mellitus and its association with Type 2 diabetes. Diab Med 2004;21:103-13.

[133] Banerjee M, Cruickshank JK. Pregnancy as the prodrome to vascular dysfunction and cardiovascular risk. Nat Clin Pract Cardiovasc Med 2006;3:596-603.

[134] Sobrevia L, Casanello P. Placenta. In: Pérez-Sánchez A, Donoso-Siña E (ed), Obstetricia. Santiago de Chile: Mediterráneo (Spanish), 2011, pg. 136-76.

[135] Blum A. Heart failure--new insights. Isr Med Assoc J 2009;11:105-11.

[136] Bianchi C, Penno G, Miccoli R, Del Prato S. Blood glucose control and coronary heart disease. Herz 2010;35:148-59.

[137] Das Evcimen N, King GL. The role of protein kinase C activation and the vascular complications of diabetes. Pharmacol Res 2007;55:498-510.

[138] Keen H. The Diabetes Control and Complications Trial (DCCT). Health Trends 1994;26:41-3.

[139] Turner RC. The U.K. Prospective Diabetes Study. A review. Diabetes Care 1998;21:C35-8.

[140] Nishikawa T, Edelstein D, Brownlee M. The missing link: a single unifying mechanism for diabetic complications. Kidney Int Suppl 2000;77:S26-30.

[141] Li JM, Shah AM. Endothelial cell superoxide generation: regulation and relevance for cardiovascular pathophysiology. Am J Physiol 2004;287:R1014-30.

[142] Valko M, Leibfritz D, Moncol J, Cronin MT, Mazur M, Telser J. Free radicals and antioxidants in normal physiological functions and human disease. Int J Biochem Cell Biol 2007;39:44-84.

[143] Selemidis S. Suppressing NADPH oxidase-dependent oxidative stress in the vasculature with nitric oxide donors. Clin Exp Pharmacol Physiol 2008; 35:1395-401.

[144] Ho FM, Lin WW, Chen BC, *et al.* High glucose-induced apoptosis in human vascular endothelial cells is mediated through NF-kappaB and c-Jun NH2-terminal kinase pathway and prevented by PI3K/Akt/eNOS pathway. Cell Signal 2006;18:391-9.

[145] Tsuneki H, Sekizaki N, Suzuki T, *et al.* Coenzyme Q10 prevents high glucose-induced oxidative stress in human umbilical vein endothelial cells. Eur J Pharmacol 2007;566:1-10.

[146] Catalano PM, Kirwan JP, Haugel-de Mouzon S, King J. Gestational diabetes and insulin resistance: role in short- and long-term implications for mother and fetus. J Nutr 2003;133:1674S-83S.

[147] De Vriese AS, Verbeuren TJ, Van de Voorde J, Lameire NH, Vanhoutte PM. Endothelial dysfunction in diabetes. Br J Pharmacol 2000;130:963-74.

[148] Nold JL, Georgieff MK. Infants of diabetic mothers. Pediatr Clin North Am 2004;51:619-37.

[149] Metzger BE, Buchanan TA, Coustan DR, *et al.* Summary and recommendations of the Fifth International Workshop-Conference on Gestational Diabetes Mellitus. Diab Care 2007; 30:S251-60.

[150] Huidobro A, Fulford A, Carrasco E. Incidence of gestational diabetes and relationship to obesity in Chilean pregnant women. Rev Med Chil 2004; 132:931-8.

[151] Belmar C, Salinas P, Becker J, *et al.* Incidence of gestational diabetes depending on different diagnosis methods and clinical consequences. Rev Chil Obstet Gynecol 2004; 69:2-7.

[152] Sobrevia L, Yudilevich DL, Mann GE. Activation of A_2-purinoceptors by adenosine stimulates L-arginine transport (system y^+) and nitric oxide synthesis in human fetal endothelial cells. J Physiol 1997; 499:135-40.

[153] Anastasiou E, Lekakis JP, Alevizaki M, *et al.* Impaired endothelium-dependent vasodilatation in women with previous gestational diabetes. Diabetes Care 1998;21:2111-5.

[154] Michiels C. Endothelial cell functions. J Cell Physiol 2003; 196:430-43.

[155] Vásquez R, Farías M, Vega JL, *et al.* D-glucose stimulation of L-arginine transport and nitric oxide synthesis results from activation of mitogen-activated protein kinases p42/44 and Smad2 requiring functional type II TGF-beta receptors in human umbilical vein endothelium. J Cell Physiol 2007; 212:626-32.

[156] Ding H, Hashem M, Triggle C. Increased oxidative stress in the streptozotocin-induced diabetic apoE-deficient mouse: changes in expression of NADPH oxidase subunits and eNOS. Eur J Pharmacol 2007; 561:121-8.

[157] Biri A, Onan A, Devrin E, Babacan F, Kavutcu M, Durak I. Oxidant status in maternal ans cord plasma and placental tissue in gestational diabetes. Placenta 2006; 27:327-32.

[158] Chaudhari L, Tandon OP, Vaney N, Agarwal N. Lipid peroxidation and antioxidant enzymes in gestational diabetics. Indian J Physiol Pharmacol 2003; 47: 441-6.

[159] Madazli R, Tuten A, Calay Z, Uzun H, Uludag S, Ocak V. The incidence of placental abnormalities, maternal and cord plasma malondialdehyde ans vascular endothelial growth factor levels in women with gestational diabetes mellitus and nondiabetic controls. Gynecol Obstet Invest 2008; 65:227-232.

[160] Long J, Liu C, Sen L, Gao H, Lui J. Neuronal mitochondrial toxicity of malondialdehyde: inhibitory effect on respiratory function and enzyme activities in rat brain mitochondria. Neurochem Res 2009;34:786-94.

[161] Kharb S. Lipid peroxidation in pregnancy with preeclampsia and diabetes. Gynecol Obstet Invest 2000;50:113-6.

[162] Peuchant E, Brun JL, Rigalleau V, Dubourg L, Thomas MJ, Daniel JY, Leng JJ, Gin H. Oxidative and antioxidative status in pregnant women with either gestational or type 1 diabetes. Clin Biochem 2004;37:293-8.

[163] Kamath U, Rao G, Raghothama C, Rai L, Rao P. Erytrocyte indicator of oxidative stress in gestational diabetes. Acta Paediatr 1998;87:676-9.

[164] Moley KH. Hyperglycemia and apoptosis: mechanisms for congenital malformations and pregnancy loss in diabetic women. Trends Endocrinol Metab 2001;12:78-82.

[165] Gow AJ, Farkouh CR, Munson DA, POsencheg MA, Ischiropoulos H. Biological significance of nitric oxide-mediated protein modification. Am J Physiol 2004;287:L262-8.

[166] Kossenjans W, Eis A, Sahay R, Brockman D, Myatt L. Role of peroxynitrite in altered fetal-placental vascular reactivity in diabetes or preeclampsia. Am J Physiol 2000;278:H1311-9.

[167] Patcher P, Obrosova IG, Mabley JG, Szabo C. Role of nitrosative stress and peroxinitrite in the pathogenesis of diabetic complications. Emerging new therapeutical strategies. Curr Med Chem 2005;12:267-75.

[168] Goldenberg RL, Culhane JF, Iams JD, Romero R. Epidemiology and causes of preterm birth. Lancet 2008;371:75-84.

[169] Cunningham DS, Christie TL, Evans EE, McCaul JF. Effect of the HELLP syndrome on maternal immune function. J Reprod Med 1993;38:459-64.

[170] Moore RM, Mansour JM, Redline RW, Mercer BM, Moore JJ. The physiology of fetal membrane rupture: insight gained from the determination of physical properties. Placenta 2006; 27:1037-51.

[171] Pandey V, Jaremko K, Moore RM, *et al.* The force required to rupture fetal membranes paradoxically increases with acute *in vitro* repeated stretching. Am J Obstet Gynecol 2007; 196:e161-67.

[172] El Khwad M, Pandey V, Stetzer B, *et al.* Fetal membranes from term vaginal deliveries have a zone of weakness exhibiting characteristics of apoptosis and remodeling. J Soc Gynecol Invest 2006;13:191-5.

[173] Woods JR. Reactive oxygen species and preterm premature rupture of membranes - A review. Placenta 2001; 22:S38-44.

[174] Wall PD, Pressman EK, Woods JR. Preterm premature rupture of the membranes and antioxidants: the free radical connection. J Perinat Med 2002; 30:447-457.

[175] Simon HU, Haj-Yehia A, Levi-Schaffer F. Role of reactive oxygen species (ROS) in apoptosis induction. Apoptosis 2000; 5:415-418.

[175] Longini M, Perrone S, Vezzosi P, *et al.* Association between oxidative stress in pregnancy and preterm premature rupture of membranes. Clin Biochem 2007; 40:793-797.

[177] Lappas M, Permezel M, Reti NG, Rice GE. The activity of antioxidant enzymes is decreased in supracervical amnion. Placenta 2007; 28:A75.

[178] Sobrevia L. Preface. Placenta 2011; 32:S78-80.

[179] Sobrevia L. Programme and abstracts of the 6th world congress on Developmental Origins of Health and Disease. J Develop Origins Health Dis 2009; 1:1-350.

CHAPTER 9

Diabetes, Developmental Programming and Oxidative Stress

Marie Saint-Faust, Isabelle Ligi, Farid Boubred and Umberto Simeoni[*]

Div Neonatology, Assistance Publique Hôpitaux de Marseille University Hospital, INSERM UMR608, France

Abstract: Incidence of Type 2 *diabetes mellitus* (T2DM) is increasing worldwide. Diabetes during pregnancy, as adverse intrauterine environment, has been shown to induce long term effects and play a crucial role in developmental programming in offspring. *In utero* exposure to increased maternal blood glucose concentrations is associated with cardio-vascular alterations, including hypertension and increased risk for obesity and T2DM at adulthood. Early programming of later dysfunction and disease in offspring may result from a combination of mechanisms acting at organ, tissue, cellular and molecular levels. Impaired glucose-insulin metabolism programmed during the critical window of perinatal development may contribute to epigenetic changes in gene expression. This disadvantageous intrauterine environment has been recently emphasised by the role of genetic pathways and in particular, perinatal disturbance of the oxidative state. This chapter examines the epidemiologic and mechanistic issues involved in the developmental programming of long term consequences in offspring of diabetic mothers, with a particular focus on oxidative stress. It also emphasises the mechanisms of hypertension, obesity and insulin resistance. In that considerable concern and because maternal diabetes may be a contributor to the current worldwide epidemic of T2DM, interventions aimed at optimizing maternal blood glucose concentrations during pregnancy should significantly impact T2DM epidemiology.

Keywords: Type 2 diabetes mellitus, maternal blood glucose, early programming, impaired glucose-insulin metabolism, critical window of perinatal development, oxidative state, epigenetic changes, intrauterine environment.

INTRODUCTION

The incidence of Type 2 *diabetes mellitus* (T2DM) is increasing worldwide. Cardio-vascular disease and the metabolic syndrome are the leading causes of mortality in western society. These reliable evidences are becoming a major challenge to global human health [1]. The age of onset of T2DM is falling, now seen in adolescents and even in children, probably because of increasing incidence of obesity [2]. Obesity and pregnancy are known factors which increase the risk for DM. The incidence of diabetes in pregnancy is as high as 5 to 8% of pregnancies in the US and in Europe, and reaches 15-20% in parts of the developing world. The roots of this epidemic are generally considered to reside in the aging world population and in environmental factors, including inappropriate nutrition and physical inactivity. However, perinatal influences, as adverse intrauterine environment, also play a crucial role.

Increasing evidence from both epidemiologic and animal studies shows that *in utero* exposure to maternal diabetes is associated with increased risk for obesity and T2DM at adulthood. Moreover, recent data, in particular those from the HAPO (Hyperglycemia and Adverse Pregnancy Outcomes) study, demonstrate that high maternal glucose concentrations in the absence of DM, adversely influence neonatal outcomes [3]. Furthermore impaired glucose-insulin metabolism programmed during the critical window of perinatal development may be transmitted to the next generation [4], possibly through epigenetic changes in gene expression. The literature recently emphasised the role of genetic pathways and in particular, disturbance of oxidative stress.

1. THE DEVELOPMENTAL ORIGINS OF ADULT HEALTH AND DISEASE (DOHAD)

Since the Barker's hypothesis had demonstrated that low birth weight is associated to increased cardio-vascular mortality rate, the development of T2DM and the metabolic syndrome, numerous epidemiologic and experimental studies have confirmed these associations [5,6]. The adverse effects of low birth weight are worsening if growth is marked by accelerated weight gain after the age of two years [7, 8].

*Address correspondence to Umberto Simeoni: Chair on Infancy, Environment and Health, The University Foundation, Université de la Méditerranée, Marseille, France; E-mail: umberto.simeoni@ap-hm.fr

Bashir M. Matata and Maqsood M. Elahi (Eds.)

These conclusions have led to the concept of the developmental "programming" of physiological and metabolic alterations which lead to disease in later life. Programming may be defined as the phenomenon whereby a stimulus occurring during a critical "window of development", namely the prenatal and early postnatal periods, can cause lifelong changes in the structure and function of the body. Intra-uterine malnutrition and growth restriction, and preterm birth are two of the influences that can induce such effects [9]. Both cause low birth weight, and share some long term physiologic consequences, including hypertension and T2DM. The thrifty phenotype hypothesis proposes that "thrifty" metabolic and physiologic responses to undernutrition in early life allow survival and protect brain growth. Such responses occur during a critical prenatal and perinatal window of sensitivity, but the changes in structure and function that accompany them persist through life [10]. The thrifty metabolism acquired *in utero* becomes disadvantageous. At any level of overweight or obesity people whose birth weights were towards the lower end of the normal range are more likely to develop T2DM and the metabolic syndrome. The thrifty phenotype is one manifestation of the general phenomenon of "developmental plasticity": a single genotype (all the genes acquired at conception) is able to produce a range of different phenotypes according to the environmental conditions experienced during development [11].

Increasing information suggests that altered intra-uterine glucose environment is able to disrupt the development trajectory and alter homeostatic regulatory mechanisms on the long term [6]. Exposure to increased glucose concentrations and to maternal diabetes during pregnancy, which generally lead to large body size at birth can induce long term cardio-vascular and metabolic disease [12]. Thus, there is a U-shaped relation between birth weight and T2DM, an observation first made in studies of the Pima Indians in the US.

2. EPIDEMIOLOGY AND CLINICAL EVIDENCE

A previous prospective study more than a decade ago revealed that the prevalence of impaired glucose tolerance in the offspring of diabetic mothers was 6 fold higher than the prevalence among controls at ages between 10 and 16 years [7]. Offspring of mothers with pre-gestational or gestational *diabetes mellitus* (GDM) had also a higher body mass index (BMI) than controls and higher arterial blood pressure [7-9]. A higher frequency of impaired glucose tolerance in offspring of mothers who had pre-gestational type 1 *diabetes mellitus* (T1DM) or T2DM or GDM has also been recorded [10]. Prospective data from the Framingham Offspring study show that the risk for impaired glucose tolerance is higher in offspring of mothers with early onset diabetes, which is consistent with an effect of intra-uterine exposure to maternal high glucose concentrations [11].

Pima Indians have an exceptionally high prevalence of T2DM. Abundant and reliable information is available from glucose tolerance tests which have been performed periodically in Pima women, including during pregnancy. The prevalence of T2DM in offspring of Pima women increases up to 6 fold in those with diabetic or pre-diabetic mothers, and while during childhood and adolescence, diabetes occurred almost exclusively among the offspring of diabetic and pre-diabetic mothers. This shows the importance of intra-uterine exposure to impaired maternal glucose metabolism, even within a population that may have increased genetic susceptibility to T2DM [13, 14].

The prevalence of obesity was higher in offspring exposed *in utero* to diabetes [15]. Indeed, even in normal birth weight offspring from diabetic pregnancies, the risk for obesity during childhood was increased [16]. A study performed in newborns has suggested an early alteration of fat metabolism in offspring, due to antenatal exposure to even mild increased glucose concentrations [17].

A systematic review of the long term effects of diabetes in pregnancy concluded that the factors related to the development of metabolic syndrome in children included: maternal GDM, maternal glycaemia in the 3rd trimester, maternal obesity, neonatal macrosomia, and childhood obesity [18].

Although environmental factors have been widely incriminated, genetic factors are considered as a possible explanation of the association between *in utero* exposure to high glucose concentrations and long term metabolic and cardio-vascular disease. According to this hypothesis, mothers with early onset diabetes or with GDM may have a particular genotype that transmits high susceptibility to T2DM to the offspring. The data strongly favour a predominant role for the intra-uterine environment. An excess of maternal diabetes has been found in several studies, both in patients with T2DM and GDM [19-21]. But most studies were retrospective and relied on the family history of diabetes [22]. In this population, 45% of offspring of mothers who were diabetic during pregnancy had diabetes in early adult life compared to 9% of offspring of mothers in whom diabetes began after the index pregnancy [23]. The prevalence of diabetes has been compared in siblings born before and after their mother developed diabetes. In diabetic offspring, the odds ratio (OR) for being born after *vs* before the onset of maternal diabetes was 3.0, while no difference was noted when comparing siblings born before and after their father developed diabetes [24].

The incidence of long term metabolic and cardio-vascular alterations in the offspring of diabetic mothers is seemingly not dependent on the type of maternal diabetes, whether T1DM or T2DM, or GDM. Therefore, recent studies show that GDM may be less disadvantageous than pre-gestational DM. The risks for overweight and obesity during childhood or at adulthood seem to follow similar profiles in offspring of T1DM and T2DM mothers [9, 25]. The predisposition to impaired glucose tolerance also seems independent on maternal diabetes type, but is related to the level of maternal hyperglycaemia [10; 26]. In an attempt to differentiate between the effects of intra-uterine exposure to hyperglycaemia and to genetic susceptibility to DM, Clausen *et al.,* [27] recently found that in type 1 diabetic mother's offspring, the risk of type 2 diabetes/pre-diabetes was significantly associated with elevated maternal blood glucose in late pregnancy.

However, genetic susceptibility to diabetes may act as a predisposing or aggravating factor in determining the risk of later diabetes in the offspring of diabetic parents. An example of a combined role of genetic and intra-uterine environmental factors has been found in maturity-onset diabetes of the young -3 (MODY3) patients, whose disease is a single-gene disorder affecting hepatocyte nuclear factor-1α gene. Mody-3 is diagnosed earlier in patients whose mother developed diabetes before pregnancy, compared to offspring of mothers whose diabetes developed after the pregnancy [28].

The frequency of short term neonatal adverse outcomes increases gradually with the level of maternal hyperglycaemia. The HAPO data suggest that high maternal sugar concentrations lead to adverse neonatal outcomes such as macrosomia, low glucose and high insulin levels, whether actual GDM is present or not. Gradually increasing adverse short term neonatal outcomes have been found with increasing maternal fasting or stimulated glucose concentrations, with no identifiable threshold of glucose concentration [29].

Maternal hyperglycaemia associated with insulin resistance (more than hyperglycaemia alone) during pregnancy are associated with an increased incidence of overweight and specific markers of the metabolic syndrome during childhood and adolescence, even though the children's fasting blood glucose concentrations and 2-hours glucose tolerance test were still normal [30, 31]. In Pima Indians, the risk of T2DM in the offspring was associated with the 2 hour plasma glucose concentration even among mothers with normal glucose tolerance. This suggests that high glucose concentrations *in utero* exert a long term effect in the absence of maternal diabetes [32].

3. PATHOPHYSIOLOGY

3.1. General Mechanisms Involved in DOHAD

Early developmental programming of adult disease and long-life dysfunction results from a combination of mechanisms acting at organ, tissue, cellular and molecular levels. Organs or systems such as kidney or vasculature are at risk, as they achieve full quantitative development during late gestation and the perinatal period. Environmental factors alter this process by reducing this quantitative, organ-specific endowment, for example the number of nephrons in kidney. Such alterations, which may be the price paid for survival, only compromise function later in life, when increasing physiologic requirements and over-solicitation of insufficient organ mass start to induce organ damage. The role of such mechanisms has been characterized in the developmental programming of hypertension [33].

Glucose crosses the placenta and maternal hyperglycaemia during pregnancy results in increased glucose concentrations in the fetus. Concerning the long term effects of *in utero* exposure to a continuous range of high glucose concentrations throughout pregnancy, the hypothesis of a fuel-mediated toxicity (Freinkel's hypothesis) is widely accepted [34]. According to such a concept, the fetus experiences a "tissue culture" environment, composed of the metabolic fuels that are delivered from the maternal blood through the placenta. Depending on the various stages of fetal tissue development and organisation, altered fuel environment may lead to "fuel-mediated teratogenicity" during the first trimester of pregnancy by a seemingly direct toxic effect of high glucose concentrations. *In vitro* studies on isolated metanephroï have shown that growth of the explants is considerably altered by excess glucose concentrations in the culture medium [35]. Later in pregnancy, in particular under the influence of inappropriately high glucose concentrations, altered brain cells, and later pancreatic beta-cells, adipose and muscle cells, and nephron development may occur, leading to long term consequences throughout life.

Changes at the molecular level, able to affect durably gene expression, are likely to be involved as a background molecular memory in the wider spectrum of developmentally acquired adult disease. Epigenetic mechanisms of altered gene expression may well be involved as they allow durable, life-long changes in gene transcription through DNA methylation on CpG islets or histones methylation or acetylation, in the absence of any change in the gene DNA sequence. Such changes are mitotically transmitted and can be passed to the next generations. Moreover, epigenetics are the molecular mechanism of parental imprinting of genes which are involved during early embryonic and fetal development, and are keys in silencing DNA sequences according to the pattern of early cellular differentiation. Epigenetics may intervene in the evolutionary process in so far as this cannot be exclusively explained by natural, genetic selection. Mechanisms such as hypoxia and oxidative stress, especially through the pathway of hexosamine biosynthesis, might be involved in diabetes embryopathy, by inducing apoptosis during critical phases of organ development [36-39].

3.2. Focus on Oxidative Stress

Numerous studies have demonstrated that oxidative stress and chronic inflammation are widely involved in atherosclerosis development and progression. Oxidative stress plays also a pivotal role in the pathogenesis of vascular disease induced by diabetes [40]. In that concern, pregnancy represents a particular state of oxidative stress. Perinatal disturbance of the oxidative state or oxidative/anti-oxidative balance, as in gestational DM or maternal DM, might be disadvantageous for foetuses and infants with long-term consequences. Many authors are trying to demonstrate existence of a hypothetical bridge between the adverse intrauterine environment in diabetes and programming of the offsprings toward DNA damage. It has been speculated a role of a placental mitochondrial dysfunction, which may generate excessive numbers of reactive oxygen species (ROS), oxidative modifications and alterations in vascular functions, also causative in cardiovascular disease and diabetes in offspring [41]. ROS production by placental mitochondria are released into fetal circulation and damage vascular mitochondrial DNA [42]. Through this pathway, increased intracellular ROS might be responsible for defective angiogenesis, activate a number of proinflammatory processes, and cause long-lasting epigenetic changes [43]. Recent published data have demonstrated an important role of fetal oxidative DNA damage, resulting in a senescent phenotype in young adult offspring of a maternal history of pre-gestational or gestational diabetes [44], Increased oxidative stress and oxidative damage to fetal DNA and vascular endothelium are implicated in a range of embryopathies, spontaneous abortion and perinatal death. In addition, there is a recent evidence of a positive association between oxidative stress, obesity and pre-diabetic state in childhood. The mechanisms underlying are unknown, but many hypotheses have been suggested, such as intrauterine chromosomal telomere attrition or activation of apoptosis signaling pathway.

Inflammatory Markers and Oxidative/Anti-Oxidative State

It has been recently reported that young adults in offspring of pre-gestational DM have a proinflammatory phenotype. An inflammatory state in the embryo has been suggested, where proinflammatory cytokines act to downregulate the principal anti-oxidative enzymes and systems. *In utero* programming of endothelial cell dysfunction, as a result of chronic exposure to oxidative stress and inflammation, has already been postulated, in particular in IUGR models. Young adults in offspring of at risk pregnancies also develop this proinflammatory state. Recent studies have demonstrated elevated soluble adhesion molecules concentrations such as sICAM-1, sVCAM-1 and E-selectin [44, 45]. Increased plasma concentrations of sICAM-1 in population may be an independent marker of increased vascular risk, a marker of endothelial dysfunction and a genetic component of systemic inflammation [46]. Elevated markers as high sensitivity C-reactive protein, interleukin-6 cord blood concentrations and TNFα concentration in embryos are also demonstration of the inflammatory state [47]. Although lipid peroxidation is already documented in the placenta in normal pregnancy, the process seems to be exacerbated in pregnancies complicated by preeclampsia or diabetes. In those cases, ROS and antioxidant system biomarkers are elevated in placental tissue of pregnant women, but also in maternal plasma and umbilical cord blood. Animal studies have found decreased embryonic prostaglandin E2 (PGE2) concentration and decreased COX-2 activity in offspring of maternal diabetes [48]. PGE2 and COX-2 may play a role in the developmental perturbations. It has been shown that high glucose levels and COX inhibitors cause severe embryonic damage and inversely. ROS excess-related and arachidonic acid deficiency-related teratological pathways are linked.

Long-term exposure to high glucose creates embryonic ROS excess either from increased ROS production or from diminished antioxidant defence capacity. ROS excess may be likely to vary with gestational time and nutritional status. Deficient antioxidant defence mechanisms have been described in individuals with low birth weight, revealing higher generation of ROS. Few data exist regarding oxidative stress in large for gestational age (LGA) children. Chiavaroli *et al.* have demonstrated a positive correlation between oxidant/antioxidant status and body mass index (BMI), and in particular with SGA and LGA children [49]. Measures of isoprostanes (PGF-2α), a prostaglandin-like compound generated by ROS-derived oxidation of arachidonic acid in cellular membranes (marker of lipid peroxidation), revealed a tendency toward higher levels in the LGA group in their study, and also independently correlated to insulin resistance. Wentzel *et al.* have demonstrated in rats that high glucose concentration *in vivo* and diabetes *in vitro* causes increased concentration of isoprostanes [48]. This indicates an embryonic increase in lipid peroxidation rate. Lipid peroxidation may induce developmental disturbance in structural lipids of mitochondrial and cellular membranes, and may also induce teratogenic pathways [50]. It has been recently found that oxidative stress is already present during the pre-pubertal age in this targeted population [49]. Several studies have assessed the relationship between birth weight and oxidative stress in SGA children, but children in offspring of gestational diabetes born LGA or AGA have not been studied yet.

DNA Damage by Telomere Attrition

Telomeres are tandem repeats of the DNA sequence (6-15 kb) at the end of chromosomes. Necessary for DNA replication and chromosomal activity, telomeres shorten at each cell division, at a rate determined by oxidative stress and DNA damage, and once shortened to a critical length, cells are triggered into senescence. It has recently been shown that telomere length is shorter in T2DM subjects and also in healthy offspring with an increased familial risk of coronary artery disease [51]. In offspring of maternal diabetes, increased oxidative stress and oxidative damage to feto-placental DNA and vascular endothelium might lead to increased intrauterine telomeric DNA damage. Cross *et al.,* have found increased cord blood telomere attrition, directly linked to the degree of oxidative DNA damage [47]. In their study, although cord blood telomere length was similar in case of maternal diabetes *vs* control, activity of cord blood mononuclear cell telomerase (a reverse transcriptase involved in the maintenance of telomere length) was significantly higher in the T1DM and GDM groups, which suggest an upregulation of telomerase activity *in utero* as a telomere length maintenance response. This result could indicate a response to potential or actual telomere damage *in utero*, a perturbation of cellular senescence "programming" and might be a crucial advance in understanding fetal programming as an epigenetic phenomenon.

Activation of Apoptosis Signalling Pathway

Maternal diabetes leads to higher frequency of congenital malformations in offspring. It has been suggested that oxidative stress, inducing excessive embryonic cell apoptosis, is the primary mechanism of diabetic embryopathy (in particular, neural tube defect). Indeed, the state of oxidative stress may directly enhance apoptosis in the embryonic and fetal tissue. Although this mechanism is unclear, it has been found recently that maternal diabetes and c-Jun N-terminal kinase (JNK) 1/2 activation in the embryos and yolk sacs are correlated with embryonic dysmorphogenesis [50]. JNK 1/2 is a, stress-activated protein kinases, member of mitogen-activated protein kinases. It specifically responds to cell stress signals, including oxidative stress and mediate regulation of apoptosis. ROS are potent inducers of JNK activation in many other systems, leading to apoptosis. P66Shc is a mediator of oxidative stress-induced apoptosis and a downstream effector of JNK activation [52]. So, the JNK-p66Shc pathway mediates oxidative stress and induces apoptosis. It may play an important role in diabetic embryopathy. A mouse model has shown a dramatic increase of JNK in malformed embryos from diabetic/hyperglycaemic mice. Dramatic increase in cleaved caspase 3 was also seen in malformed embryos. Activation of caspases (family of proteases) is the hallmark of apoptosis, as critical step. Many investigators have also found that excessive apoptosis occurs in malformed embryos and their corresponding yolk sacs under maternal hyperglycaemic conditions. Excessive apoptosis, as excessive oxidative injuries, is one of the mechanisms which might underlie the long-term risk of developing vascular and metabolic diseases.

4. PROGRAMMING OF ADULT DISEASE

4.1. Hypertension

The vascular alterations associated with *in utero* exposure to diabetes have been scarcely described. In Pima Indians, the offspring of mothers who suffered diabetes during pregnancy had higher systolic arterial blood pressure at adolescence, compared to offspring of mothers who developed T2DM, after the pregnancy [14]. Increased systolic and mean arterial blood pressure at ages 10-14 years has been found in the offspring from diabetic pregnancies in the Chicago study [9]. Mechanisms of the early programming of elevated blood pressure are complex [53]. Current knowledge is largely confined to renal and vascular mechanisms.

Renal Mechanisms

In our own laboratory and others, intra-uterine growth restriction, induced in experimental animals by maternal food restriction or uterine artery ligation, has been shown to cause glucose intolerance and hypertension in the offspring [53]. Nephrogenesis occurs during the second part of gestation and ends before birth in humans, after a definitive nephron number endowment has been achieved. Low birth weight due to maternal low protein diet during gestation is associated with reduced nephron number, and altered gene expression in the rat placenta and kidney [54, 55].

Streptozotocin-induced diabetes in pregnant rodents also reduces nephron number in neonates [35], although changes in nephron number have not been found at young adults in one study [56]. Nephron number reduction is known to increase single nephron glomerular filtration rate in the remaining nephrons, followed by glomerular hypertension, proteinuria, and activation of the renin-angiotensin system. According to Brenner's hypothesis, this leads to a vicious circle of rising blood pressure and further renal damage [57].

Interestingly, exposure to transiently high blood glucose concentrations in the mother also leads to reduced nephron number in the pups [35]. Apoptosis and increased activity of the intra-renal RAS and of nuclear factor (NF)-kappa B signalling pathway seem to be involved, as caspase–3 activity and NF-kappa B p50 and p65 components, as well as renal angiotensinogen and renin mRNAs are upregulated in the offspring of diabetic mice [58]. Increased expression of IGF-2/mannose-phosphate receptor has also been demonstrated in fetal kidneys after exposure to maternal diabetes [59].

In humans, increased urinary albumin excretion has been found in adult offspring of Pima Indians mothers with diabetes, which suggests early glomerular injury, possibly related to a similar mechanism of nephron number reduction [60].

Vascular Mechanisms

Examination of the neonatal aorta by ultrasounds as well as post-mortem studies in fetuses and infants suggests that perinatal factors such as intrauterine growth restriction, maternal hypercholesterolemia, and macrosomia due to maternal diabetes mellitus are associated with alterations that may reflect early atherosclerosis [61].

Altered angiogenesis is a key component of the later development of vascular dysfunction and disease, while the endothelium plays a major role in the development of the vasculature. The adherent endothelium undergoes a continuous renewal from tissue and circulating progenitor cells that originate in the bone marrow. In turn, circulating endothelial cells and microparticles are released from the adherent endothelium. Different patterns of circulating microparticles have been described in T1DM and T2DM patients [62]. Hyperglycaemia has been shown to alter angiogenesis in various experimental models, possibly through decreased proliferation and increased apoptosis of endothelial cells, and dysregulation of the angiogenic factor VEGF [63, 64]. Early endothelial dysfunction may well pave the way for later hypertension, as reduced vascular density and increased vascular resistance are considered to be among the early alterations that lead hypertension.

The endothelium is involved in triggering elastin synthesis by shear stress. Elastin content in the extra-cellular matrix of the arterial media is a major factor of arterial compliance. Elastin accumulates in arteries mostly during fetal and early perinatal life: little synthesis occurs during adulthood. Elastin half-life may reach several decades, thus insufficient elastin content due to low birth weight or short duration of pregnancy may be an important factor in the developmental programming of hypertension [65].

Ingram *et al.* recently showed that endothelial progenitor cells from the offspring of diabetic mothers display altered angiogenic functions [66]. Such early endothelial dysfunction consisted of reduced colony formation and self-renewal capacity, and capillary-like tube formation, due to reduced proliferation and accelerated senescence. Interestingly high glucose concentrations *in vitro* were responsible for similar effects. As seen below, concentrations of circulating soluble markers of endothelial function, such as adhesion molecules ICAM-1, VCAM-1 and E-selectin, have been found to be increased in offspring of type-1 diabetic mothers compared to offspring from non diabetic pregnancies [47, 67].

Another aspect of endothelial dysfunction is altered endothelium-dependent vasodilatory capacity. The endothelium is involved in a number of vasodilatory functions, through its capacity to generate locally acting vasoactive mediators such as nitric oxide, which relax adjacent vascular smooth muscle cells. Endothelium-dependent vasodilatory function can be assessed by ultrasound measurements of variations in brachial artery diameter during post-ischaemic hyperaemia, or it can be measured *in vitro* using vascular material obtained from animal models of gestational diabetes. Endothelium-dependent vasodilatory capacity of the mesenteric artery in response to acetylcholine has been shown to be reduced in rat offspring of diabetic mothers, while reactivity to sodium nitroprusside was preserved, which suggests that the L-Arginine-nitric oxide pathway is specifically altered [56, 68]. Furthermore, resistance arteries in rat offspring of diabetic dams show increased vasoconstrictive responses to norepinephrine [55].

4.2. Type 2 Diabetes and Obesity

Both insufficient insulin production and insulin resistance might be the mechanisms underlying the long term development of DM and obesity in offspring of hyperglycaemic pregnancies. Although the available information resulting from animal models is complex, these models clearly demonstrate that the risk for diabetes at adulthood is acquired by *in utero* exposure to high maternal glucose concentrations [69]. Furthermore, various animal studies have shown that T2DM susceptibility can be transmitted to the second and third generations.

Insufficient Insulin Production

In Pima Indians, the adult offspring of mothers who developed diabetes before the onset of the index pregnancy have decreased insulin response to glucose infusion, even in the absence of impaired glucose tolerance as measured by euglycaemic hyperinsulinaemic clamp technique [70]. However, in the adult offspring of type-1 diabetic mothers, there is reduced insulin secretion and an increased incidence of impaired glucose tolerance [26].

Animal models of moderate hyperglycaemia during gestation, obtained either by streptozotocin administration at various stages of gestation or pre-conceptionally, or by infusion of varying amounts of glucose during gestation, lead to increased or normal birth weight in the offspring, as a result of transient hyper-insulinism, but in adult life insulin production is decreased both *in vivo* and *in vitro*, despite a usually normal β cells mass [71-73].

Current knowledge on the development of the pancreas in humans suggests that it may be particularly sensitive to an altered glucose and amino-acid environment during the second half of pregnancy. Reduced β cells mass has been shown in rat fetuses of hyperglycaemic mothers, with reduced expression of IGF-2 [74].

Hyper-Insulinism and Insulin Resistance

Contrasting information on the role of insulin resistance in the development of T2DM in the adult offspring of diabetic mothers has been reported. High insulin-glucose ratios, at fasting or after glucose challenge, have been found in some studies, while other investigations in children and adolescent offspring point at confounding factors such as the concurrent development of obesity. Overweight and adiposity are characterized by increased body fat mass respect to lean, muscular mass and thus contribute as an independent factor to hyper-insulinism.

Experimental data showing reduced insulin sensitivity at adulthood in rat offspring of diabetic dams are derived principally from studies that involved severe maternal hyperglycaemia. Fetal growth is typically restricted in such models, which lead to low birth weight pups. At adulthood the size of the endocrine pancreas and the β cell mass are increased, and the *in vitro* insulin response to glucose is augmented. These studies show nevertheless a reduction of insulin action assessed by the euglycemic hyper-insulinemic clamp technique.

Hyper-insulinism *per se* has been suggested to contribute to the early programming of long term impaired glucose tolerance. In the offspring of diabetic dams early exposure to excess concentrations of insulin and leptin alters the long term orexigenic and anorexigenic neurons function in the arcuate nucleus of the hypothalamus. The regulation of appetite is thus mal-programmed in the offspring, with increased immunopositivity of orexigenic neuropeptide Y and agouti-related peptide, and decreased positivity of the anorexigenic melanocyte-stimulating hormone, both contributing to excess food intake and overweight (the "functional teratogenesis" hypothesis) [75, 76]. Epigenetic factors are likely to be involved in such changes in gene expression [75].

Excess fetal growth and fetal fat mass characterize offspring of diabetic mothers. Elevation of fetal hormones, insulin and leptin, has been found to be associated with maternal GDM. Insulin, whose action leads to increased adiposity, and leptin, which is involved in the down-regulation of appetite, is linked through the adipo-insular axis, which connects the brain and the pancreas with leptin- and insulin-sensitive peripheral tissues. Elevated insulin levels have been shown to be related with the later development of obesity. An interesting hypothesis is thus that pregnancy diabetes may lead to an increased secretion of insulin, which is insufficiently balanced by raised leptin concentrations, and the development of obesity [77].

CONCLUSION

T2DM and obesity is increasing worldwide, which is highly suggestive of the role of environmental factors such as societal changes and increased environmental and nutritional affluence. Genetic factors are unlikely to explain such a drastic evolution. Strong arguments support a perpetuating, vicious cycle of developmental programming of T2DM and cardio-vascular disease in the offspring of GDM mothers, due to *in utero* exposure to high glucose concentrations. Although the mechanisms are multiple and incompletely understood, they rely on injuries in the critical, congenital endowment of specific tissues and organs involved in cardio-vascular physiology and metabolism, and on the epigenetic memory of the stimuli, as oxidative stress and damage, that occur during the early window of susceptibility.

Increasing data show that *in utero* exposure to elevated maternal glucose concentrations affect the offspring, in the presence or absence of GDM. Interventions during pregnancy, aimed at a close monitoring of maternal blood glucose concentrations are thus likely to have an impact not only on maternal and neonatal health, but also on the epidemic of T2DM. Given the current knowledge of the importance of childhood nutrition and weight gain on lifelong health, follow-up of neonates and infants born to mothers who had GDM should receive enhanced attention, taking into account the early closure of the window of opportunity. Breastfeeding and avoidance of overfeeding in early childhood may be key firsts step in this approach. Finally, a better understanding of the cellular and molecular mechanisms of the developmental programming of hypertension, T2DM and eventually obesity by *in utero* exposure to diabetes in pregnancy may unveil pharmacological and nutritional targets for early prevention. A wide area for future research has opened.

REFERENCES

[1]   Song SH, Hardisty CA. Early-onset Type 2 diabetes mellitus: an increasing phenomenon of elevated cardiovascular risk. Expert Rev Cardiovasc Ther 2008; 6: 315-322.

[2]   Shaw J. Epidemiology of childhood type 2 diabetes and obesity. Pediatr Diabetes 2007; 8 Suppl 9: 7-15.

[3]   Metzger BE, Lowe LP, Dyer AR, *et al.* Hyperglycemia and adverse pregnancy outcomes. N Engl J Med 2008; 358: 1991-2002.

[4]   Pinheiro AR, Salvucci ID, Aguila MB, Mandarim-de-Lacerda CA. Protein restriction during gestation and/or lactation causes adverse transgenerational effects on biometry and glucose metabolism in F1 and F2 progenies of rats. Clin Sci (Lond) 2008; 114: 381-392.

[5]   Barker DJ, Winter PD, Osmond C, Margetts B, Simmonds SJ. Weight in infancy and death from ischaemic heart disease. Lancet 1989; 2: 577-580.

[6]   Ross MG, Desai M, Khorram O, McKnight RA, Lane RH, Torday J. Gestational programming of offspring obesity: a potential contributor to Alzheimer's disease. Curr Alzheimer Res 2007; 4: 213-217.

[7]   Silverman BL, Metzger BE, Cho NH, Loeb CA. Impaired glucose tolerance in adolescent offspring of diabetic mothers. Relationship to fetal hyperinsulinism. Diabetes Care 1995; 18: 611-617.

[8]   Silverman BL, Rizzo TA, Cho NH, Metzger BE. Long-term effects of the intrauterine environment. The Northwestern University Diabetes in Pregnancy Center. Diabetes Care 1998; 21 Suppl 2: B142-149.

[9]   Silverman BL, Rizzo T, Green OC, Cho NH, Winter RJ, Ogata ES *et al.* Long-term prospective evaluation of offspring of diabetic mothers. Diabetes 1991; 40 Suppl 2: 121-125.

[10]   Plagemann A, Harder T, Kohlhoff R, Rohde W, Dorner G. Glucose tolerance and insulin secretion in children of mothers with pregestational IDDM or gestational diabetes. Diabetologia 1997; 40: 1094-1100.

[11]   Meigs JB, Cupples LA, Wilson PW. Parental transmission of type 2 diabetes: the Framingham Offspring Study. Diabetes 2000; 49: 2201-2207.

[12]   Simeoni U, Barker DJ. Offspring of diabetic pregnancy: long-term outcomes. Semin Fetal Neonatal Med 2009; 14(2): 119-124

[13]   Dabelea D, Pettitt DJ. Intrauterine diabetic environment confers risks for type 2 diabetes mellitus and obesity in the offspring, in addition to genetic susceptibility. J Pediatr Endocrinol Metab 2001; 14: 1085-1091.

[14]   Bunt JC, Tataranni PA, Salbe AD. Intrauterine exposure to diabetes is a determinant of hemoglobin A(1)c and systolic blood pressure in pima Indian children. J Clin Endocrinol Metab 2005; 90: 3225-3229.

[15]   Pettitt DJ, Baird HR, Aleck KA, Bennett PH, Knowler WC. Excessive obesity in offspring of Pima Indian women with diabetes during pregnancy. N Engl J Med 1983; 308: 242-245.

[16]   Pettitt DJ, Knowler WC, Bennett PH, Aleck KA, Baird HR. Obesity in offspring of diabetic Pima Indian women despite normal birth weight. Diabetes Care 1987; 10: 76-80.

[17]   Catalano PM, Thomas A, Huston-Presley L, Amini SB. Increased fetal adiposity: a very sensitive marker of abnormal *in utero* development. Am J Obstet Gynecol 2003; 189: 1698-1704.

[18]   Vohr BR, Boney CM. Gestational diabetes: The forerunner for the development of maternal and childhood obesity and metabolic syndrome? J Matern Fetal Neonatal Med 2008; 21: 149-157.

[19]   Dorner G, Mohnike A, Steindel E. On possible genetic and epigenetic modes of diabetes transmission. Endokrinologie 1975; 66: 225-227.

[20]   Dorner G, Mohnike A. Further evidence for a predominantly maternal transmission of maturity-onset type diabetes. Endokrinologie 1976; 68: 121-124.

[21]   Martin AO, Simpson JL, Ober C, Freinkel N. Frequency of diabetes mellitus in mothers of probands with gestational diabetes: possible maternal influence on the predisposition to gestational diabetes. Am J Obstet Gynecol 1985; 151: 471-475.

[22]   Alcolado JC, Laji K, Gill-Randall R. Maternal transmission of diabetes. Diabet Med 2002; 19: 89-98.

[23]   Pettitt DJ, Aleck KA, Baird HR, Carraher MJ, Bennett PH, Knowler WC. Congenital susceptibility to NIDDM. Role of intrauterine environment. Diabetes 1988; 37: 622-628.

[24]   Dabelea D, Hanson RL, Lindsay RS, *et al.* Intrauterine exposure to diabetes conveys risks for type 2 diabetes and obesity: a study of discordant sibships. Diabetes 2000; 49: 2208-2211.

[25]   Weiss PA, Scholz HS, Haas J, Tamussino KF, Seissler J, Borkenstein MH. Long-term follow-up of infants of mothers with type 1 diabetes: evidence for hereditary and nonhereditary transmission of diabetes and precursors. Diabetes Care 2000; 23: 905-911.

[26]   Sobngwi E, Boudou P, Mauvais-Jarvis F, *et al.* Effect of a diabetic environment *in utero* on predisposition to type 2 diabetes. Lancet 2003; 361: 1861-1865.

[27]   Clausen TD, Mathiesen ER, Hansen T, *et al.* High prevalence of type 2 diabetes and pre-diabetes in adult offspring of women with gestational diabetes mellitus or type 1 diabetes: the role of intrauterine hyperglycemia. Diabetes Care 2008; 31: 340-346.

[28]   Stride A, Shepherd M, Frayling TM, Bulman MP, Ellard S, Hattersley AT. Intrauterine hyperglycemia is associated with an earlier diagnosis of diabetes in HNF-1alpha gene mutation carriers. Diabetes Care 2002; 25: 2287-2291.

[29]   Jensen DM, Korsholm L, Ovesen P, Beck-Nielsen H, Molsted-Pedersen L, Damm P. Adverse pregnancy outcome in women with mild glucose intolerance: is there a clinically meaningful threshold value for glucose? Acta Obstet Gynecol Scand 2008; 87: 59-62.

[30]   Buzinaro EF, Berchieri CB, Haddad AL, Padovani CR, de Paula Pimenta W. Overweight in adolescent offspring of women with hyperglycemia during pregnancy. Arq Bras Endocrinol Metabol 2008; 52: 85-92.

[31]   Keely EJ, Malcolm JC, Hadjiyannakis S, Gaboury I, Lough G, Lawson ML. Prevalence of metabolic markers of insulin resistance in offspring of gestational diabetes pregnancies. Pediatr Diabetes 2008; 9: 53-59.

[32]   Franks PW, Looker HC, Kobes S, *et al.* Gestational glucose tolerance and risk of type 2 diabetes in young Pima Indian offspring. Diabetes 2006; 55: 460-465.

[33]   Tauzin L, Rossi P, Giusano B, *et al.* Characteristics of arterial stiffness in very low birth weight premature infants. Pediatr Res 2006; 60: 592-596.

[34]   Freinkel N. Banting Lecture 1980. Of pregnancy and progeny. Diabetes 1980; 29: 1023-1035.

[35]   Amri K, Freund N, Vilar J, Merlet-Benichou C, Lelievre-Pegorier M. Adverse effects of hyperglycemia on kidney development in rats: *in vivo* and *in vitro* studies. Diabetes 1999; 48: 2240-2245.

[36]   Loeken MR. Advances in understanding the molecular causes of diabetes-induced birth defects. J Soc Gynecol Investig 2006; 13: 2-10.

[37]   Zhao Z, Reece EA. Experimental mechanisms of diabetic embryopathy and strategies for developing therapeutic interventions. J Soc Gynecol Investig 2005; 12: 549-557.

[38]   Horal M, Zhang Z, Stanton R, Virkamaki A, Loeken MR. Activation of the hexosamine pathway causes oxidative stress and abnormal embryo gene expression: involvement in diabetic teratogenesis. Birth Defects Res A Clin Mol Teratol 2004; 70: 519-527.

[39]   Li R, Chase M, Jung SK, Smith PJ, Loeken MR. Hypoxic stress in diabetic pregnancy contributes to impaired embryo gene expression and defective development by inducing oxidative stress. Am J Physiol Endocrinol Metab 2005; 289: E591-599.

[40]   Fatehi-Hassanabad A, Chan CB, Furman BL. Reactive oxygen species and endothelial function in diabetes. Eur J Pharmacol 2010 ; 636 : 8-17

[41]   Foster W, Myllynen P, Winn LM, Ornoy A, Miller RK. Reactive Oxygen Species, Diabetes and Toxicity in the placenta. A workshop report. Placenta 2008; 29(22): S105-S107

[42]   Leduc L, Levy E, Bouity-Voubou M, Delvin E. Fetal programming of atherosclerosis: possible role of the mitochondria. Eur J Obstet Gynecol Reprod Biol 2010; 149(2): 127-30

[43]   Giacco F, Brownlee M. Oxidative stress and diabetic complications. Circ Res 2010; 107(9): 1058-70

[44]   Cross JA, Brennan C, Gray T, *et al.* Absence of telomere shortening and oxidative DNA damage in the young adult offspring of women with pre-gestational type 1 diabetes. Diabetologia 2009; 52: 226-234

[45]   Nelson SM, Sattar N, Freeman DJ, Walker JD, Lindsay RS. Inflammation and endothelial activation is evident at birth in offspring of mothers with type 1 diabetes. Diabetes 2007; 56: 2697-2704

[46]   Witte DR, Broekmans WMR, Kardinaal AFM, Klöpping-Ketelaars IA, van Poppel G, Bots ML *et al.* Soluble intercellular adhesion molecule 1 and flow-mediated dilatation are related to the estimated risk of coronary heart disease independently from each other. Atherosclerosis 2003; 170: 147-153

[47]   Cross JA, Temple RC, Hughes JC, *et al.* Cord blood telomere, telomerase activity and inflammatory markers in pregnancies in women with diabetes or gestational diabetes. Diabet Med 2010; 27(11): 1264-70

[48]   Wentzel P, Welsh N, Eriksson UJ. Developmental damage, increased lipid peroxidation, diminished cyclooxygenase-2 gene expression, and lowered prostaglandin E2 levels in rat embryos exposed to a diabetic environment. Diabetes 1999; 48: 813-820

[49]   Chiavaroli V, Giannini C, D'Adamo E, de Giorgis T, Chiarelli F, Mohn A. Insulin resistance and oxidative stress in children born small and large for gestational age. Pediatrics 2009; 124: 695-702

[50]   Eriksson UJ. Congenital anomalies in diabetic pregnancy. Semin Fetal Neonatal Med 2009; 14: 85-93

[51]   Adaikalakoteswari A, Balasubramanyam M, Ravikumar R, Deepa R, Mohan V. Association of telomere shortening with impaired glucose tolerance and diabetic macroangiopathy. Atherosclerosis 2007; 195: 83-89

[52]   Yang P, Zhao Z, Reece EA. Activation of oxidative stress signaling that is implicated in apoptosis with a mouse model of diabetic embryopathy. Am J Obstet Gynecol 2008; 198(1): 130.e1-7

[53]   Boubred F, Buffat C, Feuerstein JM, Daniel L, Tsimaratos M, Oliver C, Lelievre-Pegorier M, Simeoni U. Effects of early postnatal hypernutrition on nephron number and long-term renal function and structure in rats. Am J Physiol Renal Physiol 2007; 293: F1944-1949.

[54]   Buffat C, Mondon F, Rigourd V, *et al.* A hierarchical analysis of transcriptome alterations in intrauterine growth restriction (IUGR) reveals common pathophysiological pathways in mammals. J Pathol 2007; 213: 337-346.

[55]   Buffat C, Boubred F, Mondon F, *et al.* Kidney gene expression analysis in a rat model of intrauterine growth restriction reveals massive alterations of coagulation genes. Endocrinology 2007; 148: 5549-5557.

[56]   Rocha SO, Gomes GN, Forti AL, *et al.* Long-term effects of maternal diabetes on vascular reactivity and renal function in rat male offspring. Pediatr Res 2005; 58: 1274-1279.

[57]   Brenner BM, Garcia DL, Anderson S Glomeruli and blood pressure. Less of one, more the other? Am J Hypertens 1988; 1: 335-347.

[58]   Tran S, Chen YW, Chenier I, *et al.* Maternal diabetes modulates renal morphogenesis in offspring. J Am Soc Nephrol 2008; 19: 943-952.

[59] Amri K, Freund N, Van Huyen JP, Merlet-Benichou C, Lelievre-Pegorier M 2001 Altered nephrogenesis due to maternal diabetes is associated with increased expression of IGF-II/mannose-6-phosphate receptor in the fetal kidney. Diabetes 50: 1069-1075.

[60] Nelson RG, Morgenstern H, Bennett PH. Intrauterine diabetes exposure and the risk of renal disease in diabetic Pima Indians. Diabetes 1998; 47: 1489-1493.

[61] Skilton MR. Intrauterine risk factors for precocious atherosclerosis. Pediatrics 2008; 121: 570-574.

[62] Sabatier F, Darmon P, Hugel B, *et al.* Type 1 and type 2 diabetic patients display different patterns of cellular microparticles. Diabetes 2002; 51: 2840-2845.

[63] Larger E, Marre M, Corvol P, Gasc JM. Hyperglycemia-induced defects in angiogenesis in the chicken chorioallantoic membrane model. Diabetes 2004; 53: 752-761.

[64] Pinter E, Haigh J, Nagy A, Madri JA. Hyperglycemia-induced vasculopathy in the murine conceptus is mediated via reductions of VEGF-A expression and VEGF receptor activation. Am J Pathol 2001; 158: 1199-1206.

[65] Martyn CN, Greenwald SE. Impaired synthesis of elastin in walls of aorta and large conduit arteries during early development as an initiating event in pathogenesis of systemic hypertension. Lancet 1997; 350: 953-955.

[66] Ingram DA, Lien IZ, Mead LE, *et al. In vitro* hyperglycemia or a diabetic intrauterine environment reduces neonatal endothelial colony-forming cell numbers and function. Diabetes 2008; 57: 724-731.

[67] Manderson JG, Mullan B, Patterson CC, *et al.* Cardiovascular and metabolic abnormalities in the offspring of diabetic pregnancy. Diabetologia 2002; 45: 991-996.

[68] Holemans K, Gerber RT, Meurrens K, *et al.* Streptozotocin diabetes in the pregnant rat induces cardiovascular dysfunction in adult offspring. Diabetologia 1999; 42: 81-89.

[69] Fetita LS, Sobngwi E, Serradas P, *et al.* Consequences of fetal exposure to maternal diabetes in offspring. J Clin Endocrinol Metab 2006; 91: 3718-3724.

[70] Gautier JF, Wilson C, Weyer C, *et al.* Low acute insulin secretory responses in adult offspring of people with early onset type 2 diabetes. Diabetes 2001; 50: 1828-1833.

[71] Aerts L, Sodoyez-Goffaux F, Sodoyez JC, *et al.* The diabetic intrauterine milieu has a long-lasting effect on insulin secretion by B cells and on insulin uptake by target tissues. Am J Obstet Gynecol 1988; 159: 1287-1292.

[72] Bihoreau MT, Ktorza A, Kinebanyan MF, Picon L. Impaired glucose homeostasis in adult rats from hyperglycemic mothers. Diabetes 1986; 35: 979-984.

[73] Aerts L, Vercruysse L, Van Assche FA. The endocrine pancreas in virgin and pregnant offspring of diabetic pregnant rats. Diabetes Res Clin Pract 1997; 38: 9-19.

[74] Serradas P, Goya L, Lacorne M, *et al.* Fetal insulin-like growth factor-2 production is impaired in the GK rat model of type 2 diabetes. Diabetes 2002; 51: 392-397.

[75] Plagemann A. 'Fetal programming' and 'functional teratogenesis': on epigenetic mechanisms and prevention of perinatally acquired lasting health risks. J Perinat Med 2004; 32: 297-305.

[76] Franke K, Harder T, Aerts L, *et al.* 'Programming' of orexigenic and anorexigenic hypothalamic neurons in offspring of treated and untreated diabetic mother rats. Brain Res 2005; 1031: 276-283.

[77] Dabelea D The predisposition to obesity and diabetes in offspring of diabetic mothers. Diabetes Care 2007; 30 Suppl 2: S169-174.

Index

www.ingramcontent.com/pod-product-compliance
Lightning Source LLC
Chambersburg PA
CBHW041715210326
41598CB00007B/668